PREVENTIVE CARDIOLOGY

CONTEMPORARY CARDIOLOGY

CHRISTOPHER P. CANNON

SERIES EDITOR

PREVENTIVE CARDIOLOGY

Strategies for the Prevention and

Treatment of Coronary Artery Disease

Edited by

JoANNE MICALE FOODY, MD

Yale University School of Medicine
New Haven, CT

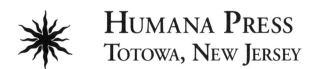

HUMANA PRESS
TOTOWA, NEW JERSEY

© 2001 Humana Press Inc.
999 Riverview Drive, Suite 208
Totowa, New Jersey 07512

Due diligence has been taken by the publishers, editors, and authors of this book to assure the accuracy of the information published and to describe generally accepted practices. The contributors herein have carefully checked to ensure that the drug selections and dosages set forth in this text are accurate and in accord with the standards accepted at the time of publication. Notwithstanding, since new research, changes in government regulations, and knowledge from clinical experience relating to drug therapy and drug reactions constantly occur, the reader is advised to check the product information provided by the manufacturer of each drug for any change in dosages or for additional warnings and contraindications. This is of utmost importance when the recommended drug herein is a new or infrequently used drug. It is the responsibility of the treating physician to determine dosages and treatment strategies for individual patients. Further, it is the responsibility of the health care provider to ascertain the Food and Drug Administration status of each drug or device used in their clinical practice. The publishers, editors, and authors are not responsible for errors or omissions or for any consequences from the application of the information presented in this book and make no warranty, express or implied, with respect to the contents in this publication.

This publication is printed on acid-free paper. ∞

ANSI Z39.48-1984 (American National Standards Institute) Permanence of Paper for Printed Library Materials.

Cover design by Patricia F. Cleary.

For additional copies, pricing for bulk purchases, and/or information about other Humana titles, contact Humana at the above address or at any of the following numbers: Tel: 973-256-1699; Fax: 973-256-8341; E-mail: humana@humanapr.com or visit our website at http://humanapress.com

Printed in the United States of America. 10 9 8 7 6 5 4 3 2 1

Library of Congress Cataloging-in-Publication Data

Preventive cardiology : strategies for the prevention and treatment of coronary artery disease / edited by
    JoAnne Micale Foody.
      p. ; cm. -- (Contemporary cardiology)
    Includes bibliographical references and index.
    ISBN 0-89603-811-4 (alk. paper)
      1. Coronary heart disease--Prevention. 2. Coronary heart disease--Risk factors. 3. Coronary heart disease--
    Pathophysiology. I. Foody, JoAnne Micale. II. Contemporary cardiology (Totowa, N.J.)
    [DNLM: 1. Coronary Disease--prevention & control. 2. Coronary Disease--therapy. WG 300 P9457 2000l]
    RC685.C6 P675 2000l
      616.1'23--dc21   00-037004

PREFACE

Preventive cardiology is a newly emerging field that places emphasis on the prevention and treatment of coronary disease. *Preventive Cardiology: Strategies for the Prevention and Treatment of Coronary Artery Disease* is intended for clinical cardiologists, internists, and allied health care professionals who wish to extend their knowledge and expertise in the rapidly expanding field of Preventive Cardiology. It is the mission of this book to provide clinicians with the understanding and tools necessary to practice prevention in their daily practices.

Recent changes in the delivery of health care in the United States, in conjunction with new scientific evidence supporting the role of preventive strategies in the maintenance of cardiovascular health, have focused new attention and efforts on the field of cardiovascular disease prevention. The field of cardiology is thus making a gradual transition from the technology-driven, intervention-oriented perspective of the last several decades to a new, preventive, molecular-based perspective. As fresh evidence amasses that preventive measures produce a considerable decrease in the incidence of both primary and secondary cardiac events and mortality, there is growing, widespread acknowledgment that health care providers from all arenas must initiate preventive strategies in the management and care of their patients.

Preventive Cardiology as a field has only come into its own in the last several years in response to striking new evidence that preventive strategies may prove to be the best interventions in treatment and prevention of cardiovascular disease.

Cardiovascular disease currently claims the lives of 500,000 men and women each year and, despite our best efforts, these numbers will continue to increase. Over the past century, technical advances have provided significant improvements in the treatment of existing coronary artery disease and have come to generate annual cardiovascular health care expenditures in the United States that exceed $100 billion, largely resulting from hospitalizations and revascularization procedures. Cardiology continues to be focused on acute care. Currently, for every dollar spent on cardiovascular disease in this country, only six cents of out-of-hospital medical therapy is spent on reinforcing healthy lifestyles. Increasing costs of medical care have led, in the field of cardiovascular medicine, to cost shifting and a reevaluation of clinical outcomes, cost-effectiveness, and the development of effective health care delivery systems. The incorporation of preventive cardiology strategies into the practice of cardiovascular medicine will be of paramount importance as we begin this new millennium. It is critical to assess the effectiveness of our current clinical strategies and to direct health care efforts and resources toward the *prevention* of the atherosclerotic process itself.

Preventive Cardiology: Strategies for the Prevention and Treatment of Coronary Artery Disease hopes to provide the clinicians with both the knowledge and the impetus to incorporate preventive strategies into their everyday practices. It will not only provide practical information for the management of patients at risk for cardiovascular disease, but also offers an overview of the new paradigms in the pathophysiology of coronary artery disease. The first part of the book will focus on the unstable atherosclerotic plaque and new strategies for modification of plaque constituents, the important and central role of the endothelium in the maintenance of cardiovascular health, and the emerging roles of oxidative stress, infection, and inflammation in coronary artery disease (CAD). This part will provide novel current perspectives on important emerging concepts in the pathophysiology of coronary atherosclerosis.

The book's second part focuses on traditional cardiovascular risk factors and also provides insights into the gender-specific aspects of CAD risk. These offer thorough, concise reviews of these various risk factors with preventive strategies outlined for the clinician. A significant body of evidence exists that strategies incorporating risk modification provide substantial benefits in patients at risk for or with coronary disease. Coronary atherosclerosis and its sequelae may be largely preventable if aggressive multidisciplinary strategies are implemented. Risk modification may prove to be one of the most significant "interventions" that any physician can perform for their patients with acute coronary syndromes.

The final part of the book provides an overview of strategies for the identification of patients at risk for CAD events, a detailed chapter on pharmacologic therapies for easy reference, as well as a review of antiplatelet agents in the prevention of coronary events. Finally, given the imperatives of cost-containment and health care resource allocation, a chapter on the pharmacoeconomics of preventive strategies as well as the implementation of a preventive cardiology clinic are included. The goal of *Preventive Cardiology: Strategies for the Prevention and Treatment of Coronary Artery Disease* is to provide an overview of the exciting opportunities to prevent the progression, and in some instances to regress the process, of coronary atherosclerosis and to incorporate these strategies into the daily practice of clinical medicine.

JoAnne Micale Foody, MD

CONTENTS

Part I New Paradigms in the Pathophysiology of Coronary Artery Disease

Part II Risk Factors and Their Management in Coronary Artery Disease

Part III Strategies for Prevention

CONTRIBUTORS

ARTHUR AGATSTON, MD • *Director, Mount Sinai Cardiac Prevention Center, Mount Sinai Medical Center of Greater Miami; Associate Professor of Medicine, The University of Miami School of Medicine, Miami, FL*

GORDON G. BLACKBURN, PHD • *Director, Cardiac Health Improvement and Rehabilitation Program, Department of Cardiology, The Cleveland Clinic Foundation, Cleveland, OH*

ROBYN BERGMAN BUCHSBAUM, MHS, CHES • *Education Coordinator, The Heart Center, The Cleveland Clinic Foundation, Cleveland OH*

JEFFREY CRAIG BUCHSBAUM MD, PHD • *Department of Radiation Oncology, The Cleveland Clinic Foundation, Cleveland OH*

CHRISTOPHER R. COLE, MD • *Department of Cardiology, The Cleveland Clinic Foundation, Cleveland OH*

RON COREY, PHD, MBA, RPH • *Global Director, Economic Strategies, Pharmacia Corporation, Peapack, NJ*

JOANNE MICALE FOODY, MD • *Yale University School of Medicine, New Haven, CT*

JOSEPH P. FROLKIS, MD, PHD • *Staff Physician, Sections of Preventive Cardiology and Preventive Medicine, Division of Medicine, The Cleveland Clinic Foundation; Assistant Professor, Department of Medicine, Case Western Reserve University School of Medicine, Cleveland, OH*

MARGARITA R. GARCES, MD • *Division of Cardiology, Mount Sinai Medical Center, Miami Beach Florida and University of Miami School of Medicine, Miami, FL*

BYRON J. HOOGWERF, MD • *Section of Preventive Cardiology, Department of Cardiology, Department of Endocrinology, and Division of Internal Medicine, The Cleveland Clinic Foundation, Cleveland OH*

MICHAEL A. LAUER, MD • *Department of Cardiology, Borgess Medical Center Research Institute, Kalamazoo, MI*

MICHAEL S. LAUER, MD • *Department of Cardiology, The Cleveland Clinic Foundation, Cleveland, OH*

ERIC H. LIEBERMAN, MD • *Division of Cardiology, Mount Sinai Medical Center, Miami Beach Florida and University of Miami School of Medicine, Miami, FL*

FRANCISCO LOPEZ-JIMENEZ, MD, MSC • *Division of Cardiology, Mount Sinai Medical Center, Miami Beach Florida and University of Miami School of Medicine, Miami, FL*

R. PRESTON MASON, PHD • *Membrane Biophysics Laboratory, Departments of Biochemistry and Medicine, Cardiovascular and Pulmonary Research Institute, MCP Hahnemann University School of Medicine, Allegheny Campus, Pittsburgh, PA*

WILLIAM F. MCGHAN, PHARMD, PHD • *Professor and Director, Graduate Program in Pharmacy Administration, University of the Sciences, Philadelphia, PA*

MICHAEL A. MILITELLO, PHARMD • *Department of Pharmacy, The Cleveland Clinic Foundation, Cleveland OH*

SCOTT A. MOORE, MD • *Department of Cardiology, Wilford Hall Medical Center, San Antonio, TX*

SIMONE NADER, MD • *Department of Cardiology, The Cleveland Clinic Foundation, Cleveland, OH*

KRISTINE NAPIER, MPH, RD • *Section of Preventive Cardiology, The Department of Cardiology, The Cleveland Clinic Foundation, Cleveland OH*

STEVEN E. NISSEN, MD • *Vice-Chairman, Department of Cardiology, Director Intravascular Ultrasound Core Laboratory, Department of Cardiology, The Cleveland Clinic Foundation, Cleveland, OH*

MELANIE OATES, PHD, MBA, RN • *Philadelphia College of Pharmacy, University of the Sciences, Philadelphia, PA*

CYNTHIA PORDON, DO • *Department of Cardiology, The Cleveland Clinic Foundation, Cleveland OH*

KILLIAN ROBINSON, MD • *Department of Cardiology, The Cleveland Clinic Foundation, Cleveland OH*

THERESA H. SEO, PHARMD • *Department of Pharmacy, The Cleveland Clinic Foundation, Cleveland OH*

STEVEN R. STEINHUBL, MD • *Department of Cardiology, Wilford Hall Medical Center, San Antonio, TX*

DONALD G. VIDT, MD • *Department of Nephrology and Hypertension, Cleveland Clinic Foundation, Cleveland, OH; Professor of Internal Medicine, Ohio State University, Columbus, OH*

I

New Paradigms in the Pathophysiology of Coronary Artery Disease

1   The Unstable Plaque
Implications and Opportunities for Prevention

*JoAnne Micale Foody, MD
and Steven E. Nissen, MD*

CONTENTS

INTRODUCTION

Over this past decade, clinical trials have added to our understanding of the pathophysiology and prevention of coronary atherosclerosis. Evidence is accumulating that cholesterol lowering has immediate consequences that may favorably affect the coronary atheroma and subsequent coronary events. Intravascular ultrasound provides a new modality by which to better understand the atheroma.

CORONARY HEART DISEASE: *AN OVERVIEW*

In the United States, approximately 14 million adults have a current diagnosis of coronary heart disease (CHD) *(1)*. One-third of the 1.5 million individuals who experience myocardial infarctions each year will die. The estimates of the financial costs (i.e., treatment and lost wages) that are associated with CHD in Americans range between $50

From: *Contemporary Cardiology: Preventive Cardiology:
Strategies for the Prevention and Treatment of Coronary Artery Disease*
Edited by: J. Foody © Humana Press Inc., Totowa, NJ

billion and \$100 billion per year *(1,2)*. Although the incidence of death from CHD has decreased in the United States, the total number of deaths from CHD has recently begun to increase after a prior steady decline. Most likely, this is the result of the increased number of middle-aged and elderly people in the population. Clearly, more effective primary and secondary CHD prevention measures are required. CHD prevention in the future will be the result of the ground-breaking research that has been conducted over the past 25 years. For example, in the 1970s, data from the Framingham Epidemiological Study demonstrated that increases in serum cholesterol levels in the general population were associated with an increased risk of death from CHD *(3–5)*. In 1988, the National Cholesterol Education Program (NCEP) identified elevated low-density lipoprotein cholesterol (LDL-C) as a primary risk factor for CHD *(6)*. In the 1993 NCEP Adult Treatment Panel II Report, this conclusion was further strengthened by the addition of aggressive dietary and drug therapy recommendations for patients with known CHD *(2)*. In 1995, Gould and associates reported meta-analysis data on 35 randomized clinical trials that lasted more than 2 years and were designed to reduce serum cholesterol levels *(7)*. They concluded that for every 10 percentage points of cholesterol lowering, CHD mortality was reduced by 13% ($p < 0.002$) and total mortality by 10% ($p < 0.03$). According to the most recently reported US National Health and Nutrition Examination Survey (NHANES III), an estimated 5.5 million Americans with CHD should be treated with lipid-lowering medications under the NCEP guidelines *(8)*. Presently, less than one-third of those CHD patients who require lipid-lowering medications actually receive treatment, and only a small proportion of those who do receive treatment achieve NCEP target levels *(1)*. In controlled clinical trials, HMG-CoA reductase inhibitors have been shown to lower total and LDL-C levels, decrease CHD-related morbidity and mortality in patients with CHD, slow progression of, and, in some cases, cause regression of coronary atherosclerosis *(1,7,9,10)*.

Over the past decade, new scientific evidence strongly supporting the role of preventive interventions in the maintenance of health has focused much needed attention and efforts on cardiovascular prevention. New trials of lipid lowering have added to our understanding of the pathophysiology and prevention of coronary atherosclerosis. As this new evidence is amassing, there is widespread acknowledgment that lipid lowering with statins should be a mainstay of treatment for the patient with chronic CAD. Intravascular ultrasound is a new imaging study that provides the opportunity to more directly view the atheroma and study its response to risk factor modification.

PATHOGENESIS OF CORONARY ARTERY DISEASE

Classic theory on the pathogenesis of acute coronary syndromes taught that the atherosclerotic process led to plaque formation and subsequent coronary artery luminal narrowing (Fig. 1). At some point, these lesions developed an overlying platelet-containing thrombus that acutely diminished coronary perfusion and resulted in an acute coronary syndrome. A new paradigm for acute coronary syndromes has emerged. New data suggest that most acute coronary syndromes involve coronary artery segments that do not have high-grade anatomic stenoses documented by recent coronary angiograms *(27)*. Moreover, it appears that less stenotic lesions characterized by thin fibrous caps, large concentrations of soft lipid accumulations, large numbers of monocytes and macrophages, and depletion of smooth muscle cells cause the majority of acute events (Fig. 2). These

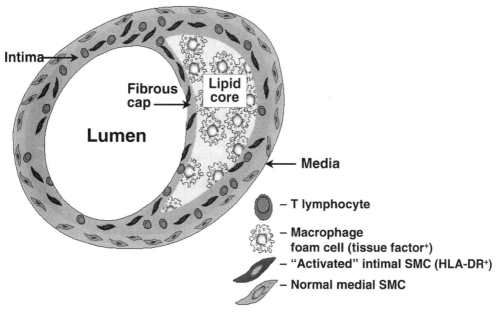

Fig. 1. Unstable plaque. Adapted from National Lipid Education Council, www.lipidhealth.org, from Libby P. Lancet. 1996;348:S4–S7.

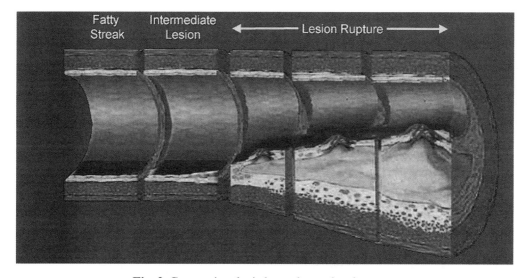

Fig. 2. Conventional wisdom: plaque development.

"vulnerable plaques" appear highly prone to rupture, thereby allowing blood to come in contact with highly thrombogenic substances found in the lipid plaque (*27–29*). Reduction of cholesterol may not only decrease the lipid content of the plaque, but can also reduce the accumulation of monocytes and macrophages, thereby helping to transform these "vulnerable" into a less active or "quiescent" plaque (*19,28,29*) (Fig. 3).

This proposed mechanism of plaque stabilization may help to explain why numerous clinical trials using lipid-lowering regimens in patients with CHD have shown that reductions in rates of coronary events and mortality are far greater than would be expected from

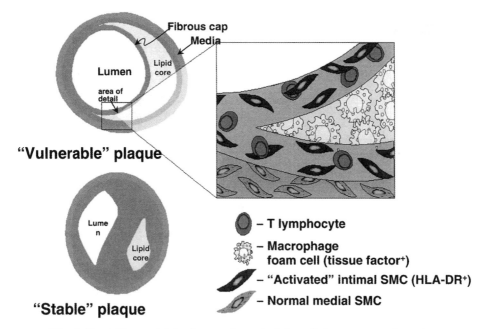

Fig. 3. Unstable vs. stable plaque; characteristics of plaques prone to rupture.

the results of lesion regression analysis performed using quantitative coronary angiography (*4,13,27,30*). For example, in the Familial Atherosclerosis Treatment Study (FATS), intensive lipid-lowering therapy improved stenosis severity by <2% and only 12% of lesions showed regression (*31*). Although the decrease in minimum diameter of the coronary artery was only a fraction of a millimeter, the risk of coronary events decreased by over 70%. These types of data strongly suggest that the beneficial effects of lipid-lowering therapy on atherosclerotic plaques are complex and dependent on multiple synergistic processes.

CORONARY ARTERY
REMODELING IN ATHEROSCLEROSIS

The phenomenon known as "coronary artery remodeling" was first described by Glagov and co-workers (*43*) (Fig. 4). This process results in outward displacement of the external vessel wall in segments with atherosclerosis (*43–46*). In the early stages of coronary disease, this adventitial enlargement prevents the atheroma from encroaching on the lumen ("positive remodeling"), thereby concealing the presence of a lesion on contrast angiography. According to pathology studies, lumen reduction may not occur until the plaque occupies more than 40% of the total vessel cross-sectional area (*43*). Although such lesions do not restrict blood flow, observational studies demonstrate that minimal, nonobstructive angiographic lesions represent an important substrate for acute coronary syndromes (*47*). It has recently been suggested that coronary lumen reduction can occur either by plaque accumulation that has exceeded the capacity of the adventitia to expand (i.e., exhaustion of "remodeling" potential) or by failure of the adventitia to expand in the presence of small or moderate plaque burden (i.e., "negative remodeling") (*48–50*).

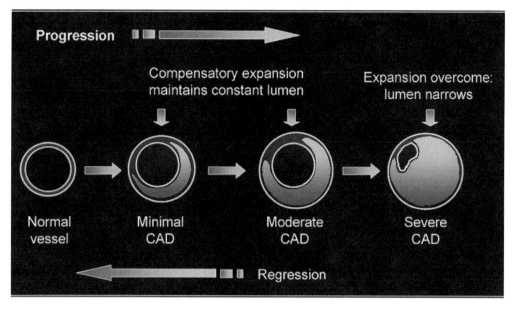

Fig. 4. Glagov's coronary remodeling hypothesis. Adapted from Glagov et al. N Engl J Med 1987; 316:1371–1375.

QUANTITATIVE ANALYSIS OF CORONARY ATHEROSCLEROSIS: *THE LIMITS OF OUR CURRENT GOLD STANDARD FOR CHARACTERIZING CAD*

The quantification of progression, regression, or development of new coronary atherosclerotic lesions has traditionally been determined by quantitative coronary angiography *(51,52)*. However, coronary angiography provides information about the atherosclerotic plaque only when the luminal dimensions of the coronary artery are substantially reduced (Fig. 5). Therefore, subtle changes in atheroma are not detectable. Several multicenter, randomized lipid lowering trials using both angiographic criteria and clinical assessments have shown improvement in luminal caliber of only 1–3%. Yet these same studies demonstrated 25–75% reduction in acute events, including myocardial infarction *(3,53–55)*.

Comparisons of angiography and postmortem specimens have documented that angiography significantly underestimates the extent of atherosclerosis as compared to postmortem histologic examination *(56–59)*. Several inherent properties in the methodology can explain the inaccuracy and large observer variability of coronary angiography. Angiography is a two-dimensional imaging modality, depicting complex coronary cross-sectional anatomy as a planar silhouette of the contrast-filled arterial lumen. However, necropsy and intravascular ultrasound studies demonstrate that coronary lesions are often highly complex, exhibiting markedly distorted or eccentric shapes. Accordingly, arbitrary viewing angles may misrepresent the true extent of luminal narrowing. Although orthogonal angiograms should accurately reflect the severity of many complex lesions, optimal imaging angles are frequently unobtainable because the vessel is obscured by side branches, disease at a bifurcation, or foreshortening *(53)*.

The method most commonly used to assess the severity of angiographic lesions employs visual or computer measurements to determine the percentage of stenosis. This approach

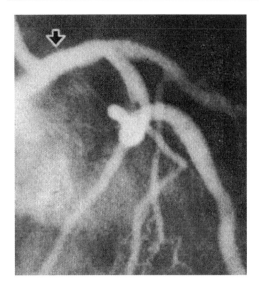 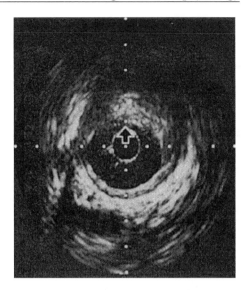

Fig. 5. Angiographically inapparent atheroma. From Nissen et al. In: Topol. Interventional Cardiology Update 1995;14.

compares the luminal diameter within the lesion to the caliber of an adjacent, uninvolved "normal" reference segment. However, necropsy and epicardial echocardiographic examinations have demonstrated that coronary atherosclerosis is often diffuse, involving long segments of the diseased vessel (*57–60*). In many patients, no truly normal segment exists, preventing accurate calculation of diameter reduction (*59,61*). In the presence of diffuse vessel involvement, determination of percent diameter stenosis will predictably underestimate true disease severity. Diffuse, concentric, and symmetrical coronary disease can affect the entire length of the vessel, resulting in an angiographic appearance of a small artery with minimal luminal irregularities. The limits of this diagnostic modality may be the reason why many of the clinical trials of lipid lowering that utilized coronary angiography as its endpoint, while having significant reductions in clinical events, were remarkably negative in relation to angiographic findings.

INTRAVASCULAR ULTRASOUND (IVUS) IMAGING OF CORONARY ARTERIES: *A NOVEL VIEW OF THE PLAQUE AND ARTERY WALL*

Until recently, atherosclerotic coronary lesions could not be visualized directly by any available imaging modality. Detection of coronary artery disease has relied on indirect methods that either evaluate the vessel lumen (angiography) or unmask the ischemic effect of coronary obstructions (nuclear or stress echocardiography). However, both methods are insensitive to the early, minimally obstructive coronary atherosclerosis, the precursor to acute coronary syndromes.

Over the last decade, an alternative imaging system, intravascular ultrasound (IVUS) has become available and is providing a radically different way to view vascular anatomy (*62–69*). The incremental value of coronary ultrasound originates from (1) the cross-sectional, tomographic perspective of the images and (2) the ability to image atheroma directly. Whereas contrast angiography depicts the complex cross-sectional anatomy of a coronary artery as a planar silhouette, ultrasound permits direct visual examination of the

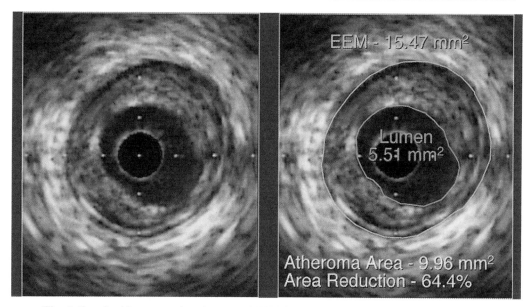

Fig. 6. Standard intravascular ultrasound (IVUS) atheroma measurements: boundaries.

vessel wall, allowing the precise measurement of atheroma size, distribution, and composition. The tomographic orientation of ultrasound enables 360° visualization of the vessel wall, rather than a two-dimensional projection of the lumen. Direct planimetry can now be performed on a cross-sectional image, which, unlike contrast angiography, is not dependent on the projection angle. Unlike angiographic stenosis sizing, which requires careful calibration of the analysis system to correct for radiographic magnification, ultrasound imaging systems overlay an internal electronic distance scale on the image. Because the velocity of sound in soft tissues is almost constant, ultrasound measurements are accurate and do not require special calibration methods *(70)* (Fig. 6).

In general, normal contrast coronary angiograms are present in 10–15% of patients undergoing angiography for suspected coronary artery disease *(71)*. However, Erbel and colleagues have observed using IVUS that atherosclerotic changes are present in 48% of patients with suspected coronary artery disease and a normal coronary angiogram *(71)*. Alfonso and co-workers have demonstrated that in patients undergoing coronary angioplasty, 80% of the angiographically normal proximal coronary segments have atheroma *(72)*. Typically, these plaques often had a semilunar shape and did not disrupt luminal contour. Often, atherosclerotic changes in coronary arteries are detected angiographically only when the plaque occupies more than 40% of the potential vessel lumen *(73)*. Therefore using IVUS, it is not surprising that the "lesion count" is often ten fold greater than by contrast angiography. As originally noted by Glagov et al., adventitial remodeling blunts changes in luminal size during progression of atherosclerosis *(43,74–77)*. IVUS can show increases or decreases in atheroma area despite changes in adventitial size *(45,46,73,75–77)*. In addition, IVUS can increase our understanding of "positive" versus "negative" remodeling on the natural history of CAD. As a result, one can expect that an in-vivo study of coronary atherosclerosis progression and/or regression can be best shown by serial IVUS examinations *(78)*. Additionally, IVUS should permit evaluation of atheroma regression or progression using a smaller sample size than would be necessary using either contrast angiography or clinical events.

LIPID LOWERING AND REGRESSION:
THE LIMITS OF ANGIOGRAPHIC TRIALS

A number of small trials have evaluated the effect of aggressive lipid lowering on actual vessel blockage. These so-called regression trials assessed the degree of atherosclerotic progression and regression by either ultrasonography of the carotid arteries or, more often, by coronary angiography. Two important observations have been made from these trials. First, although lesion regression was uncommon, the rate of lesion progression was often slowed appreciably. Second, the modest degree of change in vascular endpoints has been disproportionate to the substantial reductions in clinical events observed in some regression trials. These observations suggest that mechanisms beyond change in lumen size may account for impressive clinical benefits. Several factors may mediate the risk for plaque rupture, including the functional state of the vascular endothelium and the morphologic and biochemical makeup of the atherosclerotic plaque.

The small changes in luminal narrowing observed with lowering total cholesterol are unlikely to be the principal mechanism by which lipid lowering achieves a reduction in clinical events and revascularization rates. Endothelium-dependent vasomotor function, and the cellular characteristics of plaques that seem to be intimately related to rupture and thrombosis, are factors that might explain the clinical success from correcting the dyslipidemias.

Regression Growth Evaluation Statin Study (REGRESS)

This study *(18)* treated 885 hypercholesterolemic men with either pravastatin or a placebo for 2 yr. The 778 (88%) patients had a final angiogram adequate for quantitative coronary angiography (QCA). Patients had moderate hypercholesterolemia at entry(total cholesterol = 155–310 mg/dL). The mean segment diameter worsened by 0.10 mm in the placebo group and worsened by 0.06 mm in the pravastatin group, which represents a significant ($p = 0.02$) reduction in the rate of progression. The median minimum obstruction diameter decreased 0.09 in the placebo group vs. 0.03 mm in the pravastatin group ($p = 0.001$). Patients in the lowest quartile of LDL-C (85–147 mg/dL) had the greatest reduction in progression of atherosclerotic disease. At the end of the follow-up period, 89% of the pravastatin patients and 81% of the placebo patients were without new cardiovascular events. A 57% reduction in the need for PTCA in the pravastatin treated group ($p < 0.001$). It may be concluded from the REGRESS study that, in symptomatic men with significant CHD and normal to moderately elevated serum cholesterol, small but significant changes by QCA were noted. There was less progression of coronary atherosclerosis and fewer new cardiovascular events in the group treated with pravastatin than in the placebo group.

Pravastatin Limitation of Atherosclerosis in the Coronary Arteries (PLAC I)

The study was conducted in 480 male patients with CHD documented by coronary angiography *(19)*. These patients with LDL-C ≥130 mg/dL, but <190 mg/dL (mean LDL-C = 164 mg/dL), were treated with either pravastatin or placebo for 3 yr. Pravastatin decreased total cholesterol by 19% and LDL-C by 28% ($p ≤ 0.001$ vs. placebo for both). Pravastatin reduced progression of atherosclerosis by 40% for minimal vessel diameter ($p = 0.04$), particularly in lesions with <50% stenosis at baseline. There were fewer new lesions in patients assigned pravastatin compared to placebo ($p < 0.03$).

Primary Prevention	Secondary Prevention
WOSCOPS	4S
AFCAPS/TexCAPS	CARE LIPID

LDL-c

Fig. 7. Lipid-lowering trials.

Table 1
Major Primary and Secondary Prevention Trials, Endpoints, and Risk Reduction

Study	Intervention	Endpoint		Risk reduction (%)
Primary Prevention Trials				
WOSCOPS	Pravastatin	Fatal CAD/nonfatal MI		31
		Total mortality		22
AFCAPS/TEXCAPS	Mevacor	Fatal CAD/nonfatal MI		36

Study	Intervention	Endpoint	Event rate/5yr (%)		Risk reduction (%)
Secondary Prevention Trials					
4S	Simvastatin	Total mortality	11.5	8.2	30
		Fatal CAD/nonfatal MI	28.0	19.0	44
CARE	Pravastatin	Fatal CAD/nonfatal MI	13.2	10.2	24
LIPID	Pravastatin	CAD mortality	n/a	n/a	34

Although no significant difference was evident for change in mean vessel diameter and percent vessel diameter stenosis between pravastatin and placebo groups, a striking 60% reduction in risk of MI was noted during active treatment ($p < 0.05$) with the benefit beginning to emerge after 1 yr. Thus, in patients with CHD and mild-to-moderate cholesterol elevations, pravastatin reduces progression of coronary atherosclerosis and myocardial infarction. These effects were most marked in mild lesions (<50% diameter stenosis at baseline) and in preventing new lesion formation.

CLINICAL TRIALS OF LIPID LOWERING WITH HMG COA REDUCTASE INHIBITORS

Conclusive evidence from rigorous, large-scale, randomized clinical trials, such as the Scandinavian Simvastatin Survival Study (4S) *(11–14)*, the Cholesterol and Recurrent Events (CARE) *(16,17)* and the West of Scotland Coronary Prevention Study *(15)* has further strengthened the position of lipid lowering strategies in clinical medicine (Fig. 7; Table 1).

The landmark Scandinavian Simvastatin Survival Study (4S) *(11–14)* randomized 4,444 patients with CHD in to either simvastatin (20–40 mg/d) or placebo. Significantly, therapy with simvastain resulted in a 35% reduction in LDL-C, a 25% reduction in total cholesterol, a 42% reduction in CHD mortality, a 34% reduction in the risk of coronary events, a 37% reduction in the requirement of coronary bypass grafting or PTCA, a 30% reduction in cerebrovascular events, and, finally, an impressive 30% reduction in the risk of total mortality. Coronary event reduction was seen across all baseline LDL-C levels. The impact of simvastatin on CHD, which was evident after 1 yr of therapy, was significant at 1.5 yr and increased steadily thereafter. These results translate into a 16% reduction in CHD mortality and a 12% reduction in total mortality for each 10% reduction in levels in total cholesterol. The 4S study was the first major secondary prevention study to show a reduction in total mortality and major coronary events in CHD patients receiving lipid lowering therapy.

The West of Scotland Coronary Prevention Study (WOSCOPS) *(15)* was a primary prevention trial of 6595 men with an age range of 45–64 yr and no history of myocardial infarction randomized to either pravastatin (40 mg/d) or placebo. At entry, participants had moderate hypercholesterolemia (mean TC = 272 mg/dL; mean LDL-C = 192 mg/dL). In this study, participants receiving pravastatin had a 20% lower total cholesterol and 26% lower LDL-C, a 33% lower risk of death from CHD, a 31% reduction in the risk for the combined primary endpoint of definite nonfatal myocardial infarction and CHD death. A risk reduction of 22% was noted for total mortality ($p = 0.051$) as was a 32% risk reduction for death from all cardiovascular causes ($p = 0.033$). In this population, there was a reduction of 37% in rate of coronary revascularization procedures ($p = 0.009$). WOSCOPS was the first major study to use an HMG-CoA reductase inhibitor in primary prevention and to demonstrate the clinical benefit of lipid lowering for CHD in this population.

The Cholesterol and Recurrent Events Trial (CARE) *(16,17)* was a 5-yr study of treatment with pravastatin (40 mg/d) or placebo in 4159 patients with myocardial infarction. At entry, TC levels <240 mg/dL and LDL-C levels were between 115 and 174 mg/dL (mean = 139) representing a moderate risk population. Compared to placebo, pravastatin resulted in a 30% reduction in LDL-C (139–97 mg/dL), a 24% reduction in the primary endpoint of fatal coronary event or a nonfatal myocardial infarction ($p = 0.003$), and a 20% reduction in CHD mortality. There was also a 26% reduction in the requirement of coronary bypass grafting ($p = 0.005$) and a 23% reduction in need for PTCA ($p = 0.01$). Of note, there was a 31% reduction in cerebrovascular events ($p = 0.03$). No significant differences in overall mortality or mortality from noncardiovascular causes. The reduction in coronary events was greater in patients with higher baseline LDL-C levels. The benefits of pravastatin are first measurable 12–18 mo after initiation of therapy. The CARE trial extended the benefit of cholesterol lowering therapy with an HMG-CoA reductase inhibitor to the majority of patients with CHD who have "average" cholesterol levels.

LDL Lowering and Revascularization

The Atorvastatin versus Revascularization Treatment (AVERT) *(80)* study provides intriguing data on the role of lipid lowering in the management of patients with mild coronary atherosclerosis. It is known that lipid lowering has been effective in the reduction of percutaneous revascularization rates. In the 4S trial, PTCA was reduced by 37% with aggressive lipid lowering ($p = 0.00001$). Studies of PTCA vs. standard therapy, including ACME, MAAS, and RITA-2, have failed to demonstrate a significant reduction in coronary events. It was therefore hypothesized that, in a population with mild-to-moderate CAD under consideration for coronary revascularization via PTCA, aggressive lipid lowering would provide a significant reduction in clinical events and improved outcomes.

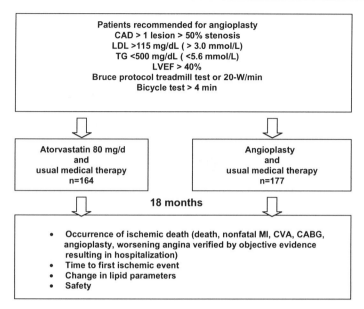

Fig. 8. The AVERT trial: Study design and inclusion criteria. From McCormick LS, et al. Am J Cardiol 1997;80:1130–1133.

The AVERT trial randomized 341 patients with CAD (one lesion of greater than or equal to 50% stenosis), LDL-C greater than 115 mg/dL, LVEF greater than 40% to either PTCA, and standard care or to medical management and aggressive lipid lowering with atorvastatin 80 mg/dL. Patients with left main or its equivalent of three-vessel CAD were excluded (Fig. 8).

The AVERT trial showed a trend toward improved outcomes with medical therapy and aggressive lipid lowering compared with PTCA and standard medical care. There was a 13% ischemic event rate in those receiving atorvastatin vs. a 21% ischemic event rate in those randomized to PTCA. This represented a 36% reduction in events in the group treated with high-dose atorvastatin, although this did not represent a statistically significant difference ($p = 0.048$) (Fig. 9). In general, high-dose atorvastatin was well tolerated with only a 2.4% incidence of AST or ALT abnormalities (>3 times normal). The AVERT trial was a small, underpowered trial with a short follow-up time. It represents a highly selected population that may not have clinical relevance. It does however, serve as an interesting hypothesis generating trial that adds insights into the role of lipid lowering in patients undergoing revascularization and points to the potential therapeutic benefits in this subset.

Given the limits of coronary angiography and the striking disparity between angiographic findings and clinical events noted in the regression trials, it is intriguing to consider the potential role of this new modality to image the atheroma. It is hypothesized that plaque composition and atheroma remodeling may constitute the beneficial effects of lipid lowering. As a two-dimensional image of the coronary lumen, angiography cannot provide a view of these changes. Intravascular ultrasound may provide a more powerful tool for understanding these intra-arterial changes. With this in mind, the recent REVERSAL study hopes to provide insight into the response of the atheroma to lipid lowering.

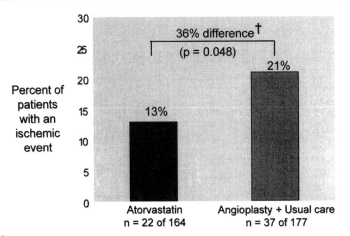

†p=0.048 (NS) (adjusted significance level p=0.045)

Fig. 9. The AVERT trial: reduction in clinical events. Presented by B. Pitt at the 71st annual AHA meeting, Dallas, Texas.

The REVERSAL study will be a multicenter, double-blind, comparative, parallel trial involving approximately 600 randomized patients at approximately 18 study sites. Patients will be randomized to daily doses of either atorvastatin 80 mg or pravastatin 40 mg (approx 300 patients per treatment group). Patients, male or female, ages 30–75 yr who require diagnostic coronary angiography or interventional percutaneous coronary procedures are eligible to participate if they meet all inclusion and exclusion criteria.

REFERENCES

1. Eisenberg DA. Cholesterol lowering in the management of coronary artery disease: the clinical implications of recent trials. Am J Med 1998;104(2A):2S–5S.
2. Expert Panel on Detection, Evaluation, and Treatment of High Blood Cholesterol in Adults. Summary of the second report of the national cholesterol education program (NCEP) expert panel on detection, evaluation, and treatment of high blood cholesterol in adults (Adult Treatment Panel II). JAMA 1993; 269:3015–3023.
3. Kannel WB. The Framingham Study: An epidemiological investigation of cardiovascular disease, Section 30. Some characteristics related to the incidence of cardiovascular disease and death: the Framingham Study. 18-year follow-up. Dept. of Health, Education and Welfare, Washington, DC, Publication No. (NIH) 74-599, 1974.
4. Kannel WB. Range of serum cholesterol values in the population developing coronary artery disease. Am J Cardiol 1995;76:69C–77C.
5. Kannel WB, Castelli WP, Gordon T, et al. Lipoprotein cholesterol in the prediction of atherosclerotic disease: new perspectives based on the Framingham Heart Study. Ann Int Med 1979;90:85–91.
6. Report of the National Cholesterol Education Program on detection, evaluation, and treatment of high blood cholesterol in adults. Arch Int Med 1988;148:36–39.
7. Gould AL, Rossouw JE, Santanello NC, Heyse JF, Furberg CD, et al. Cholesterol reduction yields clinical benefit: a new look at old data. Circulation 1995;91:2274–2282.
8. Sempos CT, Cleeman JI, Carrol MD, et al. Prevalence of high blood cholesterol among US adults. An update based on guidelines from the second report of the National Cholesterol Education Program Adult Treatment Panel. JAMA 1993;269:3009–3014.
9. Hunninghake DB. Therapeutic efficacy of the lipid-lowering armamentarium: the clinical benefits of aggressive lipid-lowering therapy. Am J Cardiol 1998;104(2A):9S–13S.
10. Holme I. Cholesterol reduction and its impact on coronary artery disease and total mortality. Am J Cardiol 1995;76:10C–17C.

11. Scandinavian Simvastatin Survival Study Group. Randomized trial of cholesterol lowering in 4444 patients with coronary heart disease: the Scandinavian Simvastatin Survival Study (4s). Lancet 1994;334: 1383–1389.
12. Bertolini S, Bon GB, Campbell LM, et al. Efficacy and safety of atorvastatin compared to pravastatin in patients with hypercholesterolemia. Atherosclerosis 1997;130:191–197.
13. Tonkin AM. Management of the long-term intervention with pravastatin in ischaemic disease (LIPID) study after the Scandinavian simvastatin survival study (4s). Am J Cardiol 1995;76:107C–112C.
14. Gotto AM Jr. Risk factor modification: rationale for management of dyslipidemia. Am J Cardiol 1998; 104(2A):6S–8S.
15. Sheperd J, Cobbe SM, Ford I, et al. For the West of Scotland coronary Prevention Study Group. Prevention of coronary heart disease with pravastatin in men with hypercholesterolemia. N Engl J Med 1996; 335:1001–1009.
16. Pfeffer MA, Sacks FM, Lemuel A, et al. Cholesterol and recurrent events: a secondary prevention trial for normolipidemic patients. Am J Cardiol 1995;76:98C–106C.
17. Sacks FM, Pfeffer MA, Moye LA, et al. The effect of pravastatin on coronary events after myocardial infarction in patients with average cholesterol levels. N Engl J Med 1996;335:1001–1009.
18. Jukema JW, Bruschke AV, van Boven AJ, et al. Coronary artery disease/myocardial infarction: effects of lipid lowering by pravastatin on progression and regression of coronary artery disease in symptomatic men with normal to moderately elevated serum cholesterol levels: The Regression Growth Evaluation Statin Study (REGRESS). Circulation 1995;91:2528–2540.
19. Pitt B, Mancini GB, Ellis SG, et al. Pravastatin limitation of atherosclerosis in the coronary arteries (PLAC I): reduction in atherosclerosis progression and clinical events. J Am Coll Cardiol 1995;26: 1133–1139.
20. Stone PH. Natural history of coronary atherosclerosis using quantitative angiography in men, and implications for clinical trials of coronary regression. Am J Cardiol 1993;71:766–772.
21. Blankenhorn DH, Nessim SA, Johnson RL, et al. Beneficial effects of combined colestipol-niacin therapy on coronary atherosclerosis and coronary venous bypass grafts. JAMA 1987;257:3233–3240.
22. Sacks FM, Gibson CM, Rosner B, et al. The influence of pretreatment low density lipoprotein cholesterol concentrations on the effect of hypocholesterolemic therapy on coronary atherosclerosis in angiographic trials. Am J Cardiol 1995;76:78C–85C.
23. Nawrocki JW, Weiss SR, Davidson MH, et al. Reduction of LDL cholesterol by 25% to 60% in patients with primary hypercholesterolemia by atorvastatin, a new HMG-CoA reductase inhibitor. Arterioscler Thromb Vasc Biol 1995;15:678–682.
24. Davidson M, McKenney J, Stein E, et al. Comparison of one-year efficacy and safety of atorvastatin versus lovastatin in primary hypercholesterolemia. Am J Cardiol 1997;79:1475–1481.
25. Dart A, Jerums G, Nicholson G, et al. A multicenter, double-blind, one-year study comparing safety and efficacy of atorvastatin versus simvastatin in patients with hypercholesterolemia. Am J Cardiol 1997; 80:39–44.
26. Jones P, Kafonek S, Laurora I, et al. Comparative dose efficacy study of atorvastatin versus simvastatin, pravastatin, lovastatin, and fluvastatin in patients with hypercholesterolemia (The Curves Study). Am J Cardiol 1998;81:582–587.
27. Libby P, Schoenbeck U, Mach F. Current concepts in cardiovascular pathology: the role of LDL cholesterol in plaque rupture and stabilization. Am J Med 1998;104(2A):14S–18S.
28. Tzivoni D, Klein J. Improvement of myocardial ischemia by lipid lowering drugs. Eur Heart J 1998;19: 230–234.
29. Massy ZA, Keane WF, Kasiske BL, et al. Inhibition of the mevalonate pathway: benefits beyond cholesterol reduction? Lancet 1996;347:102–103.
30. Rossouw JE. Lipid-lowering interventions in angiographic trials. Am J Cardiol 1995;76:86C–92C.
31. Brown BG. Regression of coronary artery disease as a result of intensive lipid-lowering therapy in men with high levels of apolipoprotein B. N Engl J Med 1990;323:1289–1298.
32. Vane JR, Anggard EE, Botting RM. Regulatory functions of the vascular endothelium. N Engl J Med 1990;323:27–36.
33. Vogel RA. Coronary risk factors, endothelial function, and atherosclerosis: a review. Clin Cardiol 1997; 20:426–432.
34. Lerman A, Burnett JC Jr. Intact and altered endothelium in regulation of vasomotion. Circulation 1992; 86(Suppl III):III-12–III-19.
35. Anderson TJ, Uehata A, Gerhard MD, et al. Close relationship of endothelial function in the human coronary and peripheral circulations. J Am Coll Cardiol 1995;26:2345–2352.

36. Vogel RA. Endothelium-dependent vasodilation of coronary artery diameter and blood flow. Circulation 1992;91:325–327.
37. Penny WF, Rockman H, Long J, et al. Heterogeneity of vasomotor responses to acetylcholine along the human coronary artery. J Am Coll Cardiol 1995;25:1046–1055.
38. Anderson EA, Mark AL. Flow-mediated and reflex changes in large peripheral artery tone in humans. Circulation 1989;79:93–100.
39. Celermajer DS, Sorenson KE, Gooch VM. Non-invasive detection of endothelial dysfunction in children and adults at risk of atherosclerosis. Lancet 1993;340:1111–1115.
40. Vogel RA, Coretti MC, Plotnick GD. Changes in flow-mediated brachial artery vasoactivity with lowering of desirable cholesterol levels in healthy men. Am J Cardiol 1996;77:37–40.
41. Corretti, MC, Plotnick GD, Vogel RA. Effect of treadmill exercise on flow-mediated brachial artery vasoactivity. J Am Coll Cardiol 1996;27:130A.
42. Vogel RA, Coretti MC, Plotnick GD. Effect of a single high-fat meal on endothelial function in healthy subjects. Am J Cardiol 1997;79:350–354.
43. Glagov S, Weisenberg E, Zarins CK. Compensatory enlargement of human coronary arteries. N Engl J Med 1987;316:1371–1375.
44. Zarins CK, Weisenberg E, Kolettis G. Differential enlargement of artery segments in response to enlarging atherosclerotic plaques. J Vasc Surg 1988;7:386–394.
45. Weissman NJ, Mendelsohn FO, Palacios IF, et al. Development of coronary compensatory enlargement in vivo: sequential assessments with intravascular ultrasound. Am Heart J 1995;130:1283–1285.
46. Berglund H, Luo H, Nishioka T, et al. Highly localized arterial remodeling in patients with coronary atherosclerosis: an intravascular ultrasound study. Circulation 1997;96:1470–1476.
47. Little WC, Constaantinescu M, Applegate RJ, et al. Can arteriography predict the site of a subsequent myocardial infarction in patients with mild-to-moderate coronary artery disease? Circulation 1988;78:1157–1166.
48. Pasterkamp G, Wensing PJ, Post MJ, et al. Paradoxical arterial wall shrinkage may contribute to luminal narrowing of human atherosclerotic femoral arteries. Circulation 1995;91:1444–1449.
49. Mintz GS, Kent KM, Pichard AD, et al. Contribution of inadequate arterial remodeling to the development of focal coronary artery stenoses: an intravascular ultrasound study. Circulation 1997;95:1791–1798.
50. Vavuranakis M, Stefanadis C, Toutouzas K, et al. Impaired compensatory coronary artery enlargement in atherosclerosis contributes to the development of coronary artery stenosis in diabetic patients: an in-vivo intravascular ultrasound study. Eur Heart J 1997;18:1090–1094.
51. Kane JP, Malloy MJ, Ports TA, et al. Regression of coronary atherosclerosis during treatment of familial hypercholesterolemia with combined drug regimens. JAMA 1990;264:3007–3012.
52. Brown G, Albers JJ, Fisher LD, et al. Regression of coronary artery disease as a result of intensive lipid-lowering therapy in men with high levels of apolipoprotein B. N Engl J Med 1990;323:1289–1298.
53. Topol E, Nissen SE. Our preoccupation with coronary luminology: the dissociation between clinical and angiographic findings in ischemic heart disease. Circulation 1995;92:2333–2342.
54. Brown BG, Zhao XQ, Sacco DE, et al. Arteriographic view of treatment to achieve regression of coronary atherosclerosis and to prevent plaque disruption and clinical cardiovascular events. Br Heart J 1993;69:S48–S53.
55. Scandinavian Simvastatin Survival Study Group. Randomized trial of cholesterol lowering in 4444 patients with coronary heart disease: the Scandinavian Simvastatin Survival Study. Lancet 1994;344:1383–1389.
56. Eusterman JH. Atherosclerotic disease of the coronary arteries. A pathologic-radiologic correlative study. Circulation 1962;26:1288–1295.
57. Arnett EN, Isner JM, Redwood DR, et al. Coronary artery narrowing in coronary heart disease: comparison of cineangiographic and necropsy findings. Ann Intern Med 1979;91:350–356.
58. Freudenberg H, Lichtlen PR. The normal wall segment in coronary stenoses—a postmortal study. Z Kardiol 1981;70:863–869.
59. Roberts WC. Quantitation of coronary arterial narrowing at necropsy in sudden coronary death. Am J Cardiol 1979;44:39–44.
60. McPherson DD, Hiratzka LF, Lamberth WC, et al. Delineation of the extent of coronary atherosclerosis by high-frequency epicardial echocardiography. N Engl J Med 1987;316:304–309.
61. Blankenhorn DH, Curry PJ. The accuracy of angiography and ultrasound imaging for atherosclerosis measurement: a review. Arch Pathol Lab Med 1982;106:483–490.
62. Nishimura RA, Edwards WD, Warnes CA, et al. Intravascular ultrasound imaging: in vitro validation and pathologic correlation. J Am Coll Cardiol 1990;16:145–154.

63. Fitzgerald PJ, Ports TA, Yock PG. Contribution of localized calcium deposits to dissection after angioplasty in vivo assessed by intravascular ultrasound imaging. Circulation 1992;86:74–70.
64. Siegel RJ, Chae JS, Maurer G, et al. Histopathologic correlation of the layered intravascular ultrasound appearance of normal adult human muscular arteries. Am Heart J 1993;126:872–878.
65. Hodgson JM, Reddy KG, Suneja R, et al. Intracoronary ultrasound imaging: correlation of plaque morphology with angiography, clinical syndrome and procedural results in patients undergoing coronary angioplasty. J Am Coll Cardiol 1993;21:35–44.
66. Hausmann D, Lundkvist AJ, Friedrich G, et al. Lumen and plaque shape in atherosclerotic coronary arteries assessed by in vivo intracoronary ultrasound. Am J Cardiol 1994;74:857–863.
67. Tuzcu EM, Hobbs, RE, Rincon G, et al. Occult and frequent transmission of atherosclerotic coronary disease with cardiac transplantation—insights from intravascular ultrasound. Circulation 1995;91: 1706–1713.
68. Weissman NJ, Palacios IF, Weyman AE. Dynamic expansion of the coronary arteries: implications for intravascular ultrasound measurements. Am Heart J 1995;130:46–51.
69. Takagi T, Yoshida K, Akasaka T, et al. Intravascular ultrasound analysis of reduction in progression of coronary narrowing by treatment with pravastatin. Am J Cardiol 1997;79:1673–1676.
70. De Mario C. Clinical application and image interpretation in intracoronary ultrasound. Eur Heart J 1998; 19:207–229.
71. Erbel R, Ge J, Bockisch A, et al. Value of intracoronary ultrasound and Doppler in the differentiation of angiographically normal coronary arteries: a prospective study in patients with angina pectoris. Eur Heart J 1996;17:880–889.
72. Alfonso F, Macaya C, Goicolea J, et al. Intravascular ultrasound imaging of angiographically normal coronary segments in patients with coronary artery disease. Am Heart J 1994;127:536–544.
73. Hausmann D, Johnson JA, Sudhir K, et al. Angiographically silent atherosclerosis detected by intravascular ultrasound in patients with familial hypercholesterolemia and familial combined hyperlipidemia: correlation with high density lipoproteins. J Am Coll Cardiol 1996;27:1562–1570.
74. Ge J, Erbel R, Zamorano J, et al. Coronary artery remodeling in atherosclerotic disease: an intravascular ultrasonic study in vivo. Coron Artery Dis 1993;4:981–986.
75. Hermiller JB, Tenaglia AN, Kisslo KB, et al. In vivo validation of compensatory enlargement of atherosclerotic coronary arteries. Am J Cardiol 1993;71:665–668.
76. Losordo DW, Rosenfield K, Kaufman J, et al. Focal compensatory enlargement of human arteries in response to progressive atherosclerosis. Circulation 1994;89:2570–2577.
77. Gerber TC, Erbel R, Gorge G, et al. Extent of atherosclerosis and remodeling of the left main coronary artery determined by intravascular ultrasound. Am J Cardiol 1993;73:666–671.
78. Tuzcu EM, De Franco AC, Goormastic M, et al. Dichotomous pattern of coronary atherosclerosis 1 to 9 years after transplantation: insights from systematic intravascular ultrasound imaging. J Am Coll Cardiol 1996;27:839–846.
79. Crow RS Prineas RJ, Hannan PJ, et al. Prognostic associations of the Minnesota Code Serial Electrocardiographic Change Classification with coronary heart disease mortality in the multiple risk factor intervention trial. Am J Cardiol 1997;80:138–144.
80. Pitt B, Waters D, Brown WV, Boven J, Schwartz L, et al. for the Atorvastatin vs. Revascularization Treatment Investigators. Aggressive lipid-lowering therapy compared with angioplasty in stable coronary artery disease. NEJM 1999;341:70–76.

2

Endothelial Function and Insights for Prevention

Eric H. Lieberman, MD, Margarita R. Garces, MD, and Francisco Lopez-Jimenez, MD, MSC

CONTENTS

INTRODUCTION

When William Harvey described the circulatory system in 1628, it was believed that the endothelium was an inert organ whose mere function was to line the arteries. Extensive research, however, has demonstrated that the endothelium is one of the most sophisticated organs in the system, playing a substantial role in the homeostasis of the circulatory system *(1)*. The endothelium serves as one of the largest paracrine organs in the body by playing a pivotal role in the regulation of such important tasks as vascular growth, vascular tone, and hemostasis. Additionally, it maintains the balance between opposing states: vasodilatation vs. vasoconstriction, growth promotion vs. inhibition, antithrombosis vs. fibrinolysis, antioxidation vs. oxidation, and anti-inflammation vs. proinflammation.

SUBSTANCES PRODUCED BY THE ENDOTHELIUM

In the early 1980s, Furchgott and Zawadski observed that vascular rings with intact endothelium exhibited vasodilatation in response to acetylcholine. In contrast, when the vascular rings were denuded of endothelium, administration of acetylcholine resulted in vasoconstriction *(2)*. They concluded that the endothelium produced a substance capable of causing vasodilatation, endothelium-derived relaxing factor (EDRF) *(3)*. It was subsequently shown that EDRF is nitric oxide or a substance capable of delivering nitric oxide. NO is synthesized in the endothelium by the nitric oxide synthase (NOS), which catalyzes the reduction of L-arginine to produce nitric oxide and citruline. There are three

From: *Contemporary Cardiology: Preventive Cardiology:*
Strategies for the Prevention and Treatment of Coronary Artery Disease
Edited by: J. Foody © Humana Press Inc., Totowa, NJ

isoforms of nitric oxide synthase: neuronal NOS, cytokine-inducible NOS, and endothelial NOS *(4,5)*. Activation of neuronal NOS and endothelial NOS depends on the intracellular concentrations of calcium ions, reduced NADPH, and tetrahydrobiopterin. The inducible NOS is an inducible enzyme present in neutrophils and macrophages that is activated by bacterial endotoxin and cytokines, which contains calmodulin, and is not activated by calcium *(6)*.

NO relaxes the vascular smooth muscle cells by the stimulation of soluble guanylate cyclase, a cytosolic enzyme, and the formation of cyclic guanosine monophosphate, which is associated with the inhibition of the contractile apparatus. In normally functioning endothelium, low levels of NO are released constantly to keep the blood vessel dilated. Physical and humoral stimuli modulate the release of NO. Shear stress, pulsatile stretching of the vessel wall, and low PO_2 appear to be the major physiologic factors for NO release in the normal endothelium *(7)*. Several studies have showed that increases in flow stimulate the release of NO and prostacyclin from the endothelial cells of the arteries. Endogenous substances that can stimulate the release of NO include cathecolamines, vasopressin, bradykinin, histamine, as well as serotonin, ADP and thrombin *(8)*.

Platelet aggregation and platelet adhesion are inhibited in vitro by NO. The activation of platelets, with its release of ADP, serotonin, and thrombin, leads to a massive production of NO, which activates soluble guanylate cyclase, elevates cyclic GMP in the platelets, and reduces cytosolic-free calcium, resulting in vascular smooth muscle relaxation. Platelet adhesion is also inhibited on the endothelium surface as a result of the release of NO in the vessel lumen *(9)*. Secretion of the granules of the platelets can be inhibited by nitric oxide. Gries et al. suggested that NO-dependent inhibition of platelet aggregation might be caused by a decrease in fibrinogen binding to the platelet glycoprotein IIb/IIIa *(10)*.

The endothelium has also been implicated in the regulation of smooth muscle cell proliferation through the complimentary release of growth promoters and growth inhibitors. The growth promoters include angiotensin II, endothelin, fibroblast growth factor, and platelet-derived growth factor. The growth inhibitors include NO and endothelium-derived heparinoids, the former acting as a short-term inhibitor of growth, and the latter exerting a prolonged control of growth *(11)*.

Prostacyclin and thromboxane A_2 are prostaglandins derived from arachidonic acid through the catalysis by cyclooxygenase *(12)*. Prostacyclin is formed primarily in endothelial cells in response to shear stress, hypoxia, and other mediators of NO production. Prostacyclin causes relaxation of the vascular smooth muscle by activating adenylate cyclase and increasing the production of cyclic adenosine monophosphate (cAMP). However, the contribution of prostacyclin to vasodilatation is negligible when compared with NO. In addition to its vasomotor properties, prostacyclin is released by the normal endothelium to inhibit the activation and aggregation of platelets.

Thromboxane A_2 is a potent platelet aggregator formed by the action of the enzyme thromboxane A_2 synthase on cyclic endoperoxides. It is primarily produced in the platelets, although smaller quantities are synthesized in macrophages, lungs, kidneys, and heart. Thus, the balance between the production of thromboxane A_2 and the production of prostacyclin by the endothelial cell is the primary factor in the regulation of hemostasis.

Bradykinin, a vasoactive kinin liberated through the action of kallikrein on kininogen, is a potent endothelium-dependent vasodilator, produced by endothelial cells in response to flow. It is also a potent stimulator of NO, prostacyclin, tissue plasminogen activator (t-PA), and endothelium-derived hyperpolarizing factor release *(13)*.

Endothelium-derived hyperpolarizing factor (EDHF) causes vasodilation by hyperpolarizing vascular smooth muscle through the stimulation of efflux through potassium ion channels *(14)*. In large arteries, both NO and EDHF contribute to endothelium-dependent vasodilation. Although NO predominates under normal circumstances, in these arteries EDHF can mediate near-normal, endothelium-dependent vasodilation when the release of NO is impaired.

Endothelin, the most potent vasoconstrictor known, was first isolated by Yanagisawa et al. *(15)* from porcine aortic endothelial cells. It is produced by the endothelial cells in response to stimulation by thrombin, transforming growth factor-β (TGF-β), interleukin-1, epinephrine, angiotensin II, arginine vasopressin, calcium ionophores, and phorbol ester. Endothelin production is regulated by three inhibitory mechanisms: cGMP-dependent inhibition, cAMP-dependent inhibition, and an inhibitory factor produced by vascular smooth muscle. Intravascular administration of endothelin produces vasoconstriction through the endothelin A receptors located in the smooth muscle cells. It also produces transient vasodilation due to the release of NO and prostacyclin via endothelin B receptors in the endothelial cells *(16)*. Numerous studies suggest that endothelin is a potent stimulator of endothelium hyperplasia and vascular hypertrophy. It has been shown that the endothelin mediates the synthesis of collagen type I in vascular smooth muscle cells *(17)*.

The angiotensin-converting enzyme (ACE) is found in the endothelial cell membrane. There, it converts angiotensin I to angiotensin II and degrades bradykinin. Angiotensin II is not only a strong vasoconstrictor, but also a mediator of smooth muscle growth and an enhancer of superoxide formation. In addition, angiotensin II has been found to enhance endothelin gene expression in animal endothelial cells *(18)*.

t-PA factor, a protease inhibitor that converts plasminogen to plasmin, is synthesized and released by the endothelial cell. Production of t-PA is directly related to stress, bradykinin, cytokines, and thrombin. This substance is inhibited by plasminogen activator inhibitor-1, an important modulator of fibrinolysis. A normal endothelium exhibits a delicate balance between t-PA factor and plasminogen activator inhibitor-1, where the presence of excess plasminogen activator inhibitor-1 may lead to increased thrombosis.

von Willebrand factor (vWF) is the main cofactor in the adhesion of platelets to the endothelium. It also stabilizes and binds coagulation factor VIII in plasma. vWF is produced and stored as granules in the endothelial cell and its release is regulated by histamine, vasopressin, adrenaline phorbol esters, fibrin, and vascular-endothelial growth factor *(19)*. Increased plasma levels of vWF have been associated with endothelial dysfunction *(20)*. Thrombomodulin, a protein composed by 556 amino acids is expressed in the endothelial cells and can be regulated by the exposure of the endothelium to interleukins, hypoxia, and endotoxins. It binds to thrombin and forms a complex, changing the conformation of thrombin, impeding the activation of platelets, the activation of Factor V, and the cleavage of fibrinogen.

CLINICAL MEASUREMENTS
OF ENDOTHELIAL DYSFUNCTION

Ludmer and colleagues *(21)* first demonstrated that endothelial function could be assessed in vivo in the human coronary circulation. Graded concentrations of acetylcholine were infused directly into the coronary arteries. It was found that patients with angiographically smooth coronary arteries dilated in response to acetylcholine; however, arteries that had angiographic evidence of atherosclerosis had paradoxical vasoconstriction to acetylcholine. Additional research has shown that endothelial function can also be assessed using physiologic stimuli such as increase in flow or in response to pacing. Patients with atherosclerotic coronary arteries have impaired flow-mediated dilation. Additional studies have demonstrated that atherosclerotic coronary arteries demonstrate paradoxical vasoconstriction in response to increases in heart rate induced by cardiac pacing. Administering NO synthase inhibitors such as monomethyl-L-argine can eliminate the vasodilator response to acetylcholine *(22)*.

Recently, a noninvasive technique has been used to assess flow-mediated vasodilatation in the brachial artery using high-resolution ultrasound. Various studies validated and reproduced this technique *(23)*. The technique involves locating the brachial artery above the antecubital fossa and obtaining a baseline measurement using a linear phased array transducer attached to an ultrasound machine. After a baseline measurement is taken, a blood pressure cuff is placed in the forearm and is inflated to suprasystolic pressures leading to transient ischemia of the arm. The resultant ischemia results in marked vasodilatation of the resistance vessels. Upon release of the blood pressure cuff, there is a marked increased in flow through the brachial artery. The increase in flow results in the release of NO from the brachial artery and subsequent vasodilatation. Endothelial function can be assessed by the degree of vasodilatation that occurs in response to this increase in flow. There is good correlation in endothelial responses of the coronary arteries testing with acetylcholine and the brachial artery using the noninvasive technique *(24)*.

FACTORS ASSOCIATED WITH ENDOTHELIAL DYSFUNCTION

Endothelial dysfunction can appear before the development of overt atherosclerosis. Furthermore, endothelial dysfunction is a diffuse and generalized process occurring in all vascular beds. The degree of endothelial dysfunction has been shown to correlate with the total number of traditional risk factors for coronary artery disease (CAD). Endothelial dysfunction generally precedes the development of clinical atherosclerosis and may be and early marker of the atherosclerotic process *(25)*.

Estrogen

Pre-menopausal women have a much lower incidence of CAD than age-matched men do. However, this difference disappears after women become menopausal. Ovarian hormones, especially estradiol, have been suggested to mediate the sex-related difference in atherogenesis *(26)*. In animal experiments, replacement of estrogen in ovariectomized monkeys has been reported to reduce the severity of coronary atherosclerosis produced by a high-cholesterol diet. Furthermore, endothelium-dependent vasodilatation varies during the menstrual cycle, and endogenous estradiol has been suggested to be responsible for that variation *(27)*. Overectomized monkeys have been shown to impair endothelial-dependent vasodilatation compared with overectomized monkeys on estrogen replacement therapy. A number of investigators have shown that estrogen can acutely improve endothelial response in postmenopausal women. In addition administration of estrogen over a period of weeks to months has also been shown to improve endothelial-dependent vasodilation *(28)*.

Smoking

Cigarette smoking is the most important modifiable risk factor for CAD and cardiovascular diseases in general. Smoking has been associated to impaired endothelial function, with a detrimental effect beginning from a young age *(29)*. Although the effect of cigarette smoking is dose dependent and is directly related to pack-years, its consequences can be seen in as little as one hour after smoking one cigarette *(30)*. Furthermore, passive smoking has also been linked to impairment in flow-mediated vasodilatation *(31)*. It has been recently demonstrated that cigar smoke can also significantly impair endothelium-dependent vasodilatation *(32)*. Smoking also potentiates the impact of other risk factors on endothelial dyfunction *(33)*.

The specific component of smoking that is responsible of the endothelial injury has not been defined. However, it is likely that the damage is the consequence of an interaction among several factors like carbon monoxide, nicotine, and tar, among others. Smokers have a higher level of oxidative stress, enhanced monocyte and platelet adherence to endothelial cells, and a lower level of plasma HDL–cholesterol level. Smoking may also increase nuclear damage to endothelial cells *(34,35)*.

Hyperlipidemia

A high cholesterol level is a widely known risk factor for CAD. Evidence from epidemiological and experimental studies support the hypothesis that high cholesterol levels induce vascular disease. Hypercholesterolemia impairs endothelial function of both the large conduit vessels and the smaller resistance vessels. The development of endothelial dysfunction precedes the development of overt atherosclerosis *(36)*. In coronary circulation, the degree of endothleial dysfunction correlates with total serum cholesterol levels *(37)*.

The mechanisms by which hypercholesterolemia impairs endothelial function is multifactorial. In general, the possible mechanisms include reduced synthesis of EDRF, impaired release of EDRF, or increased destruction of EDRF *(38–42)*. Oxidized low-density lipoprotein (LDL) has been shown to induce the expression of endothelial adhesion molecules like vascular cell adhesion molecule (VCAM-1), P-selectine and enhance the production of endothelial production of chemokines. In addition, oxidized LDL particles induce monocyte recruitment and macrophage formation with the subsequent production of cytokines and growth factors *(43)*. Hypercholesterolemia also reduces the bioavailability of endothelium-derived NO probably by reduced availability of L-arginine, the precursor of NO. It has been shown that abnormal vascular response in patients with hypercholesterolemia could be corrected by intravenous administration of L-arginine *(44,45)*. Other mechanisms by which hypercholesterolemia impairs endothelial function are by reducing the expression of endothelial NOS and also inactivating NO by superoxide anions or lipoproteins who were oxidized *(46)*. Years before the macroscopic features of atherosclerosis appear, hyperlipidemia causes abnormal conductance and resistance of the vessels.

Hypercholesterolemia induces endothelial dysfunction many years before clinical manifestations of CAD are present. A study showed that children with familiar hypercholesterolemia have endothelial dysfunction early in life when compared with healthy controls *(47)*. A study in young adults showed that subjects in the upper quartile of normal cholesterol level had much worst endothelium-dependent vasodilatation than patients in the lowest quartile of cholesterol level *(48)*.

Early studies of the beneficial effect of lipid-lowering therapy on endothelial function had a clinical confirmation of effectiveness few months later *(49)*. Anderson showed that a medical regimen with lovastatin combined with antioxidant therapy reduced cholesterol levels and improved endothelial-dependent vasomotor responses to acetylcholine after 1 yr of treatment *(50)*. Similarly, Treasure and colleagues, showed improved endothelium mediated vasodilator response to acetylcholine after a mean of only 5.5 mo of therapy with lovastatin administered to hypercholesterolemic patients *(51)*. Furthermore, full restoration of endothelial functions *(52)* was shown in patients with hypercholesterolemia receiving fluvastatin for 1 yr. Simultaneously, clinical trials showed that statins reduced the risk of total and cardiovascular death, as well as the incidence of coronary events after several years of treatment. This fact emphasizes the reliability of endothelial dysfunction assessment for early identification of potentially beneficial interventions to prevent the development and progress of atherosclerosis.

Hypertension

Hypertension is a well-known risk factor for CAD. Endothelial dysfunction occurs as a consequence of high blood pressure, probably mediated by reduction of NO, phenomenon that has been demonstrated in most forms of experimental hypertension models. Hypertension decreases the release or activity of NO. In addition to endothelial dysfunction, hypertension is also associated with vascular remodeling that leads to medial hypertrophy of the vessels. It is likely that the increase in smooth muscle mass may increase the degree of vasoconstriction in response to neurohormones, accentuating systemic vascular resistance and perpetuating hypertension. Whether the reduction in systemic blood pressure correlates with improvement in endothelial function is still controversial *(53–55)*. It is likely that experimental models of hypertension oversimplify a very complex vascular and metabolic disorder like hypertension. A clinical trial showed that after 6 mo of treatment with quinapril, hypertensive patients improved their endothelium-mediated coronary vasodilatation when compared with patients receiving placebo. It has been suggested that the beneficial effect of ACE-I on patients with history of CAD may not be limited to inhibition of ACE but also to improvement in endothelial function.

Diabetes Mellitus

Cardiovascular disease is highly prevalent in patients with diabetes mellitus. Endothelial function is abnormal in experimental models of diabetes and also in patients with the disease *(56,57)*. The principal mediator of injury in diabetics may be hyperglycemia *(58)*. In an experimental model with rings of isolated rabbit aorta, abnormal relaxation to acetylcholine is induced after exposure to high concentrations of glucose in vitro. The glucose-induced endothelial dysfunction occurs as a consequence of several factors. Hyperglycemia increases the synthesis of sorbitol, which acts as an osmolyte, resulting in cell swelling and damage. Furthermore, endothelial dysfunction induced by hyperglycemia may be also associated with an increased release of prostanoids like thromboxane A_2 and prostaglandin F2α.

The impairment of endothelial function in diabetics may be also related to abnormal intracellular signaling mechanisms, inducing the release of vasoactive mediators by the endothelial cell. Protein kinase C activation using phorbol esters induces an impaired endothelium-dependent relaxation similar to the one seen in diabetics. Other mechanisms through which hyperglycemia may induce endothelial dysfunction include an increased production of oxygen-derived free radicals, a decreased Na-K-ATPase activity level, and the presence of advanced glycosylation end products, which has been shown to inhibit NO in vitro.

Other Risk Factors

Age is an independent risk factor for the development of CAD. The effect of age is not only dependent on a longer exposure time to other directly harmful factors, but also through degeneration and aging of endothelial cells *(59,60)*. The estimated life span of a human endothelial cell is around 30 yr, after which the cell is replaced by regenerated endothelium. These regenerated cells tend to lose their capacity of releasing NO in response to platelet aggregation and thrombin.

Homocysteine is an amino acid formed during metabolism of methionine. Hyperhomocysteinemia is an independent risk factor for atherosclerosis and thrombosis. A graded response has also been demonstrated between homocysteine plasma level and the risk for CAD. The atherogenic propensity associated with hyperhomocysteinemia may be partially explained by its deleterious effect on endothelial function. Endothelium-dependent vasodilatation of the brachial artery in patients with a mean homocysteine level of 35 (mol/L was 40% lower than the dilatation seen in patients with average homocysteine level *[61]*). Whether normalization of the plasma homocysteine level is followed by improvement in endothelial function or by a risk reduction for cardiovascular events is still to be defined. Several ongoing clinical trials will help to clarify this issue.

Epidemiological evidence suggests that diets high in fruits and vegetables are associated with a reduced risk for atherosclerosis. One of the many potential mechanisms by which vitamin-enriched diets improve cardiovascular outcomes is restoring endothelial function. Vitamins are antioxidants: therefore, they have a protective effect against free radicals derived from reactive oxygen species. Administration of antioxidants, including vitamins C and E, has shown to improve endothelium-dependent vasodilatation in humans *(62,63)*. Because folic acid decreases homocysteine level, it may possibly reduce the risk of coronary events for the mechanisms explained previously. Furthermore, vitamins may prevent LDL cholesterol oxidation, thereby producing and antiatherogenic effect. Additionally, a high-fat diet can impair endothelial function acutely *(64)*, and the impairment can be prevented with concurrent intake of vitamin C.

CLINICAL APPLICATIONS
OF ASSESSMENT OF ENDOTHELIAL DYSFUNCTION

Assessment of endothelial function is primarily limited to research studies. Endothelial function testing has proven to useful in assessing the response to risk modification in a number of studies. The utility of endothleial function testing in the clinical arena remains unclear. However, it is likely that in the near future assessment of endothelial function will be a useful marker in determining the risk for cardiovascular clinical events and as a measurement of efficacy of medical interventions intended to reduce the cardiovascular risk.

REFERENCES

1. Luscher TF, Rubanyi GM, Masaki T, Vane JR, Vanhoutte PM. Endothelial control of vascular tone and growth. Circulation 1993;87(Suppl V):VI–V2.
2. Furchgott RF. The discovery of endothelium-dependent relaxation. Circulation 1993;87(Suppl V):V3–V8.

3. Furchgott RF, Zawadrki JV. The obligatory role of endothelial cells in the relaxation of arterial smooth muscle by acetylcholine. Nature 1980;288:373–376.

4. Vanhoutte PM, Perrault LP, Vilaine JP. Endothelial dysfunction and vascular disease. In: Rubanyi GM, Dzau VJ, eds. The Endothelium in Clinical Practice. Source and Target of Novel Therapies. Marcel Dekker, New York, 1997, pp. 265–289.

5. Parkinson IF, Phillips GB. Nitric oxide synthases: enzymology and mechanism-based inhibitors. In: Rubanyi GM, Dzau VJ, eds. The Endothelium in Clinical Practice. Source and Target of Novel Therapies. Marcel Dekker, New York, 1997, pp. 95–123.

6. Ikeda U, Shimada K. Nitric oxide and cardiac failure. Clin Cardiol 1997;20:837–841.

7. Busse R, Mulsch A, Fleming I, Hecker M. Mechanisms of nitric oxide release from the vascular endothelium. Circulation 1993;87(Suppl V):V18–V25.

8. Pohl U, Holte J, Busse R, Bassenge E. Crucial role of endothelium in the vasodilator response to increase to increase flow in vivo. Hypertension 1986;8:37–44.

9. Vanhoutte PM, Shimokawa H. Endothelium-derived relaxing factor and coronary vasospasm. Circulation 1989;80:1–9.

10. Gries A, Bode C, Peter K, et al. Inhaled nitric oxide inhibits platelet aggregation, P-selectin expression, and fibrinogen in vitro and in vivo. Circulation 1998;97:1481–1487.

11. Scoft-Burden T, Vanhoutte PM. The endothelium as a regulator of vascular smooth muscle proliferation. Circulation 1993;87(Suppl V):V51–V55.

12. Mehta JL, Yang BC. Prostacyclin and thromboxane: role in ischemic heart disease. In: Rubanyi GM, Dzau VJ, eds. The Endothelium in Clinical Practice. Source and Target of Novel Therapies. Marcel Dekker, New York, 1997, pp. 45–69.

13. Groves P, Kurz S, Hanjorg J, Drexler H. Role of endogenous bradykinin in human coronary vasomotor control. Circulation 1995;92:3424–3430.

14. Campbell WE, Gebredmedhin D, Pratt PF, Harder DR. Identification of oxyeicosatrienoic acids as endothelium-derived hyperpolarizing. Circ Res 1996;78:415–423.

15. Yanagisawa M, Kurihara H, Kimura S, Tomobe Y, Kobayashi M, Mitsui Y, Yazaki Y, Goto K, Masaki T. A novel potent vasoconstrictor peptide produced by vascular endothelial cells. Nature 1988;332:411–415.

16. Masaki T. Overview: reduced sensitivity of vascular response to endothelin. Circulation 1993;87(Suppl V):V33–V35.

17. Stewart D. Impact of endothelin-1 on vascular structure and function. A symposium: endothelial function and cardiovascular disease: potential mechanisms and interventions. Am J Cardiol 1998;82:14S–15S.

18. Luscher TF, Boulanger CM, Yang Z, Noll G, Dohi Y. Interactions between endothelium-derived relaxing and contracting factors in health and cardiovascular disease. Circulation 1993;87(Suppl V):V36–V44.

19. Kalafatis M, Egan J, Maim K. Coagulation factors. In: Rubanyi GM, Dzau VJ, eds. The Endothelium in Clinical Practice. Source and Target of Novel Therapies. Marcel Dekker, New York, 1997, pp. 245–264.

20. Dormandy J, Belcher G. Clinical use of prostacyclin. In: Rubanyi GM, Dzau VJ, eds. The Endothelium in Clinical Practice. Source and Target of Novel Therapies. Marcel Dekker, New York, 1997, pp. 71–94.

21. Ludmer FL, Selwyn AP, Shook TL, et al. Paradoxical vasoconstriction induced by acetylcholine in atherosclerotic coronary arteries. N Engl J Med 1986;315:1046–1051.

22. Lefroy DC, Crake T, Uren NG, et al. Effect of inhibition of NO synthesis on epicardial coronary artery caliber and coronary flow in humans. Circulation 1993;88:43–54.

23. Uehata A, Lieberman EH, Gerhard MD, et al. Noninvasive assessment of endothelium-dependent flow mediated dilation of the brachial artery. Vasc Med 1997;2:87–92.

24. Anderson TJ, Uehata A, Gerhard MD, et al. Close relation of endothelial function in the human coronary and peripheral circulations. J Am Coll Cardiol 1995;26:1235–1241.

25. Anderson TJ, Gerhard MD, Meredith IT, et al. Systemic nature of endothelial dysfunction in atherosclerosis. Am J Cardiol 1995;75:71B–74B.

26. Celerimajer DS, Sorensen K, Spiegelhalter DJ, et al. Aging is associated with endothelial dysfunction in healthy men years before the age-related decline in women. J Am Coll Cardiol 1994;24:471–476.

27. Hashimoto M, Akishita M, Eto M, et al. Modulation of endothelium-dependent flow-mediated dilatation of the brachial artery by sex and menstrual cycle. Circulation 1995;92:3431–3435.

28. Lieberman EH, Gerhard M, Uehata A, et al. Estrogen improves endothelium dependent flow-mediated vasodilation in post menopausal women. Ann Intern Med 1994;121:936–941.

29. Panza JA, Casino PR, Kiloyne CM, Quyyumi AA. Role of endothelium-derived nitric oxide in the abnormal endothelium-dependent vascular relaxation of patients with essential hypertension. Circulation 1993;87:1468–1474.

30. Celermajer DS, Sorensen KE, Georgakopoulos D, et al. Cigarette smoking is associated 20 with dose-related and potentially reversible impairment of endothelium-dependent dilation in healthy young adults. Circulation 1993;88:2149–2155.

31. Celermajer DS, Adams MR, Clarkson P, et al. Passive smoking and impaired endothelium-dependent arterial dilation in healthy young adults. N Engl J Med 1996;334:150–154.

32. Santo-Tomas M, Lopez-Jimenez F, Aldrich HR, et al. Debunking the yuppie habit: cigars and endothelial function. J Am Coll Cardiol 1999;33:232A.

33. Heitzer T, Yla-Herttuala S, Luoma J, et al. Cigarette smoking potentiates endothelial dysfunction of forearm resistance vessels in patients with hypercholesterolemia. Role of oxidized LDL. Circulation 1996; 93:1346–1353.

34. Griendling KK, Alexander RW. Oxidative stress and cardiovascular disease. Circulation 1997;96:3264–3265.

35. Reilly M, Delanty N, Lawson JA, Fitzgerald GA. Modulation of oxidant stress in vivo in chronic cigarette smokers. Circulation 1996;94:19–25.

36. Creager MA, Cooke JP, Mendelsohn ME, et al. Impaired vasodilation of forearm resistance vessels in hypercholesterolemic humans. J Clin Invest 1990;86:228–234.

37. Zeiher AM, Drexler H, Saurbier B, et al. Correlation of endothelial dysfunction in coronary microcirculation of hypercholesterolemic patients by L-arginine. Lancet 1991;338:1546–1550.

38. Verbeuren TJ, Jordaens FH, Zonnckeyn LL, et al. Effect of hypercholesterolemia on vascular reactivity in the rabbit. Circ Res 1986;58:552–564.

39. Cohen RA, Zitnay KM, Haudenschild CC, et al. Loss of selective endothelial cell vasoactive functions caused by hypercholesterolemia in pig coronary arteries. Circ Res 1988;63:903–910.

40. Shimokawa H, Vanhoutte RM. Impaired endothelium-dependent relaxation to aggregating platelets and related vasoactive substances in porcine coronary arteries in hypercholesterolemia and atherosclerosis. Circ Res 1989;64:900–914.

41. Galle J, Mulsch A, Busse R, et al. Effects of native and oxidized low density lipoproteins on formation and inactivation of EDRF. Arterioscler Thromb 1991;11:198–203.

42. Tagawa H, Tomoike H, Nakamura M. Putative mechanisms of the impairment of endothelium-dependent relaxation of the aorta with atheromatous plaque in heritable hyperlipidemic rabbits. Circ Res 1991; 68:330–337.

43. Steinberg D. Oxidative modification of LDL and atherogenesis. Circulation 1997;95:1062–1071.

44. Cooke JP, Dzau VJ, Creager MA. Endothelial dysfunction in hypercholesterolemia is corrected by L-arginine. Basic Res Cardiol 1991;86(Suppl 2):173–181.

45. Creager MA, Gallagher SJ, Girerd XJ, et al. L-arginine improves endothelium dependent vasodilation in hypercholesterolemic humans. J Clin Invest 1992;90(4):1248–1253.

46. Casino PR, Kilcoyne CM, Quyyumi AA, et al. The role of nitric oxide in endothelium-dependent vasodilation of hypercholesterolemic patients. Circulation 1993;88:2541–2547.

47. Sorensen KE, Celermajer DS, Georgakopoulos D, et al. Impairment of endothelium-dependent dilation is an early event in children with familiar hypercholesterolimia and is related to the lipoprotein (a) level. J Clin Invest 1994;93:50–55.

48. Steinberg PR, Bayazeed B, Hook G, et al. Endothelial dysfunction is associated with cholesterol levels in the high normal range in humans. Circulation 1997;96:3287–3293.

49. Leung WH, Lau CP, Wong CK. Beneficial effect of cholesterol-lowering therapy on coronary endothelium-dependent relaxation in hypercholesterolemic patients. Lancet 1993;341:1496–1500.

50. Anderson TJ, Meredith IT, Yeung AC, et al. The effect of cholesterol lowering and antioxidant therapy on endothelium in patients with coronary artery disease. N Engl J Med 1994;332:488–493.

51. Treasure CB, Klein JL, Weintraub WS, et al. Beneficial effects of cholesterol lowering therapy on the coronary endothelium in patients with coronary artery disease. N Engl J Med 1994;332:481–487.

52. Schmieder RE, Schobel HP. Is endothelial dysfunction reversible? Am J Cardiol 1995;76(2):117A–121A.

53. Berkenboom F, Langer I, Carpentier Y, Grosfils K, Fontaine J. Ramipril prevents endothelial dysfunction induced by oxidized low-density lipoproteins. Hypertension 1997;30:371–376.

54. Creager MA, Roddy MA. Effect of captopril and enalapril on endothelial function in hypertensive patients. Hypertension 1994;24:499–505.

55. Schlaifer JD, Wargovich TJ, O'Neill B, et al. Effects of quinapril on coronary blood flow in coronary artery disease patients with endothelial dysfunction. J Am Coll Cardiol 1997;80:1594–1597.

56. Johnstone MT, Creager SJ, Scales KM, et al. Impaired endothelium-dependent vasodilation in patients with insulin-dependent diabetes mellitus. Circulation 1993;88:2510–2516.

57. Williams SB, Cusco JA, Roddy MA, et al. Impaired nitric oxide-mediated vasodilation in patients with non-insulin-dependent diabetes mellitus. J Am Coll Cardiol 1996;27:567–574.

58. Cosentino F, Hishikawa K, Katusic ZS, Luscher TF. High glucose increases nitric oxide synthase expression and superoxide anion generation in human aortic endothelial cells. Circulation 1997;96:25–28.

59. Zeiher AM, Drexler H, Saurbier B, Just H. Endothelium mediated coronary blood flow modulation in humans: effects of age, atherosclerosis, hypercholesterolemia, and hypertension. J Clin Invest 1993;92: 652–662.

60. Barton M, Cosentino F, Brandes RP, et al. Anatomical heterogeneity of vascular aging: role of nitric oxide and endothelin. Hypertension 1997;30:817–824.

61. Woo KS, Chook F, Lolin YI, et al. Hyperhomocystein(e)imia is a risk factor for arterial endothelial dysfunction in humans. Circulation 1997;96:2542–2544.

62. Levine GN, Frei B, Koulouris SN, et al. Ascorbic acid reverses endothelial vasomotor dysfunction in patients with coronary artery disease. Circulation 1996;93:1107–1113.

63. Ting HH, Timimi FK, Boles KS, et al. Vitamin C improves endothelium-dependent vasodilation in patients with non-insulin-dependent diabetes mellitus. J Clin Invest 1996;97:22–28.

64. Vogel RA, Correti MC, Plotnick GD. Effect of a single high-fat meal on endothelial function in healthy subjects. Am J Cardiol 1997;79:350–354.

3

Role of Antioxidants in Coronary Artery Disease

R. Preston Mason, PHD

CONTENTS

INTRODUCTION

Free radicals contribute to the pathogenesis of both acute (ischemia–reperfusion injury) and chronic (atherosclerosis) cardiovascular diseases. This observation has led to the hypothesis that agents capable of inhibiting oxidative stress may be beneficial in the treatment of these diseases. In support of this hypothesis, prospective epidemiological studies have demonstrated a strong inverse relationship between serum antioxidant levels and the number of adverse events associated with coronary artery disease (CAD). The mechanistic rationale for this antioxidant benefit can be attributed to the "oxidative-modification hypothesis," a model that proposes that certain inflammatory processes associated with atherogenesis are triggered by free radical-induced modification of lipids associated with low-density lipoproteins (LDL) and vascular cell membranes. Oxidative stress is also an important feature of heart failure; increasing levels of serum malondialdehyde, a product of lipid peroxidation, can be correlated with severity of disease. Thus, a better understanding of the mechanisms by which oxygen-based free radicals alter cell structure–function relationships could lead to the development of new treatments for cardiovascular

From: *Contemporary Cardiology: Preventive Cardiology:*
Strategies for the Prevention and Treatment of Coronary Artery Disease
Edited by: J. Foody © Humana Press Inc., Totowa, NJ

disorders with greater efficacy and fewer side effects. This chapter discusses the basic mechanisms by which free radicals effect cell injury and the potential role for compounds with antioxidant activity to intervene in these disease processes.

OXYGEN PARADOX

The introduction of molecular oxygen (O_2) into the atmosphere created the opportunity for new, more complex life forms by allowing for the development of aerobic respiration, a powerful means of producing cellular energy. Oxygen also allows for the synthesis of complex molecules (e.g., hormones, neurotransmitters) that facilitated cellular differentiation. On the other hand, oxygen can be highly toxic to life under certain conditions, contributing directly to the etiology of various diseases. Excessive production of free radicals and/or a reduction in cellular antioxidant defense mechanisms lead to increased cell vulnerability because of the damaging effects of these reactive molecules on nucleic acids, proteins, and membrane phospholipids. This "oxygen paradox" has attracted considerable attention in biology as emerging data have provided compelling evidence for oxy-radical-induced cell injury in association with aging (1–4) and age-related diseases, including Alzheimer's disease (5–10), Parkinson's disease (11,12), CAD (2,13–15), and heart failure (16). The mechanisms that underlie oxy-radical cell injury and death is examined during the course of this review.

The presence of molecular oxygen in the atmosphere coincided with the rapid proliferation of photosynthetic organisms throughout the biological environment. However, the emergence of oxygen as an important chemical constituent of the atmosphere was not necessarily a welcome event: molecular oxygen has the ability to effectively oxidize biological material into useless components. But instead of blocking the development of life, biological organisms remarkably adapted and actually thrived under these new chemical conditions. As the terminal electron acceptor in mitochondrial respiration, oxygen was effectively adapted for cellular metabolism. Aerobic respiration provided these new organisms with a powerful advantage over anaerobic glycolysis in the production of chemical energy (e.g., ATP) from substrate molecules, such as glucose. In addition to its role in metabolism, oxygen was also adapted for the synthesis of new biological molecules that provided additional functional capabilities. Finally, oxygen was used as a detoxification agent for the destruction and elimination of harmful xenobiotics.

EFFECTS OF FREE RADICALS
ON BIOLOGICAL SYSTEMS

Despite the ability of biological organisms to successfully harness molecular oxygen for metabolism and synthetic processes, this compound remains a potent oxidizing agent that can effectively strip an electron (or a hydrogen atom) from biological molecules, leading to a disruption in normal cell structure and function. To appreciate the mechanisms that contribute to free radical-induced cellular injury, it is useful to review the basic chemical features of these reactive molecules.

The atomic structure of most atoms, including oxygen, contains pairs of electrons that have opposite intrinsic spin angular momentum. If a single electron is lost, then the remaining molecule with an unpaired electron becomes a highly reactive free radical that will act as a chain carrier in various chemical processes. When the free radical success-

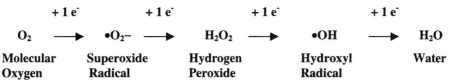

Fig. 1. Progressive reduction of oxygen by single electron transfer produces various reactive molecules, including superoxide, hydrogen peroxide and the hydroxyl free radical. Superoxide and hydroxyl radicals are oxy-radical intermediates, whereas hydrogen peroxide is considered a nonradical oxidizing agent.

fully removes an electron from another molecule, the second molecule is then oxidized, by definition. Alternatively, the radical can donate an electron, resulting in the reduction of the second molecule and oxidation of the initial free radical.

There are two primary classes of reactive free radicals present in nature: carbon-centered, alkyl radicals and oxygen-centered free radicals or oxy-radicals. The predominant oxy-radicals that mediate free radical damage in biological systems are superoxide, hydrogen peroxide, and the highly reactive hydroxyl free radical. The progressive reduction of oxygen by single electron transfer produces these various oxy-radical molecules (Fig. 1). Superoxide and hydroxyl radical molecules are considered oxy-radical intermediates while hydrogen peroxide is considered a nonradical oxidizing agent. Superoxide anions are rapidly produced by components of the mitochondrial electron transport chain that auto-oxidize molecule oxygen (O_2) as well as by enzymatic processes, such as xanthine oxidase and cytochrome P_{450}. Hydrogen peroxide is formed directly by numerous oxidases present in cytoplasmic peroxisomes.

Oxygen-based free radicals have distinct effects on cellular activities. Superoxide reacts strongly with many biological substrates, generally as a reducing agent. Superoxide can rapidly enter cells by aqueous diffusion through transmembrane anion channels and disrupt various intracellular processes. This molecule also has a beneficial role in the immune system as leukocytes produce superoxide in an effort to destroy and eliminate foreign invaders, including bacteria. Hydrogen peroxide is the product of various chemical reactions, including the breakdown of superoxide by superoxide dismutase or SOD, and can readily cross the cell membrane. In the presence of transitional metals (e.g., iron, copper), hydrogen peroxide is rapidly converted into highly reactive hydroxyl free radicals, a process referred to as the Fenton reaction.

$$Fe^{2+} + H_2O_2 \rightarrow \cdot OH + OH^- \tag{1}$$

$$Fe^{3+} + O_2^- \rightarrow Fe^{2+} + O_2 \tag{2}$$

The foregoing reaction highlights the important role of transitional metals such as iron in the development of oxy-radicals. Higher levels of stored iron may contribute to increased cardiovascular risk observed for men and postmenopausal women, by promoting the production of hydroxyl free radicals that react with biological substrates at rates limited only by free diffusion. This unstable molecule triggers a destructive chain reaction, leading to damage that is disproportionately greater than the initial event. In cellular membranes, for example, a single lipid peroxide reaction can lead to 16 additional lipid peroxide products. This process is reviewed in the following series of reactions (Eqs. 3–5), where L represents a membrane lipid molecule:

$$LH + \cdot OH \rightarrow L\cdot + H_2O \tag{3}$$

$$H_2O + L\cdot \rightarrow LOO\cdot + LH \tag{4}$$

$$LOO\cdot + LH \rightarrow L\cdot + LOOH \tag{5}$$

The cell has developed several enzymatic approaches to defending against the destructive effects of free radicals. These enzymes are designed to dismantle the primary oxygen-derived free radicals that inflict damage to the cell and include superoxide dismutase, catalase, and glutathione peroxidase. In addition to these enzymes, a number of biological chemicals are effective inhibitors of oxidative stress, including ascorbic acid, uric acid, α-tocopherol and glutathione. If prooxidant factors overwhelm the antioxidant defense systems of the cell, however, then a disequilibrium exists that results in a net increase in oxidative damage to the cell. The probability of this imbalance increases with biological aging as antioxidant defense systems deteriorate and during diseases that lead to metabolic disorders or elevations in transitional metals, such as iron.

CELLULAR TARGETS FOR FREE RADICALS AND THE ROLE OF ANTIOXIDANTS

Free radicals attack various targets within the cell in an attempt to abstract electrons and restore their internal molecular balance of electrons. The cellular targets for free-radical damage are membrane lipids, including polyunsaturated fatty acids, proteins, and nucleic acids. The process of oxidative damage, if allowed to continue unabated, will eventually effect a loss in normal cell structure and function, leading ultimately to cell death by either apoptosis or necrosis, depending on the extent of injury (2).

Antioxidants protect cells from the effects of free radicals by either interfering with their production or by attenuating their propagation once they are formed. In the first case, enzymes such as SOD or glutathione peroxidase dismantle the reactive agents that trigger free-radical damage (e.g., H_2O_2, $\cdot O_2-$), converting these reactants into chemically stable products (H_2O and O_2). The reactions mediated by these cellular enzymes are reviewed (Eqs. 6–9) as follows:

$$\text{Superoxide dismutase: } \cdot O_{2-} + \cdot O_{2-} + 2H^+ \rightarrow H_2O_2 + O_{2+} \tag{6}$$

$$\text{Catalase: } 2H_2O_2 \rightarrow 2H_2O + O_2 \tag{7}$$

$$\text{Peroxidase: } H_2O_2 + R(OH)_2 \rightarrow 2H_2O + RO_2 \tag{8}$$

$$\text{Glutathione peroxidase: } H_2O_2 + 2GSH \rightarrow GSSG + 2H_2O \tag{9}$$

Antioxidants also function by neutralizing the effects of free-radical molecules once formed, thus preventing their propagation throughout the cell. Specifically, these chemical antioxidants (e.g., α-tocopherol, probucol) function by donating an electron (or hydrogen atom) to the free-radical molecule, thus restoring the normal number of paired electrons, or by trapping the unpaired free radical into its chemical structure where it cannot cause further damage. In either case, the antioxidant is now left with an unpaired free electron and has the potential to become a prooxidant species itself. To prevent this from occurring, the antioxidant structure typically consists of chemical features that stabilize the free electron in various resonance structures (e.g., conjugated rings).

An example of a cardiovascular agent with a chemical structure that provides effective antioxidant protection is the charged dihydropyridine calcium channel blocker (CCB),

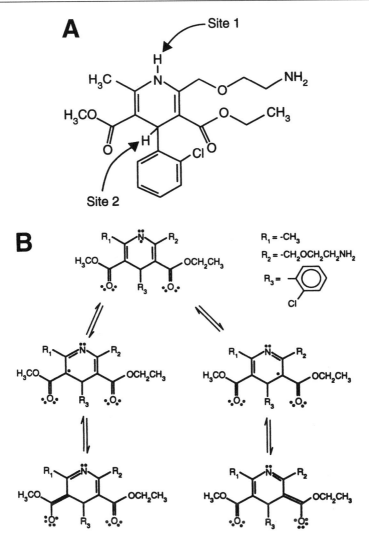

Fig. 2. Chemical antioxidant mechanisms for the charged CCB, amlodipine *(17)*. The covalent chemical structure of amlodipine includes two hydrogen atoms associated with the dihydropyridine aromatic ring that can be donated to unstable free radical molecules (**A**). Resonance stabilization structures for amlodipine at sites 1 (**B**) and 2 (**C**) are calculated.

amlodipine, a drug widely used for the treatment of hypertension and angina *(17)*. The dihydropyridine ring of amlodipine has the potential for donating two hydrogen atoms (Fig. 2). Once the hydrogen atom is abstracted, the remaining unpaired free electron can be stabilized by a number of potential resonance structures, as calculated in Fig. 2. The relatively superior antioxidant activity measured for amlodipine (Figs. 3 and 4), as compared with other antihypertensive agents, is also attributed to its high affinity for the lipid bilayer phase ($K_P > 10^4$), a primary target for oxy-radical damage *(18)*. Biophysical analyses, including differential scanning calorimetry, nuclear magnetic resonance, and X-ray diffraction, indicate that amlodipine has strong interactions with membrane phospholipid molecules due to a combination of hydrophobic and electrostatic forces, an effect that interferes with the efficient propagation of free radicals through the membrane,

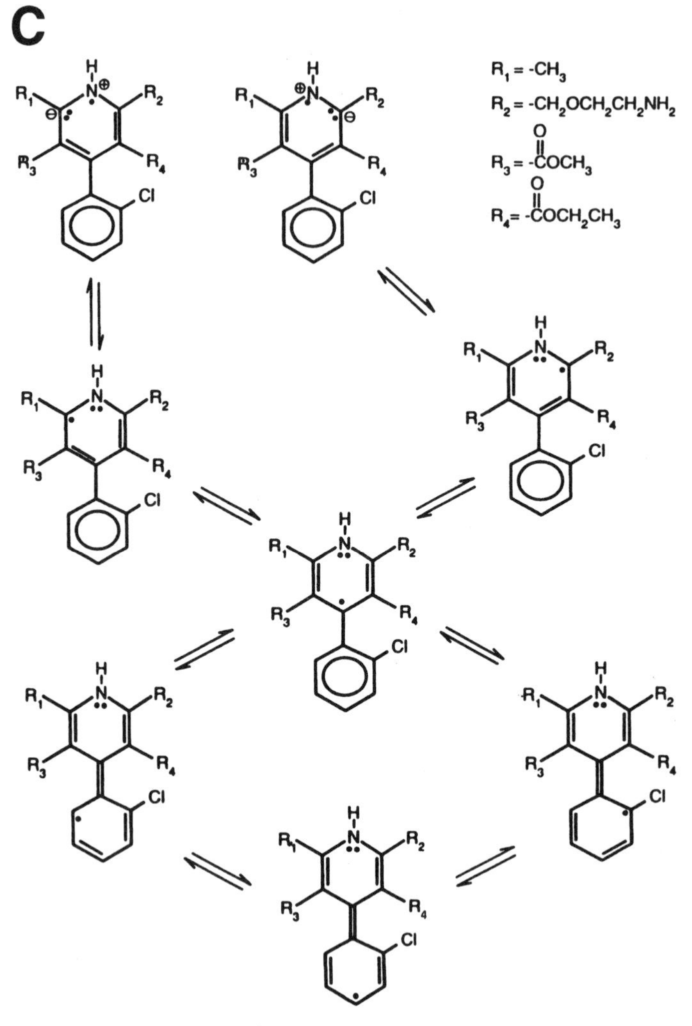

C

$R_1 = -CH_3$

$R_2 = -CH_2OCH_2CH_2NH_2$

$R_3 = -\overset{O}{\overset{\|}{C}}OCH_3$

$R_4 = -\overset{O}{\overset{\|}{C}}OCH_2CH_3$

Fig. 2. (Continued)

independent of calcium channel-binding properties (17,19,20) (Fig. 5). The strong amphiphilic nature of the amlodipine molecule also contributes to its extended duration of activity, as compared to other agents in its class, due to the combination of electrostatic and hydrophobic interactions with membrane phospholipids in the immediate environment of its receptor (18,21) (Fig. 6). Under experimental conditions in which the amlodipine molecule is rendered neutral, these distinct pharmacodynamic effects are eliminated (22). Other CCBs that do not have such high affinity for the membrane lipid bilayer do not exhibit antioxidant effects at low pharmacologic levels (<1.0 μM) (23–26).

The antioxidant activity of amlodipine may contribute to its benefit in patients with documented coronary artery disease, as recently reported in the Prospective Randomized Evaluation of the Vascular Effects of Norvasc Trial (PREVENT) (27). Patients randomized to amlodipine showed a significant reduction in angina (−33%, $p < 0.01$), major vascular procedures (−42%, $p < 0.001$), and the composite of any major event (−30%, $p > 0.01$), as compared to placebo, independent of changes in lipid levels (28). The benefits of amlodipine in CAD have not been observed with other drugs in this class, suggesting that the

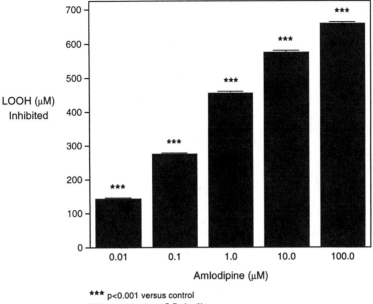

Fig. 3. Inhibition of lipid peroxide formation by amlodipine in membrane vesicles enriched with polyunsaturated fatty acids *(17)*. Lipid peroxide formation was measured as a function of amlodipine concentration (10.0 n*M* through 100.0 μ*M*) at 37°C by spectrophotometric methods. Values are expressed as mean ± SD, $n = 3$ (***$p < 0.001$ vs. control). The control level of lipid peroxide formation was 1.2 m*M*.

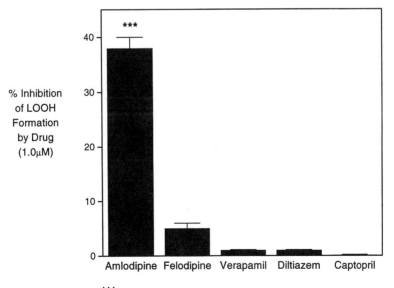

Fig. 4. Comparative effects of antihypertensive agents on inhibition of lipid peroxide formation in membrane vesicles at 37°C *(17)*. Lipid peroxide formation in DLPC vesicles was measured in the absence and presence of amlodipine, felodipine, verapamil, diltiazem, and captopril at a 1.0 μ*M* level after a 48-h incubation period. Values are expressed as mean ± SD, $n = 3$ (***$p < 0.001$ vs. control). The control level of lipid peroxide formation was 1.2 m*M*. From Mason RP, et al. J Mol Cell Cardiol 1999;31:275–281. Used with permission of Academic Press.

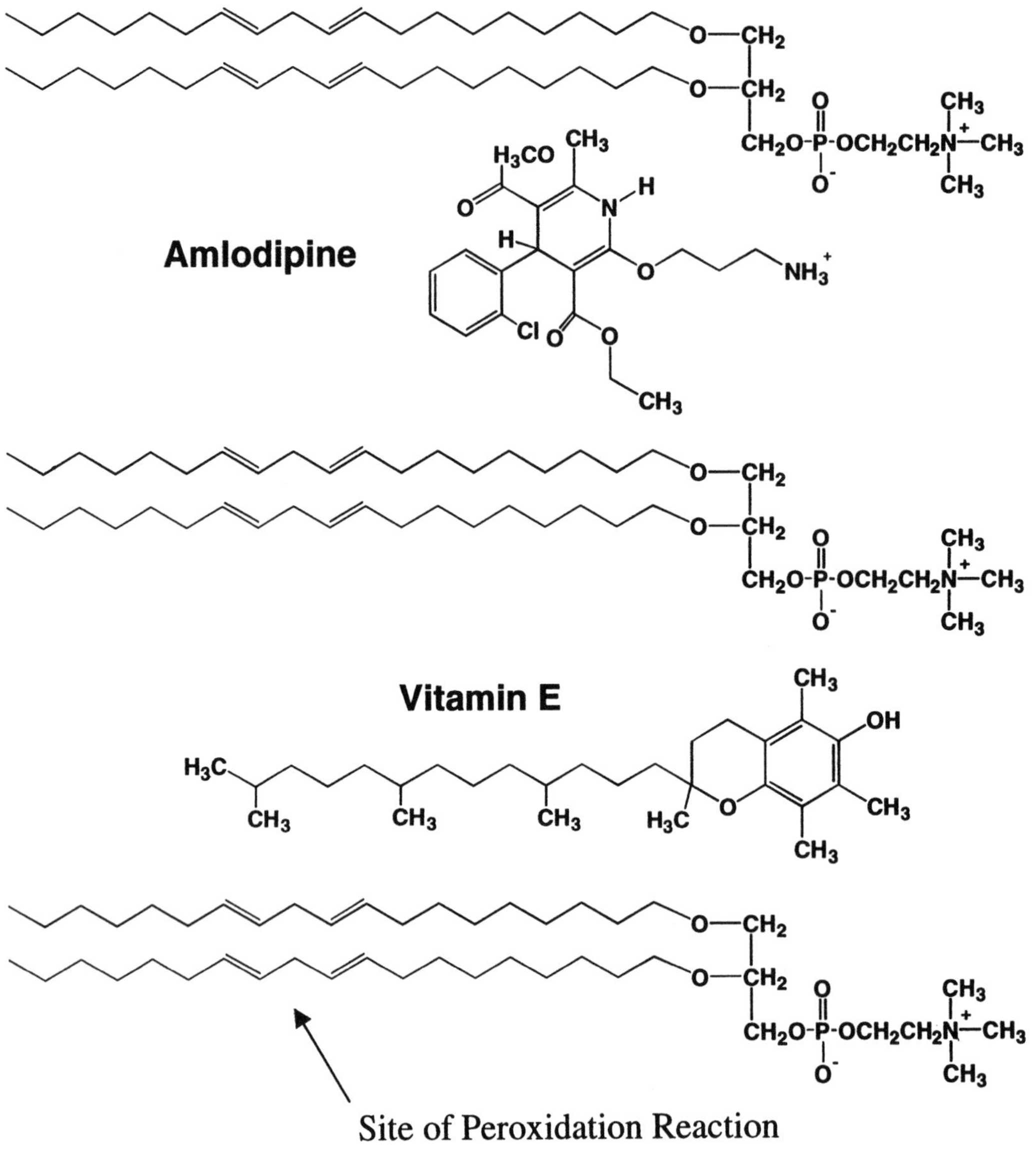

Amlodipine

Vitamin E

Site of Peroxidation Reaction

Fig. 5. Molecular model for the interactions of amlodipine and α-tocopherol with neighboring phospholipid molecules. Based on the results of the X-ray diffraction analysis, the location of amlodipine in the membrane can inhibit the propagation of free radicals by electron-donating and resonance-stabilization mechanisms.

additional antioxidant properties of this compound contribute to direct antiatherosclerotic effects (17). Antioxidant effects have also been reported for the nonselective β-adrenoceptor antagonist, carvedilol. This drug has been approved for treatment of mild to moderate congestive heart failure (CHF), a disease process characterized by progressive elevations in the levels of serum malondialdehyde, a product of lipid peroxidation (16,29,30).

In the case of the lipophilic antioxidant α-tocopherol, this compound, partitions into the cell membrane where it functions to trap or scavenge unpaired free electrons. These

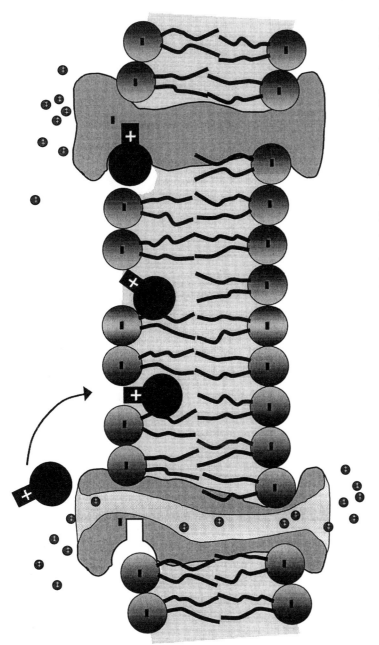

Fig. 6. Highly schematic model of the membrane and receptor physico-chemical interactions of amlodipine. In addition to mediating its strong antioxidant effects in the membrane, the amphiphilic properties of amlodipine facilitate electrostatic and hydrophobic interactions with membrane phospholipids near protein binding sites. As compared to other drugs in its class, these strong membrane interactions contribute to the intrinsic long-acting activity for amlodipine.

37

electrons are then recycled to a soluble electron acceptor at the surface of the membrane. In the absence of an agent such as ascorbic acid, α-tocopherol can eventually become a donator of free radicals or prooxidant. Thus, it is important to note that antioxidants such as α-tocopherol work in concert with other agents to effectively inhibit the chain reaction initiated by free-radical species.

The results of animal and clinical investigations have indicated an important role for lipophilic antioxidants in reducing cardiovascular morbidity and mortality, especially CAD. The rationale for this observation is attributed to the ability of these compounds to interfere with the peroxidation of lipids associated with LDL and vascular cell membranes. In particular, it has been demonstrated that LDL particles with greater resistance to oxidative damage, due to the presence of lipophilic antioxidants, have reduced cytotoxicity, interfere less with endothelium-derived nitric oxide (NO) production, and do not contribute to foam cell formation. The significance of lipid peroxidation in coronary artery disease will be discussed in greater detail as follows.

OXIDATIVE-MODIFICATION HYPOTHESIS FOR ATHEROSCLEROSIS

Peroxidation of lipids in vascular cell membranes and LDL particles represents an early and important event in the pathogenesis of atherosclerosis. The two primary products of lipid peroxidation, malondialdehyde and 4-hydroxynonenal, react strongly with various biological substrates, leading to cellular injury. Oxidative damage to polyunsaturated fatty acids of membrane phospholipids, e.g., leads to a destabilization in their intermolecular packing characteristics and subsequent loss in membrane integrity. Lipid peroxides break down into smaller molecules that either remain covalently linked to the phospholipid glycerol backbone or are released into the cytosol. Using X-ray diffraction approaches, we have directly demonstrated pronounced reductions in membrane width and alterations in phospholipid structure following oxidative stress (35). These same changes in membrane structure have been observed in cellular membranes affected by Alzheimer's disease, a neurodegenerative condition characterized by increased levels of oxidative damage (36).

According to the oxidative-modification hypothesis of atherosclerosis, LDL is mildly oxidized to a form known as minimally modified LDL. The oxidized LDL particle does not effectively bind to the high-affinity LDL receptor, thus extending its circulation and enhancing its uptake into macrophages (37,38). Modified LDL also becomes trapped in the vascular wall where it contributes to a destructive inflammatory response, including the production of granulocyte and macrophage colony-stimulating factors and the monocyte recruitment chemotactic protein 1. As more monocytes and macrophages are recruited into the developing atherosclerotic plaque, LDL undergoes additional peroxidation. Eventually, the protein component of LDL becomes fully oxidized and negatively charged. The completely oxidized LDL particle is now recognized only by macrophage scavenger receptors and internalized to form foam cells. Unlike the uptake of native LDL by the apolipoproteins B and E receptors on macrophages, the scavenger receptor pathway is not subject to negative-feedback regulation, resulting in an uncontrolled accumulation of cholesterol. The foam-cell appearance is due to the widespread presence of esterified cholesterol in intracellular vacuoles. Unless the accumulated cholesterol is eliminated, the foam cells will eventually burst and further contribute to the inflammatory response in atherosclerosis. Besides its role in foam-cell formation, oxidized LDL stimulates monocyte adhesion to the endothelium *(39)* and is directly cytotoxic to vascular cells, resulting in further release of lipids into the intimal space during the progression of atherosclerotic lesions *(40,41)*.

Several lines of evidence support the oxidative-modification hypothesis and the critical role of oxidized LDL in atherogenesis. The results of in vivo analyses indicate that patients with carotid atherosclerosis and acute myocardial infarction have higher levels of immunoreactive LDL. Antibodies to oxidized LDL have been demonstrated to selectively react with atherosclerotic plaques, as opposed to normal vessels *(42–44)*. The levels of immunoreactive LDL are also higher among patients with acute myocardial infarction than in control subjects *(44)*. Thus, the benefit associated with lipophilic antioxidants in CAD is attributed, in part, to the observation that these agents effectively incorporate into the LDL particle and increase their resistance to oxidative modification *(45)*.

Besides lipids, other basic constituents of the cell are vulnerable to free-radical-induced damage, especially nucleic acids associated with nuclear and mitochondrial DNA, and oxidizable proteins. Damage to nucleic acids by free radicals can be broadly categorized as either strand breaks or base modifications. Superoxide and hydroxyl free radicals have been shown to be potent initiators of DNA strand breaks *(46,47)*, leading directly to mutagenesis and the development of cancer. The enzymes that effect repairs to the DNA strand, which occasionally incorporate inappropriate bases into the repaired DNA molecule, facilitate this process. In addition to strand breaks, at least three modified nucleic acid bases, 8-hydroxyguanine, 5-hydroxymethyluracil, and thymine glycol, are produced by hydroxyl free-radical-induced oxidative modification *(46)*. As in the case of strand breaks, nucleic acid modification leads to mutagenesis as a result of misincorporation of bases into the DNA template during repair or replication.

In addition to lipids and nucleic acids, it is well established that oxidizable amino acids associated with cellular proteins are vulnerable to free-radical damage, leading to a loss in normal function. The products of protein oxidation are (1) residue-specific changes in the protein that can lead to a loss of normal structure and function, (2) fragmentation products, and (3) cross-linked reaction products with other molecules within the cell. The effects of any one of these processes can be highly deleterious to the cell, depending on the protein involved and extent of oxidative damage. For example, oxidation of specific amino acids on a subunit of glutamine synthetase results in a complete loss in function, leading to an abnormal increase in glutamate, an excitatory neurotoxin that contributes to the pathogenesis of stroke *(48)*. Cross-linking of membrane proteins through the formation of disulfide (S—S) bonds results in their abnormal aggregation and the formation of new ion channels. Membrane protein cross-linking can also disrupt otherwise normal proteins involved in transport or cell regulation. If a sustained source of oxy-radicals is available, then oxidative damage to cell proteins will continue unabated, leading to fundamental disruptions in cell activity.

ROLE OF ANTIOXIDANTS
IN THE TREATMENT OF ATHEROSCLEROSIS

The deleterious relationship between LDL oxidation and the development of atherosclerosis provides a compelling rationale for the use of antioxidants in the treatment of coronary disease. A number of animal studies and prospective clinical analyses that have specifically explored this question support this hypothesis. Supplementation with α-tocopherol has been shown to increase LDL resistance to oxidative modification, and thus, reduce cytotoxicity toward endothelial cells *(49)*. The lipophilic antioxidant probucol has also been demonstrated to attenuate the formation of atherosclerotic plaques in cholesterol-fed primates, an effect that correlated with an increased resistance of LDL to oxidative damage *(50)*. In addition, probucol inhibited formation of lesions in Watanabe hereditary hyperlipidemic (WHHL) rabbits, a well-characterized animal model of atherosclerosis, independent of cholesterol-lowering effects *(51)*. Consistent with these animal studies, clinical investigations have shown that probucol reduced restenosis by 47% in patients with CAD following coronary artery balloon angioplasty, presumably due to its antioxidant effects *(52)*.

Another pathological process associated with oxidized LDL is an inhibition of the constitutive release of endothelium-derived NO in the arterial wall *(53–55)*. Release of NO inhibits the abnormal adhesion of leukocytes and platelets to the endothelial surface early during the development of atherosclerosis. NO is also an important mediator of vasodilation; loss of NO can lead to vasospasm associated with acute coronary syndromes *(56)*. The interference of this process by oxidized LDL is attributed to a disruption in secondary messenger systems, including G-protein-dependent NO release *(54,55)*. Patients treated with the antioxidant probucol had improved endothelial function, as assessed by NO production, when compared to control subjects. LDL isolated from these patients showed greater resistance to oxidation in vitro and did not interfere with normal NO production from the endothelium, as compared to control LDL samples *(57)*. An important benefit associated with lipophilic antioxidants is the ability to inhibit endothelial dysfunction associated with oxidized LDL, a key early event in atherosclerosis *(15)*.

Thus, a comprehensive review of the available data provides a compelling mechanistic rationale for the use of lipophilic antioxidants to prevent cellular changes associated with CAD. By increasing the resistance of LDL to oxidative damage, agents with antioxidant activity may effectively interfere with pathologic alterations in the vessel wall during atherogenesis, including foam-cell formation, endothelial dysfunction and toxicity, leukocyte and platelet adhesion, and arterial vasospasm, secondary to a loss of normal NO production. These cellular observations also provide important insights into the results of recent clinical studies demonstrating a benefit associated with antioxidant use by reducing the expression of established CAD despite an absence of pronounced changes in atherosclerotic lesion development *(58)*. Indeed, the results of epidemiological analyses have provided direct evidence for an inverse association between the serum levels of antioxidants (e.g., vitamins E and C) and adverse outcomes associated with coronary disease. These studies will be reviewed in the next section.

EPIDEMIOLOGICAL STUDIES THAT LINK
ANTIOXIDANTS TO REDUCED CARDIOVASCULAR DISEASE

Epidemiological findings suggest a beneficial role for antioxidants in the reduction of cardiovascular morbidity and mortality associated with CAD. Large prospective cohort studies, including the Nurses' Health Study *(59)* and the Health Professionals' Follow-up Study *(60)*, have reported a 35–40% reduction in major coronary events (nonfatal myocardial infarction and death from cardiac causes) in subjects receiving the highest quintile of α-tocopherol (100–250 IU supplementation) over a 4–8 yr period, as compared to

Table 1
Prospective Epidemiology Studies on the Relationship
Between Antioxidant Intake and Coronary Artery Disease

Study	Study population	Findings
Nurses' Health Study[a]	87,245 U.S. female nurses	Inverse association between CAD and α-tocopherol intake
Health Professionals' Follow-up Study[b]	39,910 U.S. male health professional	Inverse association between CAD events and α-tocopherol intake
NHANES Study[c]	11,349 U.S men and women	Inverse association between cardiovascular mortality and ascorbic acid intake
Losonczy et al. [d]	11,178 elderly U.S. citizens	Fewer CAD events in subjects taking α-tocopherol than in those not taking it

[a] Stampfer et al. *(59)*.
[b] Rimm et al. *(60)*.
[c] Enstrom et al. *(61)*.
[d] Losonczy et al. *(66)*.

subjects in the lowest quintile (Table 1). In both of these studies, supplementation with ascorbic acid did not improve major coronary outcomes. In a separate study, however, an intake of at least 50 mg/d of ascorbic acid was associated with a significantly lower rate of cardiovascular mortality *(61)*. These findings are consistent with case-control studies that showed that patients with angina pectoris had lower plasma concentrations of α-tocopherol than subjects with normal levels of the antioxidant *(62)*. In addition, it was observed that reduced levels of ascorbic acid in leukocytes were predictive of documented coronary disease *(63)*.

A review of randomized trails designed to investigate a causal relationship between antioxidant intake and a reduction in CAD have provided further insights into this issue. Results from The Cambridge Heart Antioxidant Study demonstrated a 77% reduction in nonfatal myocardial infarctions for those patients with angiographic evidence of coronary disease that received α-tocopherol (400–800 IU/d), as compared to placebo. A benefit was also associated with beta carotene supplementation in the Physicians Health Study *(64)*. In the Alpha-Tocopherol, Beta Carotene Cancer Prevention Study, however, Finnish smokers assigned to beta carotene, α-tocopherol, or both, showed a lack of benefit with either compound over a period of 5–8 yr *(65)*. But it should be noted that the dose of α-tocopherol used (50 mg/d) was less than that required to produce a reduction in events in both the Nurse's Health Study and Health Professionals' Follow-up Study *(59,60)*. The use of α-tocopherol was also shown to be beneficial in CAD among older patients *(66)*.

Thus, a review of descriptive, case-control, and prospective cohort studies indicate an inverse relationship between the clinical manifestations of CAD and the intake of certain antioxidant vitamins. These studies support the "oxidative-modification hypothesis" of atherosclerosis, suggesting a central role for oxidative stress in the etiology of coronary artery disease. Up to now, randomized trials have shown an absence of consistent benefit with beta carotene supplementation but an apparent benefit with α-tocopherol. Further randomized trials are currently underway to address this important question as a function of antioxidant type and concentration. Beyond heart disease, a therapeutic role for α-tocopherol has been explored in other age-related disease that are linked causally to oxidative stress, including Alzheimer's disease *(5–10)*. The results of a prospective clinical study showed that the antioxidant vitamin E (2000 IU daily) slowed the progression of the disease in Alzheimer's disease patients with moderately severe impairment *(67)*. The beneficial activity of vitamin E ($p < 0.001$) was similar to that reported for the selective monoamine oxidase inhibitor *(67)*. Although the changes were modest, vitamin E did slow the clinical deterioration among patients whom had already been diagnosed with this disease.

CONCLUSION

The appearance of molecular oxygen into the earth's atmosphere coincided with the development of new and more complex life forms that effectively harnessed this complex molecule for the efficient production of cellular energy and in the synthesis of novel biomolecules. Paradoxically, oxygen also poses a serious threat to life as it oxidizes important chemical bonds, leading to alterations in cellular structure and function. In CAD, the oxidative-modification hypothesis proposes that increased vulnerability of LDL to oxidation contributes significantly to plaque development and instability. In support of this hypothesis, animal and clinical investigations have indicated that agents with antioxidant activity protect against the cytotoxic effects of oxidized LDL, including endothelium dysfunction, monocyte adhesion, platelet activation, and loss of endothelium-derived NO activity. Epidemiological studies also support a beneficial role for specific antioxidants in reducing the clinical manifestations associated with CAD. Data collected on this subject to date provide compelling support for the hypothesis that agents that increase the resistance of cells to oxidative damage may have an important role in the treatment of various age-related disorders, especially diseases of the cardiovascular system.

ACKNOWLEDGMENTS

The author acknowledges research support from a Nathan Shock Award (NIA/NIH), Gordon Biomedical Research Institute and PPG HL22633 (NHLBI/NIH). The author expresses his appreciation to Pamela E. Mason, M.S., for valuable discussions related to this manuscript. The author also thanks Robert F. Jacob and Carrie M. Blawas for assistance in preparing this manuscript.

REFERENCES

1. Porta EA. Role of oxidative stress in the aging process. In: Chow CK, ed. Cellular Antioxidant Defense Mechanisms, vol. 3. CRC Press, Boca Raton, 1988, pp. 1–52.
2. Rubin E, Farber JL. Cell injury. In: Rubin E, Farber JL, eds. Pathology, 2nd ed. JB Lippincott, Philadelphia, 1994, pp. 1–31.
3. Farber JL, Kyle ME, Coleman JB. Biology of disease: mechanisms of cell injury by activated oxygen species. Lab Invest 1990;62:670–679.
4. Choi JH, Yu BP. Brain synaptosomal aging: free radicals and membrane fluidity. Free Radic Biol Med 1995;8:133–139.
5. Lovell MA, Ehmann WD, Butler SM, Markesbery WR. Elevated thiobarbituric acid-reactive substances and antioxidant enzyme activity in the brain in Alzheimer's disease. Neurology 1995;45:1594–1601.
6. Smith CD, Carney JM, Starke-Reed PE, et al. Excess brain protein oxidation and enzyme dysfunction in normal aging and in Alzheimer disease. Proc Natl Acad Sci USA 1991;88:10,540–10,543.
7. Behl C, Davis J, Cole GM, Schubert D. Vitamin E protects nerve cells from amyloid b-protein toxicity. Biochem Biophys Res Commun 1992;186:944–950.

8. Behl C, Skutella T, Lezoualc'h F, et al. Neuroprotection against oxidative stress by estrogens: structure-activity relationship. Mol Pharmacol 1997;51:535–541.
9. Hensley K, Carney JM, Mattson MP, et al. A model for β-amyloid aggregation and neurotoxicity based on free radical generation by the peptide: relevance to Alzheimer disease. Proc Natl Acad Sci USA 1994; 91:3270–3274.
10. Benzi G, Moretti A. Are reactive oxygen species involved in Alzheimer's disease? Neurobiol Aging 1995;16:661–674.
11. Youdim MB, Riederer P. Understanding Parkinson's disease. Sci Am 1997;276:52–59.
12. Gerlach M, Ben-Shachar D, Riederer P, Youdim MB. Altered brain metabolism of iron as a cause of neurodegenerative diseases? J Neurochem 1994;63:793–807.
13. Diaz MN, Frei B, Vita JA, Keaney JF. Antioxidants and atherosclerotic heart disease. N Engl J Med 1997;337:408–416.
14. Steinberg D. Antioxidants and atherosclerosis: a current assessment. Circulation 1991;84:1420–1425.
15. Ross R. Atherosclerosis—an inflammatory disease. N Engl J Med 1999;340:115–126.
16. Diaz-Velez CR, Garcia-Castineiras S, Mendoza-Ramos E, Hernandez-Lopez E. Increased malondialdehyde in peripheral blood of patients with congestive heart failure. Am Heart J 1996;131:146–152.
17. Mason RP, Walter MF, Trumbore MW, et al. Membrane antioxidant effects of the charged dihydropyridine calcium antagonist amlodipine. J Mol Cell Cardiol 1999;31:275–281.
18. Mason RP, Rhodes DG, Herbette LG. Reevaluating equilibrium and kinetic binding parameters for lipophilic drugs based on a structural model for drug interaction with biological membranes. J Med Chem 1991;34:869–877.
19. Mason RP, Campbell SF, Wang SD, Herbette LG. Comparison of location and binding for the positively charged 1,4-dihydropyridine calcium channel antagonist amlodipine with uncharged drugs of this class in cardiac membranes. Mol Pharmacol 1989;36:634–640.
20. Bauerle HD, Seelig J. Interaction of charged and uncharged calcium channel antagonists with phospholipid membranes. Binding equilibrium, binding enthalpy, and membrane location. Biochemistry 1991; 30:7203–7211.
21. Burges RA, Gardiner DG, Gwilt M, et al. Calcium channel blocking properties of amlodipine in vascular smooth muscle and cardiac muscle *in vitro*: evidence for voltage modulation of vascular dihydropyridine receptors. J Cardiovasc Pharmacol 1987;9:110–119.
22. Kass RS, Arena JP. Influence of pH on calcium channel block by amlodipine, a charged dihydropyridine compound. Implications for location of the dihydropyridine receptor. J Gen Physiol 1989;93:1109–1127.
23. Mak IT, Weglicki WB. Comparative antioxidant activities of propranolol, nifedipine, verapamil, and diltiazem against sarcolemmal membrane lipid peroxidation. Circ Res 1990;66:1449–1452.
24. Mak IT, Boehme P, Weglicki WB. Antioxidant effects of calcium channel blockers against free radical injury in endothelial cells: correlation of protection with preservation of glutathione levels. Circ Res 1992;70:1099–1103.
25. Janero DR, Burghardt B, Lopez R. Protection of cardiac membrane phospholipid against oxidative injury by calcium antagonists. Biochem Pharmacol 1988;37:4197–4203.
26. Ondrias K, Misik V, Gergel D, Stasko A. Lipid peroxidation of phosphatidylcholine liposomes depressed by the calcium channel blockers nifedipine and verapamil and by the antiarrhythmic-antihypoxic drug stobadine. Biochim Biophys Acta 1989;1003:238–245.
27. Byington RP, Miller ME, Herrington D, et al. Rationale, design, and baseline characteristics of the Prospective Randomized Evaluation of the Vascular Effects of Norvasc Trial (PREVENT). Am J Cardiol 1997;80:1087–1090.
28. Byington RP, Chen J, Furberg CD, Pitt B. Effect of amlodipine on cardiovascular events and procedures. J Am Coll Cardiol 1999;33:314A.
29. Yue TL, Cheng HY, Lysko PG, et al. Carvedilol, a new vasodilator and beta-adrenoceptor antagonist, is an antioxidant and free radical scavenger. J Pharmacol Exp Ther 1992;263:92–98.
30. Lysko PG, Lysko KA, Webb CL, et al. Neuroprotective activities of carvedilol and a hydroxylated derivative. Biochem Pharmacol 1998;56:1645–1656.
31. Packer M, O'Connor CM, Ghali JK, et al. Effect of amlodipine on morbidity and mortality in severe chronic heart failure. Prospective Randomized Amlodipine Survival Evaluation Study Group. N Engl J Med 1996;335:1107–1114.
32. Mason RP, Leeds PR, Jacob RF, et al. Inhibition of excessive neuronal apoptosis by the calcium antagonist amlodipine and antioxidants in cerebellar granule cells. J Neurochem 1999;72:1448–1456.
33. Olivetti G, Abbi R, Quaini F, et al. Apoptosis in the failing human heart. N Engl J Med 1997;336: 1131–1141.

34. Narula J, Haider N, Virmani R, et al. Apoptosis in myocytes in end-stage heart failure. N Engl J Med 1996;335:1182–1189.

35. Mason RP, Walter MF, Mason PE. Effect of oxidative stress on membrane structure: Small angle x-ray diffraction analysis. Free Radic Biol Med 1997;23:419–425.

36. Mason RP, Shoemaker WJ, Shajenko L, et al. Evidence for changes in the Alzheimer's disease brain cortical membrane structure mediated by cholesterol. Neurobiol Aging 1992;13:413–419.

37. Steinberg D, Parthasarathy S, Carew TE, Khoo JC, Witztum JL. Beyond cholesterol. Modifications of low-density lipoprotein that incease its atherogenicity. N Engl J Med 1989;320:915–924.

38. Steinbrecher UP, Lougheed M, Kwan WC, Dirks M. Recognition of oxidized low density lipoprotein by the scavenger receptor of macrophages results from derivatization of apolipoprotein B by products of fatty acid peroxidation. J Biol Chem 1989;264:15,216–15,223.

39. Frostegard J, Haegerstrand A, Gidlund M, Nilsson J. Biologically modified LDL increases the adhesive properties of endothelial cells. Atherosclerosis 1991;90:119–126.

40. Schwartz CJ, Valente AJ, Sprague EA, et al. The pathogenesis of atherosclerosis: an overview. Clin Cardiol 1991;14:I1–I16.

41. Cathcart MK, Morel DW, Chisolm GM, III. Monocytes and neutrophils oxidize low density lipoprotein making it cytotoxic. J Leukoc Biol 1985;38:341–350.

42. Palinski W, Rosenfeld ME, Yla-Herttuala S, et al. Low density lipoprotein undergoes oxidative modification in vivo. Proc Natl Acad Sci USA 1989;86:1372–1376.

43. Salonen JT, Yla-Herttuala S, Yamamoto R, et al. Autoantibody against oxidised LDL and progression of carotid atherosclerosis. Lancet 1992;339:883–887.

44. Holvoet P, Perez G, Zhao Z, et al. Malondialdehyde-modified low density lipoproteins in patients with atherosclerotic disease. J Clin Invest 1995;95:2611–2619.

45. Reaven PD, Parthasarathy S, Beltz WF, Witztum JL. Effect of probucol dosage on plasma lipid and lipoprotein levels and on protection of low density lipoprotein against in vitro oxidation in humans. Arterioscler Thromb 1992;12:318–324.

46. Floyd RA, Carney JM. Free radical damage to protein and DNA: mechanisms involved and relevant observations on brain undergoing oxidative stress. Annals of Neurology 1992;32(Suppl):S22–S27.

47. Brawn K, Fridovich I. DNA strand scission by enzymically generated oxygen radicals. Arch Biochem Biophys 1981;206:414–419.

48. Oliver CN, Starke-Reed PE, Stadtman ER, et al. Oxidative damage to brain proteins, loss of glutamine synthetase activity, and production of free radicals during ischemia/reperfusion-induced injury to gerbil brain. Proc Natl Acad Sci USA 1990;87:5144–5147.

49. Belcher JD, Balla J, Balla G, et al. Vitamin E, LDL, and endothelium. Brief oral vitamin supplementation prevents oxidized LDL-mediated vascular injury in vitro. Arterioscler Thromb 1993;13:1779–1789.

50. Sasahara M, Raines EW, Chait A, et al. Inhibition of hypercholesterolemia-induced atherosclerosis in the nonhuman primate by probucol. I. Is the extent of atherosclerosis related to resistance of LDL to oxidation? J Clin Invest.1994;94:155–164.

51. Carew TE, Schwenke DC, Steinberg D. Antiatherogenic effect of probucol unrelated to its hypocholesterolemic effect: evidence that antioxidants in vivo can selectively inhibit low density lipoprotein degradation in macrophage-rich fatty streaks and slow the progression of atherosclerosis in the Watanabe heritable hyperlipidemic rabbit. Proc Natl Acad Sci USA 1987;84:7725–7729.

52. Tardif JC, Cote G, Lesperance J, et al. Probucol and multivitamins in the prevention of restonosis after coronary angioplasty. Multivitamins and Probucol Study Group. N Engl J Med 1997;337:365–372.

53. Chin JH, Azhar S, Hoffman BB. Inactivation of endothelial derived relaxing factor by oxidized lipoproteins. J Clin Invest 1992;89:10–18.

54. Kugiyama K, Kerns SA, Morrisett JD, et al. Impairment of endothelium-dependent arterial relaxation by lysolecithin in modified low-density lipoproteins. Nature 1990;344:160–162.

55. Kugiyama K, Ohgushi M, Sugiyama S, et al. Lysophosphatidylcholine inhibits surface receptor-mediated intracellular signals in endothelial cells by a pathway involving protein kinase C activation. Circ Res 1992;71:1422–1428.

56. Levine GN, Keaney JF Jr, Vita JA. Cholesterol reduction in cardiovascular disease. Clinical benefits and possible mechanisms. N Engl J Med 1995;332:512–521.

57. Plane F, Jacobs M, McManus D, Bruckdorfer KR. Probucol and other antioxidants prevent the inhibition of endothelium-dependent relaxation by low density lipoproteins. Atherosclerosis 1993;103:73–79.

58. Stephens NG, Parson A, Schofield PM, et al. Randomised controlled trial of vitamin E in patients with coronary disease: Cambridge Heart Antioxidant Study (CHAOS). Lancet 1996;347:781–786.

59. Stampfer MJ, Hennekens CH, Manson JE, et al. Vitamin E consumption and the risk of coronary disease in women. N Engl J Med 1993;328:1450–1456.
60. Rimm EB, Stampfer MJ, Ascherio A, et al. Vitamin E consumption and the risk of coronary heart disease in men. N Engl J Med 1993;328:1450–1456.
61. Enstrom JE, Kanim LE, Klein MA. Vitamin C intake and mortality among a sample of the United States population. Epidemiology 1992;3:194–202.
62. Riemersma RA, Wood DA, Macintyre CC, et al. Low plasma vitamins E and C. Increased risk of angina in Scottish men. Ann NY Acad Sci 1989;570:291–295.
63. Ramirez J, Flowers NC. Leukocyte ascorbic acid and its relationship to coronary artery disease in man. Am J Clin Nutr 1980;33:2079–2087.
64. Hennekens CH, Buring JE, Manson JE, et al. Lack of effect of long-term supplementation with beta carotene on the incidence of malignant neoplasms and cardiovascular disease. N Engl J Med 1996;334:1145–1149.
65. The Alpha-Tocopherol BCCPSG. The effect of vitamin E and beta carotene on the incidence of lung cancer and other cancers in male smokers. N Engl J Med 1994;330:1029–1035.
66. Losonczy KG, Harris TB, Havlik RJ. Vitamin E and vitamin C supplement use and risk of all-cause and coronary heart disease mortality in older persons: The Established Populations for Epidemiologic Studies of the Elderly. Am J Clin Nutr 1996;64:190–196.
67. Sano M, Ernesto C, Thomas RG, et al. A controlled trial of selegiline, alpha-tocopherol, or both as treatment for Alzheimer's disease. The Alzheimer's Disease Cooperative Study. N Engl J Med 1997;336:1216–1222.

4

Inflammation and Infection in Coronary Artery Disease

Michael A. Lauer, MD

INTRODUCTION

It has recently been recognized that atherosclerosis in all stages of development and progression—from the fatty streak to the ruptured plaque causing a myocardial infarction—is a specialized inflammatory response. The central role of inflammation in atherosclerosis is underscored by the last two papers authored by the late Russell Ross, whose pioneering research and writing shaped much of our understanding of the pathology over the last 30 years. Both of these reviews asserted unequivocally that "atherosclerosis is an inflammatory disease" *(1,2)*.

Although the understanding of atherosclerosis as an inflammatory disease at the pathological and molecular biology levels has been well described and accepted, the development of animals models of atherosclerosis by inducing chronic inflammation is more formative. Numerous observational studies delineating clinical markers of inflammation and its relationship to the development and progression of atherosclerosis have recently been reported, although widespread acceptance and verification of these studies are ongoing. There is recent evidence that chronic infection with viral agents or bacteria such as *Chlamydia pneumoniae* may contribute to the progression of atherosclerosis. Several small trials of antibiotic therapy reducing cardiovascular events have prompted larger-scale trials. Clinical trials of treatments targeted at specific mediators in the inflammatory process as a means of interrupting the atherosclerotic process are in the formative stages.

This chapter briefly reviews the pathobiology of the atherosclerosis development and progression, emphasizing the inflammatory nature of this disease. Second, the role of markers of inflammation in detecting early or progressive atherosclerotic disease and

From: *Contemporary Cardiology: Preventive Cardiology:*
Strategies for the Prevention and Treatment of Coronary Artery Disease
Edited by: J. Foody © Humana Press Inc., Totowa, NJ

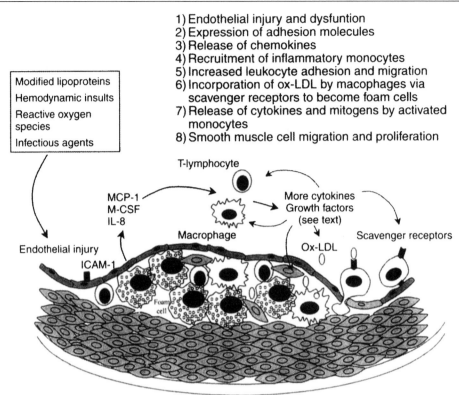

1) Endothelial injury and dysfuntion
2) Expression of adhesion molecules
3) Release of chemokines
4) Recruitment of inflammatory monocytes
5) Increased leukocyte adhesion and migration
6) Incorporation of ox-LDL by macophages via scavenger receptors to become foam cells
7) Release of cytokines and mitogens by activated monocytes
8) Smooth muscle cell migration and proliferation

Modified lipoproteins
Hemodynamic insults
Reactive oxygen species
Infectious agents

T-lymphocyte

MCP-1
M-CSF
IL-8

More cytokines
Growth factors
(see text)

Macrophage

Scavenger receptors

Endothelial injury

Ox-LDL

ICAM-1

Foam cell

Fig. 1. Inflammation and formation of fatty streak. Adapted from ref. *5*. ©1999 Lippincott Williams & Wilkins. All rights reserved. Used with permission.

potentially guiding therapy or detection of a vulnerable plaque is discussed. Finally, the evidence for infectious agents as risk factors and possible etiologic agents of atherosclerosis is presented along with a review of the current trials exploring antibiotic therapy as possible treatment and prevention of atherosclerosis. The data reviewed in this chapter are not likely to dramatically modify the current management of patients; instead, it presents a modified approach to the understanding of atherosclerosis that should provide a revised framework to consider new and revised therapies in the coming years.

ATHEROSCLEROSIS IS AN INFLAMMATORY DISEASE

Early Lesions

The fatty streak is the earliest identifiable lesion of atherosclerosis, appearing early in childhood *(3)*. The fatty streak is a purely inflammatory lesion *(4)*. The process begins when monocyte-derived macrophages and T lymphocytes, in response to a variety of insults to the vascular endothelium in the form of free radicals caused by cigarette smoking, hypertension, modified lipoproteins, glycosylation products of diabetes, or elevated homocysteine, enter the arterial wall *(1)*. The inflammatory response to these various inciting factors is generalized stereotypical response (Fig. 1) *(5)*. The first step in this inflammatory response to injury is an upregulation of intracellular adhesion molecules such as vascular cell adhesion molecule-1 (VCAM-1), intracellular adhesion molecule-1 (ICAM-1), and E-selectin *(6–9)*. These adhesion molecules along with chemoattractants secreted by the endothelium such as monocyte chemoattract protein *(2)* (MCP-1), macrophage colony-stimulating factor (M-CSF), and interleukins begin a parade of monocyte-derived macro-phages and T-lymphocytes into the arterial wall *(10)*. With the uptake of oxidized low-density lipoproteins (LDL) these macrophages become foam cells and the collection of inflammatory cells is recognizable as a fatty streak *(11)*.

Intermediate Lesions

As the monocyte-derived macrophages and T lymphocytes accumulate in the arterial wall, they secrete a variety of proinflammatory cytokines such as interleukins 1 and 6 and tumor necrosis factor alpha (TFN-α), which further upregulate the adhesion molecules as well as promote the uptake of oxidized LDL *(12)*. These cytokines, along with growth factors such as platelet-derived growth factor and fibroblast growth factor, stimulate the proliferation of smooth muscle cells that form layers between the expanding pool of macrophages and foam cells to form the intermediate plaque *(13)*. Another product of the macrophages are a group of elastases, collagenases, and proteinases known collectively as the matrix metalloproteinases. Several of these degrading enzymes have been shown to be present in developing atheroma, especially those associated with aneurysmal dis-ease. It may be that these enzymes are responsible for the degradation of the arterial wall allowing outward expansion of the developing atheroma without impinging on the lumen until a relatively late stage *(14–21)*.

Complex Lesions and Plaque Rupture

As the atherosclerotic plaque continues to develop, a thin fibrous cap consisting largely of collagen develops overlying a mixture of monocytes, extracellular matrix and lipid, smooth muscles cells, and areas of necrosis *(22)*. Thus, the fibrous cap can erode or rup-ture. Such rupture most frequently occur at the shoulder region at the edge of a plaque were the fibrous cap is often thin and shear stresses are at a maximum due to local geom-etry and the Law of LaPlace *(23,24)*. Macrophages and other inflammatory cells accu-mulate at these shoulder regions, and with the release of matrix mettaloproteinasses contribute to erosion and rupture of the vulnerable thin fibrous cap *(10,14,25,26)*. With exposure of the bloodstream to the underlying lipid core, which is highly thrombogenic, this small erosion or rupture can lead to mural thrombosis and myocardial infarction.

MARKERS OF INFLAMMATION IN ATHEROSCLEROSIS

Elevated C-Reactive Protein as a Risk Factor for Cardiovascular Events

C-reactive protein (CRP) is a protein produced solely in the liver under the influence of IL-6 and other inflammatory cytokines. It is named for its affinity for the c-polysac-charide of *Pneumonococcus* and is known to rise significantly as a marker of generalized inflammation in response to acute or chronic infection or injury. Recently, a high-sen-sitivity CRP (hs-CRP) assay has been developed that allows accurate discrimination in the high normal range associated with chronic inflammatory states *(27)*. The presence and degree of inflammation defined by CRP, fibrinogen, IL-1, IL-6, and TNF-α has been associated with an increased risk of future cardiac events.

The European Concerted Action on Thrombosis and Disabilities Angina Study Group examined 3043 patients with angina who underwent coronary angiography and were fol-lowed for 2 yr. After adjustment for the extent of coronary artery disease and other risk factors, an increased incidence of myocardial infarction or sudden death was associated

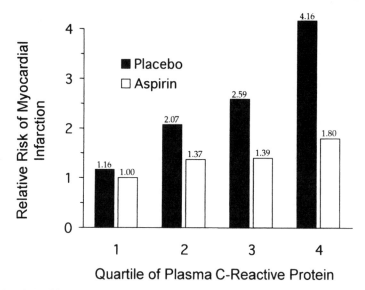

Fig. 2. Relative risk of first myocardial infarction associated with baseline plasma concentrations of c-reactive protein, stratified according to randomized assignment to aspirin or placebo therapy. From ref. *30.*

with higher baseline concentrations of fibrinogen, von Willebrand factor antigen, and tissue plasminogen activator (t-PA) antigen. The concentration of CRP was directly correlated with the incidence of coronary events, except when adjusted for fibrinogen concentration. In contrast, low fibrinogen and CRP levels were associated with a low risk of new coronary events, even in patients with elevated cholesterol *(28).* A nested case-control study of 148 case patients and 296 control patients, drawn from the 12,000 patients enrolled the Multiple Risk Factor Intervention Trial (MRFIT) followed for up to 17 yr found that the risk of coronary heart disease (CHD) death in the quartile of patients with the highest baseline levels of CRP (>3.3 mg/L) was 2.8 times that of patients in the lowest quartile of CRP levels (<1.2 mg/L). For smokers, the relative risk of CHD death in the highest quartile of CRP as compared with the lowest quartile was 4.3 (95% confidence interval 1.74–10.8) *(29).*

A study from the Physician's Health Study found that in 543 apparently healthy men baseline, the men in the quartile with the highest baseline CRP values (>2.11 mg/L) had three times the risk of myocardial infarction. The relationship between CRP and cardiovascular events was independent of other cardiovascular risk factor or homeostatic variables. Additionally, the use of aspirin was associated with significant reductions in the risk of myocardial infarction among men in the highest quartile but with only small, nonsignificant reductions among those in the lowest quartile of CRP level (Fig. 2) *(30).* These and other studies comprise fairly convincing evidence that chronic inflammation, as measured by CRP, is related clinically to the development of coronary artery disease (CAD). The differential treatment effect of aspirin in the Physician's Health Study opens the door to the clinical use of hs-CRP to help guide therapy.

A second, large observational study showing a differential treatment effect based on hs-CRP levels was a nested case-control study of 391 patients with a prior myocardial infarction in the Cholesterol and Recurrent Events (CARE) trial of pravastatin therapy who subsequently developed recurrent nonfatal myocardial infarction (MI) or a fatal

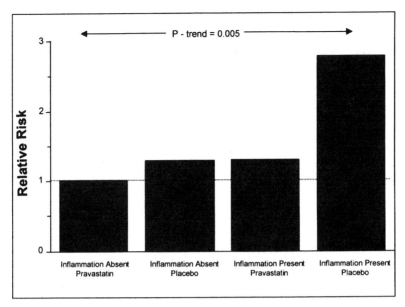

Fig. 3. Relative risk of recurrent events among postmyocardial infarction patients according to presence (both cRP and SAA levels >90th percentile) or absence (both cRP and SAA levels, 90th percentile) of evidence of inflammation and by randominzed pravastatin assignment. From ref. *31.*

coronary event and from an equal number of age- and sex-matched participants who remained free of these events during follow-up. CRP and serum amyloid A (SAA) levels at baseline were higher among cases than control subjects (for CRP $p = 0.05$; for SAA $p = 0.006$) such that individuals with levels in the highest quintile had a relative risk of recurrent events 75% higher than those with levels in the lowest quintile. The risk reduction with pravastatin was much greater (54%) in those with an elevated level of CRP than in the patients without such an elevation (25%) (Fig. 3) suggesting that a subset of patients who stand to derive particular benefit from hydroxymethylglutaryl (HMG) co-A reductase inhibitor therapy might be predicted based on an elevated hs-CRP *(31).* The mechanism behind this interaction is unclear although it has been proposed that it may be due to an interaction between inflammatory mediators and the incorporation of ox-LDL, or due to the anti-inflammatory properties of the HMG co-A reductase inhibitors *(32.33).*

Elevated C-Reactive Protein
as a Prognostic Factor in Acute Coronary Syndromes

The emergence of inflammation as central in the process of plaque rupture has prompted exploration into the pattern of increases in inflammatory markers in acute coronary syndromes. Of particular relevance to the future use of these markers in a clinical setting are whether markers such as hs-CRP can aid in the diagnosis of acute coronary syndromes as well in the determination of the prognosis of developing complications and recurrent events.

It has long been recognized that the levels CRP *(34–36)* and IL-6 *(37,38)* rise with myocardial infarction, although it was unclear if this response was anything more than a marker of inflammation associated with myocardial necrosis. More recent studies have shown that increases in CRP and IL-6 can occur prior to elevations in myocardial specific troponins or CK-MB and may indicate a poor prognosis *(39–41).*

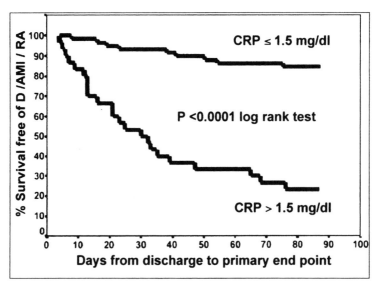

Fig. 4. Kaplan–Meier plot: cumulative freedom from risk of death, MI, or refractory angina within 90 d with CRP levels above or below 1.5 mg/dL. From ref. *46.*

In terms of diagnosis and as a predictor of in-hospital events, Liuzzo and colleagues *(39)* found that the levels of CRP and SAA protein were ≥0.3 mg/dL in 13% of 32 patients with stable angina, in angina 65% of 31 patients with unstable angina, and 76% of 29 patients with acute myocardial infarction. At the time of hospital admission, creatine kinase and cardiac troponin T levels were normal in all the patients. The 20 patients with unstable angina who had levels of CRP and SAA protein > or = 0.3 mg/dL had more in-hospital ischemic episodes and a trend toward higher rates of revascularization, MI, and death than those with levels <0.3 mg/dL *(39)*. A study of 195 patents with unstable angina found that the rate of in-hospital death, myocardial infarction, or emergency revascularization was not higher in patients with a CRP level >0.3 mg/dL *(42)*. In a study of 437 patients with non-ST elevation coronary syndromes enrolled in the Thrombolysis in Myocardial Infarction (TIMI) 11A trial, a CRP level of ≥1.55 mg/dL at presentation was correlated with an increase in 14-d mortality, even in patients with a negative rapid qualitative assay for cardiac-specific troponin T *(40)*.

There have also been several studies showing the utility of an elevated hs-CRP level as a predictor of recurrent events and late complications after admission for acute coronary syndromes. In a study of 965 patients with unstable angina or non-Q-wave MI enrolled in the Fragmin during Instability in Coronary Artery Disease (FRISC) Study, stratification by baseline CRP levels showed that there was a gradation of mortality risk at 5 mo with CRP *(43)*. In a separate study of 102 patients with unstable angina followed for 3 mo, hs-CRP was a predictor of myocardial infarction in a multivariate model and added incremental prognostic to the level of troponin T *(44)*.

Several studies have addressed whether CRP levels at discharge may be a more reliable predictor of future instability than those at admission. A study of 54 patients with unstable angina found that a CRP of >3 mg/L at discharge was most predictive of recurrent instability at 1 yr *(45)*. In a similar study of 194 patients with unstable angina including both derivation and a validation sets, the CRP level at discharge was more predictive than at admission for the combined endpoint of refractory angina, MI, or death at 90 d.

CRP at hospital discharge was the strongest independent marker of an adverse outcome with a relative risk of 3.16 (95% CI 2.0–5.2, $p = 0.0001$) (Fig. 4). A cutoff point of 1.5 mg/dL for CRP provided optimum sensitivity and specificity for adverse outcome, based on the receiver operator curves (46).

Although an elevated CRP level in patients with acute non-ST elevation coronary syndromes is fairly well established as a negative prognostic predictor at this point, the next step is to determine if this is an indicator of chronic inflammation that could potentially be treated to improve outcome. There have been several reports that the CRP levels are lower in patients who have undergone successful thrombolytic therapy as compared with those with failed thrombolysis or who did not receive reperfusion therapy (47–50), although further work is necessary to clarify this relationship. There have not been any published reports of any treatment strategies or pharmacological agents having a differential effect based on CRP levels at the time of admission for acute coronary syndromes such as those reported with aspirin and HMG co-A reducatse inhibitors in chronic atherosclerotic disease. There are several trials of anti-inflammatory or anticytokine agents in various stages of planning, and several of these may incorporate an elevated CRP level as an enrolling criterion.

DETECTION OF THE VULNERABLE PLAQUE

There has been recent interest in developing technology to localize a vulnerable plaque that may be prone to rupture and cause an acute coronary syndrome. If those patients at increased risk for plaque rupture could be determined by an increased hs-CRP or other inflammatory marker, a search for a vulnerable plaque may lead to a catheter-based treatment to stabilize such a lesion. Human atherosclerotic plaques from carotid endarterectomy specimens have been shown to display thermal heterogeneity, with areas of increased temperature correlating with clusters of macrophages (51). Macrophages have been shown to produce heat associated with increased glucose metabolism and phagocytosis (52). Clustering of macrophages have been shown to occur at the shoulder region of an atherosclerotic plaque that is most prone to rupture (23,24,53). Macrophages also play a role in restenosis following percutaneous coronary intervention (54), although in a more diffuse manner than in primary plaque rupture. Restenotic lesions are also associated with changes in temperature profile but these changes are more diffuse and of a smaller magnitude than seen in native atherosclerosis,which is consistent with a more diffuse infiltration of macrophages (55).

It has been suggested that a catheter-based means for measuring coronary artery temperature profile may offer a means of determining which plaques are most active and either responsible for an acute coronary syndrome or predict those that might cause acute events in the near future. An intravascular catheter for the in vivo thermography of coronary arteries has been developed and is used to show that the temperature heterogeneity between plaque and healthy vessel wall increases progressively from stable angina to unstable angina to acute MI (56). Further preliminary data from this same group suggest that within each diagnostic class, those percutaneous coronary intervention (PCI) targets sites with increased temperature heterogeneity are associated with worse outcomes (57). Other catheter-based systems utilizing infrared (58) or near-infrared imaging (59) to detect arterial wall temperature profile are in earlier stages of development. The development of this technology is not ready for clinical use at this time, but its development in parallel with studies of plaque stabilization pharmacological agents, which could be used either systemically or locally, is promising.

THE CASE FOR AN INFECTIOUS COMPONENT TO ATHEROSCLEROSIS

The traditional risk factors of smoking, hypertension, hyperlipidemia, diabetes, and more recently hyperhomocysteinemia only account for approximately 30–50% of cases of advanced atherosclerosis *(60)*. This implies that there may be an undetermined amount of chronic inflammation contributing to the atherosclerotic process. Several infectious agents that tend to cause chronic inflammatory states—most notably *C. pnuemoniae* and members of the herpesvirus family have recently been proposed and fervently studied as possible inciting agents in at least a portion of the these unexplained cases of atherosclerosis.

Viral Disease

The theory that infectious agents may play a role in the development of atherosclerosis dates back more than 20 yr. Fabricant and co-workers found that when chickens were infected with Marek's disease virus, an avian herpesvirus, typical atherosclerotic lesions developed in large coronary arteries, aortas, and major aortic branches of infected normocholesterolemic or hypercholesterolemic chickens *(60a,60b)*. The authors suggested that these results may have important bearing on our understanding of human arteriosclerosis since there is widespread and persistent infection in humans with up to five different herpes viruses.

Cytomegalovirus

Cytomegalovirus (CMV) antigen has been detected in atherosclerotic plaque *(61–63)*, although this may be due to an innocent bystander phenomenon. CMV has also been shown to induce arterial changes similar to early atherosclerotic lesions in a rat allograft model *(64,65)*. Although studies have linked CMV seropositivity to arterial disease, most of these studies have shown an association with transplant vasculopathy *(66–68)*, early carotid thickening *(69–72)*, or restenosis after percutaneous intervention *(69,73)*. Although a few studies have associated CMV seropositivity with native coronary disease, these associations have been rather marginal *(74,75)*. There is preliminary evidence that as multiple pathogens (including CMV, hepatitis A, herpesvirus types 1 and 2, and *C. pneumoniae*) capable of producing a chronic inflammatory response coinfect a particular patient, the CRP levels increase and coronary artery disease prevelance increases *(76–78)*.

Bacterial Agents

Helicobacter Pylori

The discovery that *Helicobacter pylori* was the causative agents for a large portion of peptic ulcer disease, a disease that for many years was not felt to be infectious or a primary inflammatory disorder, certainly laid the foundation for the theory that bacterial infections could be an etiologic agent of atherosclerosis. Several reports have reported an association between seropositivity and atherosclerosis *(79–81)*, although these associations have been fairly weak, and often diminish *H. pylori* even further with controlling other risk factors. There is some evidence to suggest that if there is an association it is due to folate deficiency associated with chronic gastric disease.

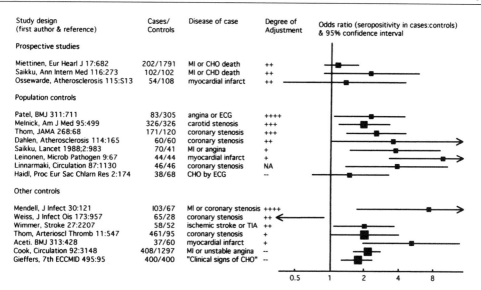

Study design (first author & reference)	Cases/ Controls	Disease of case	Degree of Adjustment	Odds ratio (seropositivity in cases:controls) & 95% confidence interval
Prospective studies				
Miettinen, Eur Hearl J 17:682	202/1791	MI or CHO death	++	
Saikku, Ann Intern Med 116:273	102/102	MI or CHD death	++	
Ossewarde, Atherosclerosis 115:S13	54/108	myocardial infarct	++	
Population controls				
Patel, BMJ 311:711	83/305	angina or ECG	++++	
Melnick, Am J Med 95:499	326/326	carotid stenosis	+++	
Thom, JAMA 268:68	171/120	coronary stenosis	+++	
Dahlen, Atherosclerosis 114:165	60/60	coronary stenosis	++	
Saikku, Lancet 1988;2:983	70/41	MI or angina	+	
Leinonen, Microb Pathogen 9:67	44/44	myocardial infarct	+	
Linnarmaki, Circulation 87:1130	46/46	coronary stenosis	NA	
Haidl, Proc Eur Sac Chlarn Res 2:174	38/68	CHO by ECG	--	
Other controls				
Mendell, J Infect 30:121	l03/67	MI or coronary stenosis	++++	
Weiss, J Infect Ois 173:957	65/28	coronary stenosis	++	
Wimmer, Stroke 27:2207	58/52	ischemic stroke or TIA	++	
Thom, Arterioscl Thromb 11:547	461/95	coronary stenosis	+	
Aceti. BMJ 313:428	37/60	myocardial infarct	+	
Cook, Circulation 92:3148	408/1297	MI or unstable angina	--	
Gieffers, 7th ECCMID 495:95	400/400	"Clinical signs of CHO"	--	

0.5   1   2   4   8

Fig. 5. Odds ratios of epidemiological studies of *C. pneumoniae* seropositivity and vascular disease. From ref. *86*.

CHLAMYDIA PNEUMONIAE

C. pneumoniae is a newly discovered third species of chlamydia shown to cause pneumonia, bronchitis, pharyngitis, and sinusitis in humans *(82)*. It was first described by Grayston and co-workers *(83)*. *C. pneumoniae* is an obligate intracellular organism that spends most of its life cycle within macrophages. Most infections are subclinical or cause only benign flulike symptoms *(84)*. The prevalence of antibodies to *C. pneumoniae* begins in late adolescence and increases with age to at least 50% in middle age U.S. adults, and as high as 80% in the elderly *(84,85)*.

Seroepidemiologic Studies. A link between *C. pneumoniae* and atherosclerosis was first suggested when Saikku and colleagues reported a small seroepidemiologic study showing a much higher rate of seropositivity in patients with acute myocardial infarction or chronic coronary disease than in patients without such history *(86)*. Saikku discovered this association after testing the antigen detection techniques that he had learned in Dr. Grayston's laboratory on a population that he thought to be normal, those admitted to the coronary intensive care unit, and found the seropositive rate to be much higher than expected. To date there have been at least 20 studies showing a relationship between seropositivity to *C. pneumoniae* and atherosclerotic disease and events, whereas there have been several which have failed to show a relationship (Fig. 5).

In a case-control study of from the Helsinki Heart Study, the 103 patients of the 4081 enrolled who suffered fatal or nonfatal MI or sudden cardiac death during the 5-yr follow-up where compared to matched controls in terms of antibodies against *C. pneumoniae* at study entry. Using a conditional logistic regression model, odds ratios for the development of coronary heart disease were 2.7 (95% CI, 1.1–6.5) for elevated IgA titers, 2.1 (CI, 1.1–3.9) for the presence of immune complexes, and 2.9 (CI, 1.5–5.4) for the presence of both factors *(87)*. Recently, longer term follow-up was reported on this same cohort with follow-up out to 8.5 yr and including baseline serology to adenovirus, enterovirus, cytomegalovirus, and herpes simplex virus as well as to *C. pneumoniae* and *H. pylori*. Antibody levels to herpes simplex type I (HSV- 1) and to *C. pneumoniae* were higher in cases than in controls, whereas the distributions of antibodies to other infectious agents were similar. Mean CRP was higher in cases (4.4 vs. 2.0 mg/L; $p = 0.001$), and high CRP increased the risks associated with smoking and with high antimicrobial antibody levels. The odds ratios in subjects with high antibody and high CRP levels were 25.4 (95% CI 2.9–220.3) for HSV-1 and 5.4 (95% CI 2.4–12.4) for chlamydia compared with subjects with low antibody levels and low CRP. High antibody levels to either HSV-1 or to *C. pneumoniae* increased the risk independently of the other, and their joint effect was close to additive *(88)*. These data support the concept that patients with evidence on chronic infection from an infectious agent, or more likely several agents, is at particular risk for events, and may be a population that may benefit from therapeutic intervention, although the details of such a strategy is yet to be worked out.

Another study that showed an association between elevated levels of antibodies to chlamydia and angiographically significant atherosclerosis was a 342-patient case control study from the Group Health Cooperative in Seattle, WA. After adjusting for age, gender, and calendar quarter of blood drawing, the OR for CAD associated with the presence of antibody was 2.6 (95% confidence interval, 1.4–4.8) *(89)*. Like the Helsiki Heart study there was an associatoin with smoking. In fact in this study, the association was limited to cigarette smokers, in whom the odds ratio (OR) was 3.5 (95% confidence interval, 1.7–7.0). Among never-smokers, the OR was 0.8 (95% confidence interval, 0.3–1.9). Some have suggested that smokers increase susceptibility to respiratory tract infections such as *C. pneumoniae* may explain part of the atherosclerotic risk associated with atherosclerosis *(90)*.

A study of particular note that failed to show an association between seropositivity to *C. pneumoniae* comes from the Physician's Health Study in which, contrary to the association between CRP and events in this population, there was no increase risk for cardiovascular events with *C. pneumoniae (91)*. Note that this study is based on antibody presence at entry into the study that include 12-yr follow-up. It is not known whether seroconversion during the follow-up period occurred more frequently in those suffering events. This study was also controlled for smoking status, hyperlipidemia, and other more traditional cardiovascular risk factors. As pointed out earlier, there may be an interaction between both hyperlipidemia and smoking with *C. pneumoniae* that would account for weakening of the association when these factors are controlled.

Antigen Detection Studies. *C. pneumoniae* or its antigens have been found in atheroma from human aorta *(92)*, carotid arteries *(93)*, and coronary arteries *(94–96)*. Although these studies are intriguing in that they show that chlamydia is able to survive within atherosclerotic plaque, it does not, however, prove a causative role as they could be present as an innocent bystander, since the organism inhabits macrophages that inhabit atherosclerotic plaque. Conversely, *C. pneumoniae* could have an effect on atherosclerosis without direct infection as it could induce a chronic inflammatory response due to chronic infection at a distance site.

Animal Studies. Although Koch's postulates cannot be fully met in a multifactorial disease such as atherosclerosis, proof for *C. pneumoniae's* role in the initiation or progression of atherosclerosis, as well as insight into the mechanism of such a role, comes from animal models of chlamydial facilitated atherosclerosis *(77)*. In apoE-deficient mice, *C. pneumoniae* infection accelerates the progression of atherosclerosis in the aortic arch *(97)*. *C. pneumoniae* was detected by direct plating, isolation, and polymerase chain reaction in alveolar macrophages and peripheral blood mononuclear cells, but not plasma, of intranasally inoculated mice *(98)*. Normocholesterolemic rabbits develop intimal altera-tions when infected with *C. pneumoniae (98a,98b)* and rabbits fed a modestly cholesterol enhanced diet have been shown by Muhlestein and colleagues *(98c)* to develop acceler-ated aortic atherosclerosis which is prevented by treatment with the macrolide antibiotic azithromycin *(99)*. *C. pneumoniae* antigen could be detected in the aortic atheroma in this model, and although treatment ameliorated the accelerated atherosclerosis, *C. pneumoniae* antigen was still detected in the atheroma following treatment. It is unclear whether this represented viable quiescent organism or merely antigenic remnants of killed organism. The coronary arteries of cholesterol fed minipigs show inflammatory changes including an increased presence of matrix metalloproteinases when infected intranasally with *C. pneumoniae (100)*. These various animal models add convincing evidence that *C. pneu-moniae* can contribute to the atherosclerotic process. Continued work with these models will be important to continue to elucidate the mechansims behind chlamydia's role in atherosclerosis and details regarding potential treatments and their timing.

The Early Clinical Trials. Two relatively small trials of macrolide antibiotics which are effective against *C. pneumoniae* showed dramatic reductions of coronary events with short courses of therapy. The ROXIS Pilot Study was an Argentinean study in which 202 patients with unstable angina or non-Q-wave MI regardless of serology status were randomized to roxithromycin 150 mg or placebo for up to 30 d. At 30 d, there was a statistically significant reduction in the combined endpoint of cardiac death, myocardial infarction, and severe recurrent ischemia (2% vs. 9%, $p = 0.03$) *(101)*. The treatment effect seem to dwindle over time, however, such that at 3 and 6 mo although there was still a difference in the combined endpoint, the difference had lost statistical significance (12.5% vs. 4.37%, $p = 0.06$ at 3 mo, 14.6% vs. 8.69%, $p = 0.26$ at 6 mo) *(102)*. It is unclear whether this lost of treatment effect is due to inadequate length of treatment, or merely a play of chance at 30 d.

The second preliminary study that drew a considerable amount of attention, despite its small size and several flaws in study design, was performed at a single center in the UK. In this study, 60 fairly stable post-MI patients who were at lest 6 mo out from their infarction and had persistently positive (>1:64) *C. pneumoniae* antibody titers were randomized to either 3- or 6-d regimens of oral azithromycin ($n = 40$) or placebo ($n = 20$). In a rather questionable analysis in which 20 patients who met study criteria but were not randomized were included in the placebo group, a fivefold reduction in a combined endpoint that included death, MI, or unstable angina requiring intravenous medical therapy or mechanical reperfusion therapy *(103)*.

When first published in 1997, these two trials generated a considerable amount of enthusiasm and reports of some practitioners beginning to prescribe macrolide antibiot-ics to their patients with unstable coronary syndromes or a history of MI. The longer-term follow-up from the ROXIS trial and warnings about possible adverse effects helped to temper some of this enthusiasm *(104)*. Even more enthusiasm was lost when the results of the ACADEMIC trial were reported. This single-center randomized trial of 302 patients with CAD was designed to examine the effect of 3 mo of azithromycin therapy on serum markers of inflammation (CRP, IL-1, IL-6, and TNF-α) and *C. pneumoniae* IgG titers. Azithromycin reduced a global rank sum score of the four inflammatory markers at 6 mo ($p = 0.011$) but not at 3 mo. Change-score ranks were significantly lower for CRP ($p = 0.011$) and IL-6 ($p = 0.043$). In contrast to the two earlier trials no reduction in clinical events was seen, although it was not powered to do so *(105)*.

Ongoing Antibiotic Trials. Based on the encouraging results of the early small-scale treatment trials of the macrolide antibiotics has lead to the organization of several large-scale multicenter randomized trials. The WIZARD (Weekly Intervention with Zithromax for Atherosclerosis and Its Related Disorders) trial has completed enrollment of 3,535 patients. Patients with a history of a myocardial infarction at least 6 wk previously without recent revascularization who had an IgG titer to *C. pneumoniae* of $> = 1{:}16$ were randomly assigned either to 600 mg/d azithromycin for 3 d then 600 mg/wk for 11 additional weeks or to placebo. The primary endpoint of the study is the time to death, MI, a revascularization procedure, or hospitalization for angina. Initial results are expected in mid-2000 *(106)*.

There is some concern that even 12 wk of therapy as given in the ACADEMIC and WIZARD trials is too short to effectively eradicate infection with *C. pneumoniae* and have a lasting impact on clinical events. This concern stems from chlamydia species being obligate intracellular organisms who spend much of their lifecycles relatively inaccessible to antibiotics, even those with excellent tissue penetration such as azithromycin. This concern of the inadequacy of relatively short courses of antibiotics will be addressed by the Azithromycin Coronary Events Study (ACES). In this trial, 4000 patients with either a history of myocardial infarction or documented CAD are being randomized to a full year of either weekly azithromycin or placebo. Dosage and endpoints are similar to the WIZARD trial. Unlike WIZARD, ACES is enrolling patients regardless of the presence of chlamydial antibodies. Enrollment should be completed in mid-2000, and will require approximately 3 yr to accumulate sufficient clinic endpoints.

There is some controversy as to whether the antiatherosclerotic effects of macrolide antibiotics in animals and preliminary clinical studies *(101,103)* are due to an antimicrobial effect or the generalized anti-inflammatory properties inherit to this class of antibiotics *(107–113)*. The ACES trial will shed some light on this issue by allowing comparison of event rates and markers of inflammation between patients who are seropositive and those who are seronegative. This matter is further complicated, however, by variable rates of the degradation of seropositivity. This rises the possibility that a certain portion of patients who are *C. pneumoniae* seronegative have persistent infection with an inadequate immune response, and are therefore particularly susceptible to the chronic effects of infection such as progression of atherosclerosis. There are a number of smaller trials that are also ongoing (Table 1). All of the current trials are secondary prevention trials, there is some recent basic and animal data that suggests that *C. pneumoniae* infection asserts its effect on the atherosclerotic early in its development, so that it may be necessary to treat much earlier in the disease in a primary prevention strategy. Such trials would be very lengthy and expensive. Efforts are also underway to develop vaccines again *C. pneumoniae*, but there is significant difficulty in developing such a vaccine due to the antigen presentation properties of the organism. Regardless of the results of the currently ongoing trials of secondary prevention, much more additional work is necessary to more complete understand the mechanisms of *C. pneumoniae*'s contribution to atherosclerosis.

CONCLUSIONS

Atherosclerosis is now clearly recognized as a chronic inflammatory disease at a basic level. Recent studies of clinical markers of this specialized inflammatory response have developed rapidly. These clinical markers can now be used to predict those patients who

Table 1
Ongoing Antibiotic Trials in Coronary Disease

Trial	Population	Endpoint	Regimen	Treatment duration (wk)	Size (enrollment)
WIZARD[1]	Post-MI	MACE	Azithro	12	3535
ACES[1]	CAD	MACE	Azithro	52	4000
MARBLE[1]	CABG-list	MACE	Azithro	12	1200
STAMINA[2]	Peri-MI	Inflammatory marker	Anti-HP	2	600
APRES[3]	Angioplasty	Restenosis	Roxithro	6	1000
ANTIBIOS[1]	Post-MI	MACE	Roxithro	6	4000
Munich[4]	Angioplasty	Restenosis	Roxithro	4	1000
ACADEMIC[1]	CAD	Inflammatory marker	Azithro	12	300
AZACS	ACS	MACE	Azithro	12	1400

All studies have a placebo arm.
Azithromycin (azithro) dosing is 600 mg once weekly for 3 mo
STAMINA uses *H. pylori* regimens [PPI/(AZ vs AMOX)/MTN]
Roxithromycin (roxithro) dosing is 300 mg qd for 4–6 weeks.
WIZARD, ACADEMIC and ANTIBIOS select on *C. pneumoniae* titer.
MACE = major adverse cardiac events (death, MI, revascularization, admission for angina)
CAD = stable CAD; post MI = history of myocardial infarction; ACS = acute coronary syndromes.

are at increased risk for the development of atherosclerosis or its complications. Chronic infections by several bacterial and viral agents have been shown to be associated with a chronic inflammatory response and with increased atherosclerotic events. In the coming years studies will be emerging that will incorporate the use of the markers of inflammation to guide therapies aimed at interrupting the development and progression of the chronic infection and inflammation. This is indeed an exciting time in which a true paradigm shift is occurring in the understanding and treatment of atherosclerosis as an inflammatory disease.

REFERENCES

1. Ross R. Atherosclerosis—an inflammatory disease. N Engl J Med 1999;340:115–126.
2. Ross R. Atherosclerosis is an inflammatory disease. Am Heart J 1999;138:S419–S420.
3. McGill HC Jr. George Lyman Duff memorial lecture. Persistent problems in the pathogenesis of atherosclerosis. Arteriosclerosis 1984;4:443–451.
4. Stary HC, Chandler AB, Glagov S, et al. A definition of initial, fatty streak, and intermediate lesions of atherosclerosis. A report from the Committee on Vascular Lesions of the Council on Arteriosclerosis, American Heart Association. Circulation 1994;89:2462–2478.
5. Morrow DA, Ridker PM. Inflammation in cardiovascular disease. In: Topol EJ, ed. Textbook of Cardiovascular Medicine Updates. Lippincott Williams & Wilkins, Cedar Knolls, NJ, 1999; 2(4):1–12.
6. Rohde LE, Lee RT, Rivero J, et al. Circulating cell adhesion molecules are correlated with ultrasound-based assessment of carotid atherosclerosis. Arterioscler Thromb Vasc Biol 1998;18:1765–1770.
7. Nakashima Y, Raines EW, Plump AS, Breslow JL, Ross R. Upregulation of VCAM-1 and ICAM-1 at atherosclerosis-prone sites on the endothelium in the ApoE-deficient mouse. Arterioscler Thromb Vasc Biol 1998;18:842–851.
8. Talbott GA, Sharar SR, Harlan JM, Winn RK. Leukocyte-endothelial interactions and organ injury: the role of adhesion molecules. New Horiz 1994;2:545–554.
9. Wood KM, Cadogan MD, Ramshaw AL, Parums DV. The distribution of adhesion molecules in human atherosclerosis. Histopathology 1993;22:437–444.

10. Libby P, Sukhova G, Lee RT, Galis ZS. Cytokines regulate vascular functions related to stability of the atherosclerotic plaque. J Cardiovasc Pharmacol 1995;25:S9–S12.
11. Aqel NM, Ball RY, Waldmann H, Mitchinson MJ. Monocytic origin of foam cells in human atherosclerotic plaques. Atherosclerosis 1984;53:265–271.
12. Mantovani A, Sozzani S, Introna M. Endothelial activation by cytokines. Ann NY Acad Sci 1997;832: 93–116.
13. Ip JH, Fuster V, Badimon L, et al. Syndromes of accelerated atherosclerosis: role of vascular injury and smooth muscle cell proliferation. J Am Coll Cardiol 1990;15:1667–1687.
14. Galis ZS, Muszynski M, Sukhova GK, et al. Enhanced expression of vascular matrix metalloproteinases induced in vitro by cytokines and in regions of human atherosclerotic lesions. Ann NY Acad Sci 1995; 748:501–507.
15. Amorino GP, Hoover RL. Interactions of monocytic cells with human endothelial cells stimulate monocytic metalloproteinase production. Am J Pathol 1998;152:199–207.
16. Galis ZS, Sukhova GK, Kranzhofer R, Clark S, Libby P. Macrophage foam cells from experimental atheroma constitutively produce matrix-degrading proteinases. Proc Natl Acad Sci USA 1995;92: 402–406.
17. Kwon HM, Kang S, Hong BK, et al. Ultrastructural changes of the external elastic lamina in experimental hypercholesterolemic porcine coronary arteries. Yonsei Med J 1999;40:273–282.
18. Newby AC, Southgate KM, Davies M. Extracellular matrix degrading metalloproteinases in the pathogenesis of arteriosclerosis. Basic Res Cardiol 1994;89:59–70.
19. Prescott MF, Sawyer WK, Linden-Reed JV, et al. Effect of matrix metalloproteinase inhibition on progression of atherosclerosis and aneurysm in LDL receptor-deficient mice overexpressing MMP-3, MMP-12, and MMP-13 and on restenosis in rats after balloon injury. Ann NY Acad Sci 1999;878: 179–190.
20. Schonbeck U, Mach F, Sukhova GK, et al. Regulation of matrix metalloproteinase expression in human vascular smooth muscle cells by T lymphocytes: a role for CD40 signaling in plaque rupture? Circ Res 1997;81:448–454.
21. Schoenhagen P, Ziada KM, Kapadia SR, et al. Extent and direction of arterial remodeling in stable versus unstable coronary syndromes: An intravascular ultrasound study. Circulation 1999;101:598–603.
22. Davies MJ. A macro and micro view of coronary vascular insult in ischemic heart disease. Circulation 1990;82:II38–II46.
23. Lendon CL, Davies MJ, Born GV, Richardson PD. Atherosclerotic plaque caps are locally weakened when macrophages density is increased. Atherosclerosis 1991;87:87–90.
24. Moreno PR, Falk E, Palacios IF, et al. Macrophage infiltration in acute coronary syndromes. Implications for plaque rupture. Circulation 1994;90:775–778.
25. Fabunmi RP, Sukhova GK, Sugiyama S, Libby P. Expression of tissue inhibitor of metalloproteinases-3 in human atheroma and regulation in lesion-associated cells: a potential protective mechanism in plaque stability. Circ Res 1998;83:270–278.
26. Galis ZS, Sukhova GK, Lark MW, Libby P. Increased expression of matrix metalloproteinases and matrix degrading activity in vulnerable regions of human atherosclerotic plaques. J Clin Invest 1994;94: 2493–2503.
27. Wilkins J, Gallimore JR, Moore EG, Pepys MB. Rapid automated high sensitivity enzyme immunoassay of C-reactive protein. Clin Chem 1998;44:1358–1361.
28. Thompson SG, Kienast J, Pyke SD, et al. Hemostatic factors and the risk of myocardial infarction or sudden death in patients with angina pectoris. European Concerted Action on Thrombosis and Disabilities Angina Pectoris Study Group [see comments]. N Engl J Med 1995;332:635–641.
29. Kuller LH, Tracy RP, Shaten J, Meilahn EN. Relation of C-reactive protein and coronary heart disease in the MRFIT nested case-control study. Multiple Risk Factor Intervention Trial. Am J Epidemiol 1996;144:537–547.
30. Ridker PM, Cushman M, Stampfer MJ, et al. Inflammation, aspirin, and the risk of cardiovascular disease in apparently healthy men. N Engl J Med 1997;336:973–979.
31. Ridker PM, Rifai N, Pfeffer MA, et al. Inflammation, pravastatin, and the risk of coronary events after myocardial infarction in patients with average cholesterol levels. Cholesterol and Recurrent Events (CARE) Investigators. Circulation 1998;98:839–844.
32. Kurakata S, Kada M, Shimada Y, et al. Effects of different inhibitors of 3-hydroxy-3-methylglutaryl coenzyme A (HMG-CoA) reductase, pravastatin sodium and simvastatin, on sterol synthesis and immunological functions in human lymphocytes in vitro. Immunopharmacology 1996;34:51–61.

33. Vaughan CJ, Murphy MB, Buckley BM. Statins do more than just lower cholesterol [see comments] [published erratum appears in Lancet 1997 Jan 18;349(9046):214]. Lancet 1996;348:1079–1082.

34. de Beer FC, Hind CR, Fox KM, et al. Measurement of serum C-reactive protein concentration in myocardial ischaemia and infarction. Br Heart J 1982;47:239–243.

35. Kushner I, Broder ML, Karp D. Control of the acute phase response. Serum C-reactive protein kinetics after acute myocardial infarction. J Clin Invest 1978;61:235–242.

36. Voulgari F, Cummins P, Gardecki TI, et al. Serum levels of acute phase and cardiac proteins after myocardial infarction, surgery, and infection. Br Heart J 1982;48:352–356.

37. Ikeda U, Ohkawa F, Seino Y, et al. Serum interleukin 6 levels become elevated in acute myocardial infarction. J Mol Cell Cardiol 1992;24:579–584.

38. Miyao Y, Yasue H, Ogawa H, et al. Elevated plasma interleukin-6 levels in patients with acute myocardial infarction. Am Heart J 1993;126:1299–1304.

39. Liuzzo G, Biasucci LM, Gallimore JR, et al. The prognostic value of C-reactive protein and serum amyloid a protein in severe unstable angina. N Engl J Med 1994;331:417–424.

40. Morrow DA, Rifai N, Antman EM, et al. C-reactive protein is a potent predictor of mortality independently of and in combination with troponin T in acute coronary syndromes: a TIMI 11A substudy. Thrombolysis in Myocardial Infarction. J Am Coll Cardiol 1998;31:1460–1465.

41. Biasucci LM, Vitelli A, Liuzzo G, et al. Elevated levels of interleukin-6 in unstable angina [see comments]. Circulation 1996;94:874–877.

42. Benamer H, Steg PG, Benessiano J, et al. Comparison of the prognostic value of C-reactive protein and troponin I in patients with unstable angina pectoris. Am J Cardiol 1998;82:845–850.

43. Toss H, Lindahl B, Siegbahn A, Wallentin L. Prognostic influence of increased fibrinogen and C-reactive protein levels in unstable coronary artery disease. FRISC Study Group. Fragmin during Instability in Coronary Artery Disease. Circulation 1997;96:4204–4210.

44. Rebuzzi AG, Quaranta G, Liuzzo G, et al. Incremental prognostic value of serum levels of troponin T and C- reactive protein on admission in patients with unstable angina pectoris. Am J Cardiol 1998; 82:715–719.

45. Biasucci LM, Liuzzo G, Grillo RL, et al. Elevated levels of C-reactive protein at discharge in patients with unstable angina predict recurrent instability. Circulation 1999;99:855–860.

46. Ferreiros ER, Boissonnet CP, Pizarro R, et al. Independent prognostic value of elevated C-reactive protein in unstable angina. Circulation 1999;100:1958–1963.

47. Pietila K, Harmoinen A, Poyhonen L, et al. Intravenous streptokinase treatment and serum C-reactive protein in patients with acute myocardial infarction. Br Heart J 1987;58:225–229.

48. Pietila K, Harmoinen A, Teppo AM. Acute phase reaction, infarct size and in-hospital morbidity in myocardial infarction patients treated with streptokinase or recombinant tissue type plasminogen activator. Ann Med 1991;23:529–535.

49. Pudil R, Pidrman V, Krejsek J, et al. The effect of reperfusion on plasma tumor necrosis factor alpha and C reactive protein levels in the course of acute myocardial infarction. Acta Med 1996;39:149–153.

50. Pietila K, Harmoinen A, Hermens W, et al. Serum C-reactive protein and infarct size in myocardial infarct patients with a closed versus an open infarct-related coronary artery after thrombolytic therapy. Eur Heart J 1993;14:915–919.

51. Casscells W, Hathorn B, David M, et al. Thermal detection of cellular infiltrates in living atherosclerotic plaques: possible implications for plaque rupture and thrombosis [see comments]. Lancet 1996; 347:1447–1451.

52. Loike JD, Silverstein SC, Sturtevant JM. Application of differential scanning microcalorimetry to the study of cellular processes: heat production and glucose oxidation of murine macrophages. Proc Natl Acad Sci USA 1981;78:5958–5962.

53. van der Wal AC, Becker AE, van der Loos CM, Das PK. Site of intimal rupture or erosion of thrombosed coronary atherosclerotic plaques is characterized by an inflammatory process irrespective of the dominant plaque morphology [see comments]. Circulation 1994;89:36–44.

54. Moreno PR, Bernardi VH, Lopez-Cuellar J, et al. Macrophage infiltration predicts restenosis after coronary intervention in patients with unstable angina. Circulation 1996;94:3098–3102.

55. Lauer MA, Zhou ZM, Forudi F, et al. The temperatures of atherosclerotic lesions in the hypercholesterolemic rabbit double injury model are elevated following angioplasty. J Am Coll Cardiol 1999;33:67A.

56. Stefanadis C, Diamantopoulos L, Vlachopoulos C, et al. Thermal heterogeneity within human atherosclerotic coronary arteries detected in vivo: a new method of detection by application of a special thermography catheter. Circulation 1999;99:1965–1971.

57. Stefanadis C, Diamantopoulos L, Vlachopoulos C, et al. Plaque temperature as a prognostic factor for long-term outcome in acute ischemic syndromes. Circulation 1999;100:I-446.
58. Guo B, Willerson JT, Bearman G, et al. Infrared fiber optic Imaging of atherosclerotic plaques. Circulation 1999;100:I-446.
59. Moreno PR, Lodder RA, O'Connor WN, et al. Characterization of vulnerable plaques by near infrared spectroscopy in an atherosclerotic rabbit model. J Am Coll Cardiol 1999;33:66A.
60. Ridker PM, Haughie P. Prospective studies of C-reactive protein as a risk factor for cardiovascular disease. J Invest Med 1998;46:391–395.
60a. Fabricant CG, Fabricant J, Litrenta MM, Minick CR. Virus-induced atherosclerosis. J Exp Med 1978; 148:335–340.
60b. Fabricant CG, Fabricant J, Minick CR, Litrenta MM. Herpesvirus-induced atherosclerosis in chickens. Fed Proc 1983;42:2476–2479.
61. Melnick JL, Hu C, Burek J, et al. Cytomegalovirus DNA in arterial walls of patients with atherosclerosis. J Med Virol 1994;42:170–174.
62. Hendrix MG, Salimans MM, van Boven CP, Bruggeman CA. High prevalence of latently present cytomegalovirus in arterial walls of patients suffering from grade III atherosclerosis. Am J Pathol 1990;136: 23–28.
63. Hendrix MG, Dormans PH, Kitslaar P, et al. The presence of cytomegalovirus nucleic acids in arterial walls of atherosclerotic and nonatherosclerotic patients. Am J Pathol 1989;134:1151–1157.
64. Lemstrom K, Koskinen P, Krogerus L, et al. Cytomegalovirus antigen expression, endothelial cell proliferation, and intimal thickening in rat cardiac allografts after cytomegalovirus infection. Circulation 1995;92:2594–2604.
65. Lemstrom KB, Bruning JH, Bruggeman CA, et al. Cytomegalovirus infection enhances smooth muscle cell proliferation and intimal thickening of rat aortic allografts. J Clin Invest 1993;92:549–558.
66. McGiffin DC, Savunen T, Kirklin JK, et al. Cardiac transplant coronary artery disease. A multivariable analysis of pretransplantation risk factors for disease development and morbid events. J Thorac Cardiovasc Surg 1995;109:1081–1089.
67. Mangiavacchi M, Frigerio M, Gronda E, et al. Acute rejection and cytomegalovirus infection: correlation with cardiac allograft vasculopathy. Transplant Proc 1995;27:1960–1962.
68. Gao SZ, Hunt SA, Schroeder JS, et al. Early development of accelerated graft coronary artery disease: risk factors and course. J Am Coll Cardiol 1996;28:673–679.
69. Zhou YF, Shou M, Guetta E, et al. Cytomegalovirus infection of rats increases the neointimal response to vascular injury without consistent evidence of direct infection of the vascular wall. Circulation 1999; 100:1569–1575.
70. Nieto FJ, Adam E, Sorlie P, et al. Cohort study of cytomegalovirus infection as a risk factor for carotid intimal-medial thickening, a measure of subclinical atherosclerosis. Circulation 1996;94:922–927.
71. Sorlie PD, Adam E, Melnick SL, et al. Cytomegalovirus/herpesvirus and carotid atherosclerosis: the ARIC Study. J Med Virol 1994;42:33–37.
72. Adam E, Melnick JL, Probtsfield JL, et al. High levels of cytomegalovirus antibody in patients requiring vascular surgery for atherosclerosis. Lancet 1987;2:291–293.
73. Zhou YF, Leon MB, Waclawiw MA, et al. Association between prior cytomegalovirus infection and the risk of restenosis after coronary atherectomy. N Engl J Med 1996;335:624–630.
74. Melnick JL, Adam E, DeBakey ME. Possible role of cytomegalovirus in atherogenesis. JAMA 1990; 263:2204–2207.
75. Dummer S, Lee A, Breinig MK, et al. Investigation of cytomegalovirus infection as a risk factor for coronary atherosclerosis in the explanted hearts of patients undergoing heart transplantation. J Med Virol 1994;44:305–309.
76. Zhu J, Quyyumi AA, Norman JE, et al. Total pathogen burden contributes incrementally to coronary artery disease risk and to C-reactive protein levels. Circulation 1998;98:I-142.
77. Epstein SE, Zhou YF, Zhu J. Infection and atherosclerosis: emerging mechanistic paradigms. Circulation 1999;100:e20–e28.
78. Wanishsawad C, Zhou YF, Epstein SE. Chlamydia pneumoniae-induced transactivation of the major immediate early promoter of cytomegalovirus: potential synergy of infectious agents in the pathogenesis of atherosclerosis. J Infect Dis 2000;181:787–790.
79. Markus HS, Mendall MA. Helicobacter pylori infection: a risk factor for ischaemic cerebrovascular disease and carotid atheroma. J Neurol Neurosurg Psychiatry 1998;64:104–107.

80. Whincup PH, Mendall MA, Perry IJ, et al. Prospective relations between Helicobacter pylori infection, coronary heart disease, and stroke in middle aged men. Heart 1996;75:568–572.
81. Patel P, Mendall MA, Carrington D, et al. Association of Helicobacter pylori and Chlamydia pneumoniae infections with coronary heart disease and cardiovascular risk factors [see comments] [published erratum appears in Br Med J 1995 Oct 14;311(7011):985]. Br Med J 1995;311:711–714.
82. Grayston JT, Aldous MB, Easton A, et al. Evidence that Chlamydia pneumoniae causes pneumonia and bronchitis. J Infect Dis 1993;168:1231–1235.
83. Grayston JT, Campbell LA, Kuo CC, et al. A new respiratory tract pathogen: Chlamydia pneumoniae strain TWAR. J Infect Dis 1990;161:618–625.
84. Saikku P. The epidemiology and significance of Chlamydia pneumoniae. J Infect 1992;25(Suppl 1): 27–34.
85. Grayston JT, Wang SP, Kuo CC, Campbell LA. Current knowledge on Chlamydia pneumoniae, strain TWAR, an important cause of pneumonia and other acute respiratory diseases. Eur J Clin Microbiol Infect Dis 1989;8:191–202.
86. Saikku P, Leinonen M, Mattila K, et al. Serological evidence of an association of a novel Chlamydia, TWAR, with chronic coronary heart disease and acute myocardial infarction. Lancet 1988;2:983–986.
86a. Danesh J, Collins R, Peto R. Chronic infections and coronary heart disease: is there a link? Lancet 1997;350:430–436.
87. Saikku P, Leinonen M, Tenkanen L, et al. Chronic Chlamydia pneumoniae infection as a risk factor for coronary heart disease in the Helsinki Heart Study. Ann Intern Med 1992;116:273–278.
88. Roivainen M, Viik-Kajander M, Palosuo T, et al. Infections, inflammation, and the risk of coronary heart disease. Circulation 2000;101:252–257.
89. Thom DH, Grayston JT, Siscovick DS, et al. Association of prior infection with Chlamydia pneumoniae and angiographically demonstrated coronary artery disease. JAMA 1992;268:68–72.
90. Hahn DL, Golubjatnikov R. Smoking is a potential confounder of the Chlamydia pneumoniae-coronary artery disease association. Arterioscler Thromb 1992;12:945–947.
91. Ridker PM, Kundsin RB, Stampfer MJ, et al. Prospective study of Chlamydia pneumoniae IgG seropositivity and risks of future myocardial infarction. Circulation 1999;99:1161–1164.
92. Kuo CC, Gown AM, Benditt EP, Grayston JT. Detection of Chlamydia pneumoniae in aortic lesions of atherosclerosis by immunocytochemical stain. Arterioscler Thrombs 1993;13:1501–1504.
93. Grayston JT, Kuo CC, Coulson AS, et al. Chlamydia pneumoniae (TWAR) in atherosclerosis of the carotid artery. Circulation 1995;92:3397–3400.
94. Kuo CC, Shor A, Campbell LA, et al. Demonstration of Chlamydia pneumoniae in atherosclerotic lesions of coronary arteries. J Infect Dis 1993;167:841–849.
95. Muhlestein JB, Hammond EH, Carlquist JF, et al. Increased incidence of Chlamydia species within the coronary arteries of patients with symptomatic atherosclerotic versus other forms of cardiovascular disease. J Am Coll Cardiol 1996;27:1555–1561.
96. Ramirez JA. Isolation of Chlamydia pneumoniae from the coronary artery of a patient with coronary atherosclerosis. The Chlamydia pneumoniae/Atherosclerosis Study Group. Ann Intern Med 1996;125: 979–982.
97. Moazed TC, Campbell LA, Rosenfeld ME, et al. Chlamydia pneumoniae infection accelerates the progression of atherosclerosis in apolipoprotein E-deficient mice. J Infect Dis 1999;180:238–241.
98. Moazed TC, Kuo CC, Grayston JT, Campbell LA. Evidence of systemic dissemination of Chlamydia pneumoniae via macrophages in the mouse. J Infect Dis 1998;177:1322–1325.
98a. Fong IW, Chiu B, Viira E, et al. Rabbit model for Chlamydia pneumoniae infection. J Clin Microbiol 1997;35:48–52.
98b. Laitinen K, Laurila A, Pyhala L, et al. Chlamydia pneumoniae infection induces inflammatory changes in the aortas of rabbits. Infect Immun 1997;65:4832–4835.
98c. Muhlestein JB, Anderson JL, Hammond EH, et al. Infection with *Chlamydia pneumoniae* accelerates the development of atherosclerosis and treatment with azithromycin prevents it in a rabbit model. Circulation 1998;97:633–636.
99. Muhlestein JB, Anderson JL, Hammond EH, et al. Infection with Chlamydia pneumoniae accelerates the development of atherosclerosis and treatment with azithromycin prevents it in a rabbit model. Circulation 1998;97:633–636.
100. Lauer MA, Mawhorter SD, Vince DG, et al. Increase in coronary artery matrix metallo-proteinases in mini-pigs induced by intranasal Chlamydia pneumoniae infection. J Am Coll Cardiol 2000;35:302A.

101. Gurfinkel E, Bozovich G, Daroca A, et al. Randomised trial of roxithromycin in non-Q-wave coronary syndromes: ROXIS Pilot Study. ROXIS Study Group. Lancet 1997;350:404–407.
102. Gurfinkel E, Bozovich G, Beck E, et al. Treatment with the antibiotic roxithromycin in patients with acute non-Q-wave coronary syndromes. The final report of the ROXIS Study [see comments]. Eur Heart J 1999;20:121–127.
103. Gupta S, Leatham EW, Carrington D, et al. Elevated Chlamydia pneumoniae antibodies, cardiovascular events, and azithromycin in male survivors of myocardial infarction. Circulation 1997;96: 404–407.
104. Grayston JT. Antibiotic treatment of Chlamydia pneumoniae for secondary prevention of cardiovascular events [editorial] [see comments]. Circulation 1998;97:1669–1670.
105. Anderson JL, Muhlestein JB, Carlquist J, et al. Randomized secondary prevention trial of azithromycin in patients with coronary artery disease and serological evidence for Chlamydia pneumoniae infection: The Azithromycin in Coronary Artery Disease: Elimination of Myocardial Infection with Chlamydia (ACADEMIC) study. Circulation 1999;99:1540–1547.
106. Dunne M. WIZARD and the design of trials for secondary prevention of atherosclerosis with antibiotics. Am Heart J 1999;138:S542–S544.
107. Fox BJ, Odom RB, Findlay RF. Erythromycin therapy in bullous pemphigoid: possible anti-inflammatory effects. J Am Acad Dermatol 1982;7:504–510.
108. Takeshita K, Yamagishi I, Harada M, et al. Immunological and anti-inflammatory effects of clarithromycin: inhibition of interleukin 1 production of murine peritoneal macrophages. Drugs Exp Clin Res 1989;15:527–533.
109. Agen C, Danesi R, Blandizzi C, et al. Macrolide antibiotics as antiinflammatory agents: roxithromycin in an unexpected role. Agents Actions 1993;38:85–90.
110. Kita E, Sawaki M, Mikasa K, et al. Alterations of host response by a long-term treatment of roxithromycin. J Antimicrob Chemother 1993;32:285–294.
111. Umeki S. Anti-inflammatory action of erythromycin. Its inhibitory effect on neutrophil NADPH oxidase activity. Chest 1993;104:1191–1193.
112. Scaglione F, Rossoni G. Comparative anti-inflammatory effects of roxithromycin, azithromycin and clarithromycin. J Antimicrob Chemother 1998;41(Suppl B):47–50.
113. Labro MT. Anti-inflammatory activity of macrolides: a new therapeutic potential? J Antimicrob Chemother 1998;41(Suppl B):37–46.

II

Risk Factors and Their Management in Coronary Artery Disease

5

Dyslipidemias
and Coronary Artery Disease
Clinical Evidence and Clinical Implications

JoAnne Micale Foody, MD

CONTENTS

INTRODUCTION
CLINICAL TRIALS IN DYSLIPIDEMIA
GUIDELINES FOR THE MODIFICATION OF LIPIDS
CLINICAL EFFICACY IN SPECIAL POPULATIONS
CONCLUSIONS
REFERENCES

INTRODUCTION

Epidemiology

Except for age, dyslipidemia is the most important predictive factor for coronary artery disease *(1)*. The strong, independent, continuous, and graded relationship between total cholesterol (TC) levels, or low-density lipoprotein (LDL) cholesterol level and the risk of coronary artery disease (CAD) events has been clearly demonstrated world wide in men and women and in all age groups *(2–6)*. High cholesterol levels are a major contributor to CAD: 38 million Americans have a TC of >240 mg/dL and 96 million are estimated to have levels above 200 mg/dL *(7)*. In general, a 1% increase in the LDL cholesterol level may lead to a 2–3% increase in CAD risk *(3,4)*. Aggressive lipid-lowering drug treatment in high-risk individuals will reduce coronary heart disease (CHD) morbidity and mortality rates and increase overall survival *(8–12)*.

Conclusive evidence from rigorous, large-scale, randomized clinical trials, such as the Scandinavian Simvastatin Survival Study (4S) *(9)*, the Cholesterol and Recurrent Events (CARE) *(8)* trial in secondary prevention, and the West of Scotland Coronary Prevention Study (WOSCOPS) *(11)* in high-risk primary prevention has given new impetus to the practice of preventive cardiology. Recent findings from the secondary prevention Long Term Intervention with Pravastatin in Ischaemic Disease (LIPID) *(12)* trial and the primary prevention Air Force/Texas Coronary Atherosclerosis Prevention Study (AFCAPS/TEXCAPS) *(13)* has further strengthened the position of lipid-lowering strategies in clinical medicine.

From: *Contemporary Cardiology: Preventive Cardiology:*
Strategies for the Prevention and Treatment of Coronary Artery Disease
Edited by: J. Foody © Humana Press Inc., Totowa, NJ

Despite national guidelines *(14)* emphasizing the importance of lipid lowering, more than two thirds of patients treated for hyperlipidemia by primary care physicians fail to reach NCEP targets. More striking is the fact that 80% of patients with established CAD, those at greatest risk, fail to reach the NCEP target *(15)*. This failure is partially due to inconsistent strategies applied toward the management of patients at risk for the development and progression of CAD.

Epidemiologic and Population Studies

TOTAL CHOLESTEROL

Cholesterol is now viewed as a crucial factor in the development of atherosclerosis 1. Initial work from the Framingham Study *(2)* as well as from the Multiple Risk Factor Intervention Trial (MRFIT) *(5,16)* have demonstrated a continuous and graded positive relationship between the level of TC and CAD mortality.

In the Framingham Study *(2,5,6)*, a stepwise increase in serum cholesterol and the associated increase in 24-yr incidence of CHD were particularly powerful factors in young men but were much less apparent in women. In the Framingham Study, 20% of myocardial infarctions (MI) occurred within a range of cholesterol that is considered "normal" by the National Cholesterol Education Program (NCEP) guidelines (<200 mg/dL). The contribution of LDL to CAD risk in young men was apparent in the Framingham study. In an older population of men and women (aged 50 to 80 yr), LDL-C was associated significantly ($p < 0.05$) with CHD after 7 yr of follow-up.

MRFIT *(5,16)* investigated the effect of risk factor interventions on the development of CHD. A total of 361,662 men were screened for the MRFIT, and a 6-yr mortality rate was calculated in relation to serum cholesterol. Of note, the risk of CAD death increased progressively in men with a serum cholesterol higher than 181 mg/dL. Men with a serum cholesterol levels in excess of 253 mg/dL had a relative risk 3.8 times greater than those men with levels lower than 181 mg/dL. Furthermore, serum cholesterol higher than the 90th percentile is often used to define "hypercholesterolemia," yet 54% of the CHD occurred in men whose levels fell below the 85th percentile. In this group of 356,222 men aged 35–57 without previous MI, there was no lower threshold below which CAD risk did not occur.

LDL CHOLESTEROL

The dyslipidemia most clearly associated with the development of CAD is hypercholesterolemia particularly due to an elevation in LDL cholesterol. Based on the known relationship between LDL-C and CAD, the treatment guidelines of the NCEP *(17)* focus on LDL cholesterol reduction for the primary and secondary prevention of CAD events. Numerous clinical trials support the importance of LDL-Cholesterol lowering in decreasing CAD risk, both in angiographic trials, which measure CAD progression, and in trials that assess morbidity and mortality.

LDL Subclasses and Clinical Implications. It is important to remember that LDL is not a homogeneous particle but consists of a set of discrete subspecies with distinct molecular properties, including size and density. In normal subjects, at least four major LDL subspecies can be identified: LDL-I is the largest and least dense, and, the smallest, LDL-IV, is the most dense. LDL size is a powerful predictor of CAD risk, independent of triglycerides (TG), HDL-C, LDL-C, and body mass index (BMI) *(18)*.

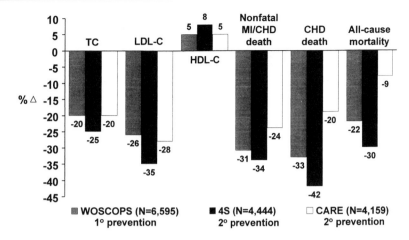

Fig. 1. Lipid lowering and clinical events in recent statin trials. N = number enrolled.

Three prospective trials that investigated the predictive nature of LDL size have been reported. The Physicians Health Study investigated the importance of LDL subclass pattern on CAD risk in 14,916 men. In 266 cases and 308 control subjects followed for 7 yr, LDL diameter was related to CAD. The Stanford Five City Project prospectively evaluated the role of LDL size in CAD in 124 matched pairs of cases and control subjects. LDL size was significantly smaller and more dense ($p < 0.001$) among CAD cases compared with control subjects. The association was graded across quintiles of LDL size. This difference was independent of HDL-C, triglycerides, smoking, blood pressure, and BMI. In this study, LDL size was the best discriminator of CAD status. The Quebec Cardiovascular Study was a prospective investigation of CAD risk factors in 2103 asymptomatic men. After 5 yr of follow-up, LDL diameter proved to be an independent predictor of CAD risk. The power of LDL size as a risk predictor was independent of age, BMI, alcohol consumption, smoking, fasting triglycerides, Apo B, and LDL and HDL cholesterol.

Although elevated LDL-C increases CAD risk, it appears that an LDL subclass distribution may be a more common and more powerful predictor of risk. It is present in 50% of men with CAD and identifies a group of people that can respond particularly well to appropriate treatment and are good arteriographic responders to treatment. Total and LDL-C are frequently within normal limits in these individuals and thus, their high-risk state is not identified on routine blood tests *(18)*.

CLINICAL TRIALS IN DYSLIPIDEMIA

LDL-C Modification

Conclusive evidence from rigorous, large scale, randomized clinical trials, such as the 4S study *(9)*, CARE *(8)*, and WOSCOPS *(11)* has given new impetus to the practice of preventive cardiology. Recent results from the LIPID trial *(12)*, in combination with landmark secondary prevention trials, have further strengthened the position of lipid-lowering strategies in clinical medicine (Fig. 1).

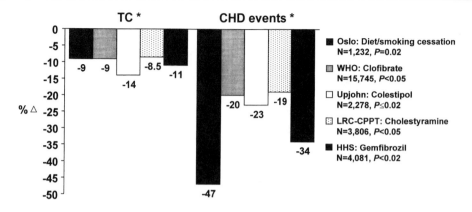

Fig. 2. Early primary-prevention trials: overview. N = number enrolled. *Net difference between treatment and control groups (P values are for events). Adapted from ref. *54.*

PRIMARY PREVENTION TRIALS

Until recently, the literature did not support protecting patients through cholesterol reduction. Early primary prevention trials tested the hypothesis that a decrease in TC leads to a decrease in cardiovascular events (Fig. 2). In the early 1980s, two additional large-scale primary trials were conducted: LRC-CPPT *(19–21)* and the HHS *(22,23)*. The LRC-CPPT was a randomized, double-blind, placebo-controlled trial of diet plus cholestyramine vs. diet and placebo. This landmark study conclusively showed that reducing cholesterol by diet and a pharmacological regimen reduced the risk of CHD in men with hypercholesterolemia. Specifically, a 10–15% reduction in serum cholesterol may result in a 20–30% reduction in risk for CHD. The HHS was a double-blind, placebo-controlled primary prevention trial that randomized men without CHD to receive either placebo or gemfibrozil. Overall, a 34% reduction in the incidence of CHD was observed. Importantly, the HHS identified a subgroup of patients with high risk for cardiac events. This group was characterized by an LDL-C: HDL-C ratio >5 and TG >200 mg/dL and experienced a 71% reduction in CHD event rate with treatment. These studies demonstrated significant reductions in lipids and an associated decrese in CHD events. They provide clear evidence of the clinical benefits associated with the primary prevention of CHD.

With the development of HMG CoA Reductase inhibitors, a new era of lipid lowering management was begun. These powerful new drugs provided significant mortality benefit in patients without overt CAD. The landmark WOSCOPS *(11)* was conducted on 6595 men between the ages of 45 and 64 with TC levels >252 mg/dL and LDL cholesterol levels between 174 and 232 mg/dL, but no clinical evidence of heart disease. Study participants were treated with dietary intervention and randomized to receive placebo or pravastatin 40 mg/d. Pravastatin reduced the risk of first heart attack by 31% and the need for coronary revascularization procedures by 37% (Fig. 3).

More recently, AFCAPS/TEXCAPS *(13)* capitalized on the increased risk of healthy subjects with low HDL and increased TC/HDL ratios. Therapy with the cholesterol-lowering drug lovastatin (Mevacor) reduced the risk of first acute major coronary events in healthy adults with average to mildly elevated cholesterol levels and low HDL by 36% (Fig. 4). The trial included 6605 healthy adults aged 45 to 73 (997 women, 487 Hispanic Americans, and 206 African-Americans) including a broad spectrum of men and women,

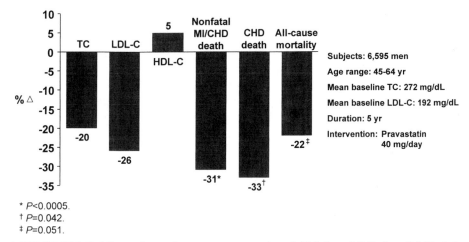

* P<0.0005.
† P=0.042.
‡ P=0.051.

Fig. 3. WOSCOPS: lipid lowering and coronary events. *p < 0.005. †p = 0.042. ‡p = 0.051. Adapted from ref. 11.

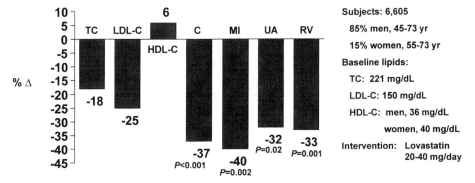

C=coronary events defined as fatal/nonfatal myocardial infarction, sudden death, and unstable angina;
MI=fatal/nonfatal myocardial infarction; UA=unstable angina;
RV=revascularizations.

Fig. 4.   AFCAPS/TEXCAPS: LDL-C lowering and coronary events. C = coronary events defined as fatal/nonfatal myocardial infarction, sudden death, and unstable angina; MI = fatal/nonfatal myocardial infarction; UA = unstable angine; RV = revascularizations. Adapted from ref. 13.

including African-Americans and Hispanic Americans. Over 20% were aged 65 and older. Inclusion criteria for the study included lack of evidence for CAD, an LDL cholesterol between 130 and 190 mg/dL, HDL less than 45 mg/dL (less than 47 mg/dL for women), and TG levels less than 400 mg/dL. Therefore, none of the participants had evidence of heart disease; 22% had hypertension, 2% had diabetes, and 12% were smokers. Participants were randomly assigned to receive either lovastatin or a placebo. Dosage of the drug began at 20 mg/d and in 50% of patients was raised to 40 mg/d in order to target the LDL cholesterol to <100 mg/dL. Before the trial was begun, the average TC level among participants was 221 mg/dL, the LDL level was 150 mg/dL and the average HDL level was 37 mg/dL. TC levels in the lovastatin group were reduced by 18.4%, LDL fell by 25% and TGs were reduced by 15%.

   Preliminary results indicate that patients taking lovastatin had reduced risk for coronary events. Their risk of first acute coronary event (sudden death, MI, unstable angina) was reduced by 36%, risk of first coronary events was reduced by 54% in women, 34%

in men, 43% in hypertensive patients and diabetic patients, and 29% in the elderly. Patients in the lovastatin group also had a 33% reduction in procedures such as angioplasty and bypass, and a 34% reduction in hospitalization due to unstable angina.

These results are particularly significant, as most of the study participants would not ordinarily have been considered candidates for cholesterol-lowering therapy based on previous NCEP guidelines. This group, however, represent the majority of persons who eventually develop heart disease. This study represents a significant advance in our understanding of the role of reducing cholesterol in preventing new onset of heart disease in apparently healthy persons.

Although the WOSCOPS study demonstrated that treatment of relatively high-risk men with profoundly elevated cholesterol levels significantly reduced risk of heart attack and death from heart disease, it is the AFCAPS/TEXCAPS study that has demonstrated benefit in those with more typical risk profiles including lower cholesterol values. It has been suggested that AFCAPS/TEXCAPS expands the number of persons in the United States by over 8 million people who are possible candidates for cholesterol-lowering drug therapy. The participants in AFCAPS/TEXCAPS would not ordinarily have been considered candidates for cholesterol-lowering therapy based on previous NCEP guidelines.

SECONDARY PREVENTION TRIALS

Scandinavian Simvastatin Survival Study (4S). The 4S *(9)* included 4444 men and women with CAD and TC 212–309 mg/dL to treatment with simvastatin (20–40 mg) or placebo for up to 6.2 yr. The mean LDL level at baseline was 188 mg/dL with a range of 130–266 mg/dL. The number of patients with major coronary events (coronary deaths or nonfatal MI) was 622 (28%) in the placebo group and 431 (19%) in the simvastatin group ($p < 0.00001$). To demonstrate the sustained efficacy and safety of simvastatin, the 4S investigators designed and implemented a 2-yr extension of 4S. Over the combined study period (7.4 yr) total mortality in the placebo group was 15.8% vs. 11.4% among patients treated with simvastatin ($p = 0.0001$) (Fig. 5). After completion of the original study, all patients in the placebo group were offered therapy with simvastatin. Nonetheless, the curves continued to separate and patients treated with simvastatin were found to benefit over the full study period. Simvastatin maintained the reduction in risk of total mortality by 30% ($p = 0.00001$) *(24)*. A recent analysis presented vascular event curves over the duration of the 4S trial, including intermittent cluadication, carotid bruits, angina, and cerebrovascular events *(25)*. Note that the curves separate at 2 yr and beyond (Fig. 6), except perhaps for carotid bruits, which appears to separate earlier.

CARE. This is a randomized controlled trial *(8)* that was designed to evaluate the effects of treatment with pravastatin in 4159 subjects who had experienced an acute MI 3–20 mo prior to randomization and had moderately elevated total cholesterol levels (mean = 209 mg/dL). Patients were randomized to either pravastatin (40 mg/dL or placebo; in addition, they followed the NCEP-recommended guidelines for diet therapy and, if their LDL levels were persistently elevated (>175 mg/dL), they received cholestyramine. Results were encouraging: over a 5-yr period, total cholesterol levels were reduced by 20%, LDL levels dropped by 28%, TG declined by 14%, and HDL increased by 5% (Fig. 7). The incidence of primary combined endpoint of CHD death or nonfatal MI was reduced by 24% ($p < 0.002$) (Fig. 8). CARE was not statistically powered to observed differences in mortality. Importantly, the benefits of pravastatin therapy in preventing recurrent coronary events were similar in the subset analysis of age, sex, ejection factor, hypertension, diabetes mellitus, and smoking.

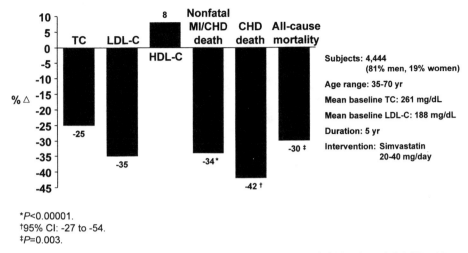

*P<0.00001.
†95% CI: -27 to -54.
‡P=0.003.

Fig. 5. 4S: Effect of LDL-C lowering and coronary events. * $p < 0.0001$. † $p = 95\%$ CI: -27 to -54. ‡ $p = 0.003$. Adapted from ref. 9.

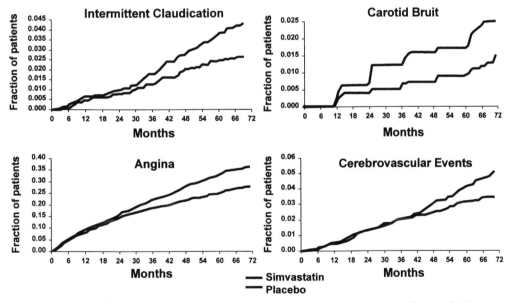

Fig. 6. 4S: Effects of cholesterol lowering ischemic endpoints. Adapted from ref. 25.

This secondary prevention trial suggests that risk reduction in this large portion of the population with only moderately elevated TC could have positive public health implications. It remains to be determined whether treatment for lower levels of LDL will be beneficial.

LIPID. This is a secondary prevention study *(12)*, performed in New Zealand and Australia. It was a double blinded randomized placebo-control study on 9014 subjects (1511 of whom were women, one-third over age 65 yr, 777 diabetics) using pravastatin 40 mg/d. Subjects age 31–75 yr, who experienced an acute MI or unstable angina within the previous 3 mo–3 yr, and had total cholesterol values from 155–270 mg/dL, triglycerides less than 445 mg/dL, were eligible for participation. A significant medical or surgical event, significant heart failure, renal or hepatic disease, uncontrolled endocrine disorders, or use of cyclosporine and/or lipid-lowering agents excluded the patients from being recruited.

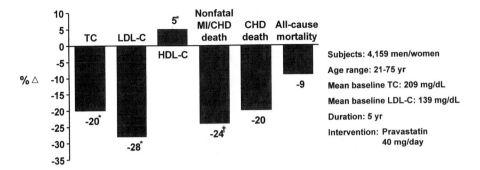

*As compared to placebo.
†P=0.003.

Fig. 7. CARE: Effect of lipid lowering on lipids and coronary events. *As compared to placebo.
†p = 0.003. Adapted from ref. 8.

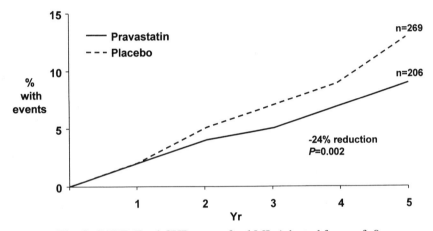

Fig. 8. CARE: Fatal CHD or nonfatal MI. Adapted from ref. 8.

Baseline levels of lipids included total cholesterol 219, LDL 150, TG 139, and HDL 37 mg/dL. Eighty-two percent of the participants were taking aspirin, whereas 47% were on beta blockers. Despite the local discretion permitted within the protocol, intent-to-treat analyses found a 25% reduction in LDL values according to original recruitment assignments. The primary endpoint, coronary mortality, was reduced by 24% ($p < 0.0005$). Secondary objectives, total mortality (reduced by 23%, $p < 0.0001$), and overall cardiac events (23% reduction, $p < 0.0001$) were also met with demonstrated positive results. The risk reduction in MI incidence was 29%, $p < 0.00001$. Procedure rates of coronary artery bypass graft (CABG) and percutaneous transluminal coronary angioplasty (PTCA) were also reduced by 24% and 18%, respectively. Stroke incidence was reduced by 20% ($p = 0.022$).

There were no major safety biochemical differences between the placebo and drug groups. Liver enzymes (ALT/AST) were mildly higher in the pravastatin group ($p = 0.01$), but was not of clinical significance. It was concluded that one cardiovascular event could be prevented through the treatment for 6 yr of 20 LIPID-equivalent patients. Furthermore, the safety of providing this medication was clear. The LIPID study was designed to determine the benefits of pravastatin in the majority of people with heart disease.

Table 1
Lipid Lowering and Plaque Regression: Monotherapy Studies

Study	Treatment group		Δ% Stenosis (p)	% Event reduction
	Regimen	LDL-C		
NHLBI II	D + R	↓31	—	33
STARS	D + R	↓36	↓7.7 (<0.01)	89
Heidelberg	D + E	↓8	↓4.0 (0.05)	−27[a]
CCAIT	D + L	↓29	↓1.2 (0.039)	—
MARS	D + L	↓38	↓0.6	—
BECAIT	D + F	↓3	↓2.55	77
LCAS	D + Fl	↓24	↓2.0 (0.043)	33
Post-CABG	D + L	↓14	↓5.4 (0.001)	—

[a] A 27% reduction means a 27% increase (NS). D = diet; R = resin; E = exercise program; F = fibrate-type drug; Fl = fluvastatin; L = lovastatin.
Data from refs. 42 and 52–54.

Table 2
Lipid Lowering and Plaque Regression: Combination Therapy Studies

Study	Treatment group		Δ% Stenosis (p)	% Event reduction
	Regimen	LDL-C		
CLAS I	D + R + N	↓43	—	25
POSCH (5y)	D + PIB ± R	↓42	—	35 (62)
Lifestyle	V + M + E	↓37	↓2.2 (0.001)	—
FATS (N+C)	D + R + N	↓32	↓0.9 (0.005)	80
FATS (L+C)	D + R + L	↓46	↓0.7 (0.02)	70
CLAS II	D + R + N	↓40	—	43
USCF-SCOR	D + R + N ± L	↓39	↓1.5 (0.04)	—
SCRIP	D + (R+N+L+F) + E, BP	↓21	—	50
HARP	D + P + N + C + F	↓41	↑2.1	33
Post-CABG	D + L + C	↓37–40	↓0.054	29

[a] C = cholestyramine; D = diet; E = exercise program; F = fibrate-type drug; L = lovastatin; M = relaxation techniques; N = nicotinic acid; P = pravastatin; PIB = partial ileal bypass; R = resin; V = vegetarian diet.
Data from refs. 53 and 54.

Although the 4S trial was the first secondary prevention trial to clearly demonstrate a reduction in total mortality, the LIPID trial had significant differences in design and hypotheses. Eighty percent of the LIPID enrollees were not candidates for 4S based on their cholesterol level, age, or history of CAD. LIPID included patients (1) over the age of 70, (2) a greater proportion of diabetics, (3) a lower baseline cholesterol range, and (4) physician discretion in lipid management. LIPID is the first study to examine the use of an HMG (hydroxymethylglutaryl) CoA reductase inhibitor in patients with a history of unstable angina. The LIPID study provides new data on noncoronary mortality (stroke) and on other groups such as women and diabetic patients, who, to date, were underrepresented in clinical trials.

Regression Trials

A number of smaller trials have evaluated the effect of aggressive lipid lowering on actual vessel blockage. These so-called regression trials (Tables 1 and 2) assessed the degree of atherosclerotic progression and regression by either ultrasonography of the carotid arteries or, more often, by coronary angiography. The Multicenter Anti-Atheroma

Table 3
Post-CABG Angiographic Outcomes

| | MRE | | Difference | |
	Moderate	Aggressive	%	p Value
Progression	39	28	28	<0.001
New occlusions	16	10	40	<0.001
New lesions	21	10	52	<0.001
	Mean lumen change in mm			
Minimum diameter	−0.38	−0.20	48	<0.001
Mean diameter	−0.34	−0.16	52	<0.001

MRE = Mean per-patient percentage of grafts.
From ref. *42*.

Study (MAAS) was a double-blind clinical trial that randomized 381 patients with documented CHD to receive dietary treatment plus simvastatin 20 mg/d or placebo over a 48-mo trial duration. Angiographic analysis showed a decrease rate of progression of luminal stenosis in the simvastatin group, with a divergence between the plotted curves of the simvastatin and placebo groups.

The St. Thomas' Arteriographic Regression Study (STARS), followed coronary arteriography in 90 men whose TCs were between 232 and 386 mg/dL and were randomized to a control group, to a group treated with a low-fat, high-fiber (3.6 g/1000 kcal pectin) diet, or to a group treated with the low-fat, high-fiber diet plus cholestyramine (16 g/d). No substantial differences were reported among the groups for HDL-C. Arteriographically defined progression was reported to have occurred in 54% of the control group, compared with 19% of the diet group and 17% of the diet + cholestyramine group, respectively. Regression occurred in 4% of the control group, compared with 42% of the diet group and 38% of the diet + cholestyramine group, respectively. Dense LDL reduction was reported to be the best predictor of arteriographic change *(158)*.

The Cholesterol Lowering Atherosclerosis Study (CLAS) involved 162 postcoronary bypass patients randomly assigned to placebo or treatment with colestipol and niacin. Following 2 yr of treatment, the average number of lesions that progressed was significantly lower ($p = 0.03$) in the drug-treatment group. The number of subjects who showed new atheroma formation in native coronary arteries ($p = 0.03$) and changes in bypass grafts ($p = 0.04$) was also significantly lower. Atherosclerosis regression was reported to have occurred in 16.2% of the drug-treated patients ($p = 0.002$). Drug treatment resulted in a 43% reduction in LDL-C, 22% reduction in TGs, and a 37% increase in HDL-C. The mean LDL-C in the treatment and control groups were 97 and 160 mg/dL, respectively. Subjects with lower TGs received no arteriographic benefit compared to the control group despite substantial blood lipid changes.

The Coronary Artery Bypass Study (CABS) investigated the effect of aggressive LDL-C reduction (goal of LDL-C 60-85 mg/dL) vs. moderate LDL-C reduction (goal LDL-C 130–140 mg/dL) for 4 yr, in 1351 subjects who had a previous CABGs. Thirty-five percent of the moderate treatment group had substantial progression of their grafts compared with 24% in the aggressive treatment group ($p < 0.001$) (Table 3). Although this indicates benefit from aggressive treatment, it also indicates that 24% of CABS patients who achieved LDL-C <100 mg/dL, continued to show arteriographic progression.

Recently reported investigations using single-statin therapy have consistently reported significant LDL-C reduction and a reduction in the rate of progression of arteriographically determined CAD *(170,171)*. MAAS treated 167 placebo and 178 simvastatin (20 mg/d) patients for 4 yr with arteriograms at baseline, 2 yr, and 4 yr *(171)*. Forty-two percent of patients were taking beta blockers, which may tend to complicate interpretation due to the effect of beta blockers on plasma lipoproteins and, in particular, small LDL *(12)*. A 32% reduction in LDL-C with simvastatin was associated with significantly less progression and more regression. Although clinical events were less in the simvastatin group, it was not statistically significant.

The Regression Growth Evaluation Statin Study (REGRESS) treated 885 hypercholesterolemic men with either pravastatin or a placebo for 2 yr. The mean segment diameter worsened by 0.10 mm in the placebo group and worsened by 0.06 mm in the pravastatin group, which represents a significant ($p = 0.02$) reduction in the rate of progression. The Pravastatin Limitation of Atherosclerosis in the Coronary Arteries (PLAC-I) study treated 408 CAD patients with either pravastatin or placebo for 3 yr. There was a trend for decreased progression ($p = 0.07$) and a significant reduction in progression for lesions <50% at baseline ($p < 0.04$). The Canadian Coronary Artery Intervention Trial (CCAIT) used lovastatin in 331 CAD patients to reduce LDL-C and impact CAD progression. Progression with no regression occurred in 48 or 146 (32.9%) of the lovastatin-treated patients and in 76 of 153 (49.7%) placebo-treated patients. Lovastatin slowed the progression of CAD in patients with a mean baseline LDL-C of 173 mg/dL, but there was no significant effect on regression. The Monitored Atheroma Regression Study (MARS) was similar to CCAIT in the treatment of CAD patients with lovastatin or placebo. Following 2 yr of treatment, the lovastatin group had a 38% reduction in LDL-C and a trend for reduced arteriographic progression (increased 2.2% placebo and increased 1.6% lovastatin, $p < 0.20$) but was significantly reduced for lesions >50% obstructed.

The Stanford Coronary Risk Intervention Project (SCRIP) used quantitative coronary arteriography to assess the effect of 4 yr of multifactorial risk intervention in a group of 300 subjects who had documented CAD randomized to a usual-care group and a special intervention group. The special intervention group received diet, exercise, weight reduction, and smoking cessation advice. Bile acid binding resins, nicotinic acid, gemfibrozil, and lovastatin were used to achieve an LDL-C goal of 110 mg/dL. Baseline plasma lipids were representative of a typical CAD population. The LDL-C was reduced approximately 18% more, and HDL-C increased approximately 7% more in the special intervention group than the usual-care group. A significantly greater ($p < 0.01$) annualized rate of minimum diameter change for diseased vessels appeared in the usual-care group (0.046 mm/yr), compared to the special intervention group (0.022 mm/yr). Coronary artery disease regression was reported to be significantly greater ($p < 0.025$) in the special intervention group (21%) than in the usual-care group (10%). For the final 3 yr of the study, significantly fewer deaths ($p < 0.006$) and nonfatal MIs occurred in the special intervention group ($n = 2$) than in the usual-care group ($n = 13$).

Two important observations have been made from these trials. First, although lesion regression was uncommon, the rate of lesion progression was often slowed appreciably. Second, the small changes in luminal narrowing observed with lowering TC are unlikely to be the principal mechanism by which lipid-lowering achieves a reduction in clinical events and revascularization rates. Endothelium-dependent vasomotor function, and the

cellular characteristics of plaques that seem to be intimately related to rupture and thrombosis, are factors that might explain the clinical success from correcting the dyslipidemias.

HDL Cholesterol

Although LDL cholesterol is considered the predominant atherogenic lipoprotein
in the development of CAD, there is significant variability in the clinical expression of
CAD at any given LDL concentration. HDL also exerts significant positive effects on the
process of coronary atherosclerosis. The NCEP identifies a low HDL-C (<35 mg/dL) as
a major independent risk factor for CAD. Consistent evidence of an inverse and continuous relationship between HDL-C and CAD exists.

The Framingham Heart Study produced compelling epidemiologic evidence that a
low level of HDL was an independent predictor of CAD (44). In fact, at all levels of LDL
cholesterol, the level of HDL cholesterol influences the risk of developing CAD. The
recent VA HDL Intervention Trial (VA-HIT) and Bezafibrate Intervention Trial (BIP)
trials have demonstrated that increasing HDL decreases CAD, the Lipid Research Clinics
Coronary Primary Prevention Trial (LRC-CPPT) (45–48) using cholestyramine and the
Helsinki Heart Study (HHS) using gemfibrozil, both have demonstrated that increasing HDL lowered CAD events independent of the effect on LDL lowering. The Adult
Treatment Panel (ATP)II of the NCEP identified low-HDL cholesterol as a major risk
factor for CAD and recommends that all healthy adults be screened for both total cholesterol and HDL cholesterol levels.

The observation that low HDL-C was associated with CAD was verified by the Framingham Study (44), which revealed HDL-C to have the strongest standard lipoprotein
relation (inverse) to CAD. In men who have HDL-C lower than 25 mg/dL, the CAD incidence over 4 yr was 180/1000 compared to 25/1000 in men who had HDL-C in excess
of 64 mg/dL. Furthermore, this relationship persisted above the age of 60 yr.

In the Tromso Heart Study, 6595 young men (20–49 yr) were followed for 2 yr. Seven-
teen suffered MIs, and each case was matched with two control subjects for age, residence,
ethnic origin, and physical activity. The HDL-C made a threefold greater contribution to
the prediction of CHD events than LDL-C in the "young" population. Total cholesterol and
triglycerides were not different between the groups. Mean LDL-C was 222 mg/dL and
190 mg/dL in the MI patients and control subjects, respectively, and HDL-C was 25.6 mg/
dL and 39.4 mg/dL, respectively.

Data from the Framingham Heart Study, Lipid Research Clinics Prevalence Mortality
Follow-Up Study (LRCF), the LRC-CPPT Placebo Group, and the MRFIT are consistent. In general, a 1-mg/dL increase in HDL-C was associated with a significant reduction
in CAD risk of 2% in men and of 3% in women. In the LRCF, in which only fatal endpoints were documented, a 1-mg/dL increase in HDL-C was associated with a significant
reduction of fatal endpoints of 3.7% in men and 4.7% in women. The HDL-C level was
unrelated to noncardiovascular disease mortality.

Triglycerides

The independent relationship between plasma triglycerides (TG) and CAD has now
been established (49). It is likely that the defective lipoprotein metabolism involved in
hypertriglyceridemia may create a vascular environment predisposed to atherogenesis.
Elevated fasting plasma triglyceride is a hallmark of insulin resistance syndrome, a meta-

bolic disorder characterized by hyperinsulinemia, glucose intolerance, decreased HDL-C, and possibly central obesity and increased production of atherogenic small dense LDL particles.

Data from the observational Prospective Cardiovascular Muenster (PROCAM) *(50)* study showed that CHD risk is high when TG exceed 200 mg/dL and the TC: HDL-C ratio is high (>5) because of low HDL-C (<35 mg/dL). In this 8-yr prospective study of 4639 German males, aged 40–65 yr, the incidence of major coronary events steadily increased to 132/1000 events per year in patients with TG levels < 800. There were 258 total events in the entire population of subjects. Patients with TG > 200 mg/dL had at least twice the coronary event rate as patients with entirely normal TG levels. Coronary events appear to increase in proportion to TG levels, with the exception of the small number of subjects having TG > 800 mg/dL. Within this same population, increased lipoprotein little A antigen [Lp(a)] levels were also an independent risk factor for coronary disease. Patients with increased levels of this lipoprotein had nearly twice the coronary event rate as outpatients with normal levels of Lp(a) *(50)*.

In the observational Paris Prospective Study *(50a)*, fasting plasma TG concentration was the only significant predictor of CHD death rate rate on multivariate analysis in 943 middle-aged men with diabetes or impaired glucose tolerance followed up for 11 yr. Variables in the analysis were fasting plasma cholesterol, fasting plasma TG, age, systolic blood pressure, smoking, body mass index (BMI), and insulin and glucose concentrations. HDL-C concentrations were not measured. The mean annual CHD mortality rate was approximately three times higher in men who had TG above the median (123 mg/dL, 1.39 mmol/L) and TC above the median (220 mg/dL, 5.7 mmol/L) than men with values below the medians. The mean annual CHD mortality rate was approximately three times higher in men who had TG above the median (123 mg/dL) and TC above the median (220 mg/dL) than in patients with values below the median. TG concentrations < 123 mg/dL seemed to obliterate the harmful effects of hypercholesterolemia; but with TG >123 mg/dL, harmful effects became noticeably worse, not only for those with elevated plasma cholesterol, but also for those with a normal cholesterol concentration.

The HHS *(51)*, conducted in hyperlipidemic men, demonstrated that increased fasting TG levels in conjunction with a high LDL-C: HDL-C ratio was associated with markedly increased risk for a CHD event. Increased risk was observed for men with elevated TG (>200 mg/dL, 2.3 mmol/L) and men with low HDL-C (<42 mg/dL, 1.08 mmol/L); however, the highest risk occurred in the subgroup of men with elevated TG (>200 mg/dL) and a high LDL-C:HDL-C ratio (>5). These results demonstrate the interdependence among the lipoprotein abnormalities—elevated TG, low HDL-C, and elevated LDL-C—for predicting CHD risk *(51)*.

Hypertriglyceridemia is almost always associated with increased coronary risk on univariate analysis. In some studies, it is also associated with increased risk on multivariate analysis, although not in other studies. This risk for CHD associated with hypertriglyceridemia may be a direct result of the influence of TG-rich lipoprotein accumulation in the circulation on the course of atherosclerotic plaque formation. Alternatively, it may be that hypertriglyceridemia, a central feature of the insulin resistance syndrome, is a simple marker for coronary risk owing to other associated conditions of insulin resistance, such as evolving type 2 diabetes, isolated low HDL-C levels, and obesity. This may explain the decline in the significance of hypertriglyceridemia on multivariate analysis.

HDL-C Intervention Trials

Clinical intervention trials have, until recently, focused on lowering LDL-C. Even with the best LDL-lowering therapies available, only one third of heart disease risk is eliminated. It is clear that CAD is caused by the combination of multiple cardiovascular risks and that a low HDL may be an important contributor to the overall progression of CAD.

Two new prospective, morbidity/mortality studies have been recently tested the hypothesis that HDL is an independent risk factor for CAD. The BIP (56), a randomized, placebo-controlled clinical trial, assessed the effects of bezafibrate vs. placebo in 8000 persons with known CAD. BIP determined whether bezafibrate reduced the endpoints of CAD death and nonfatal MI in 3122 patients with CAD who had a "normal" serum total cholesterol (180–250 mg/dL) and HDL-C <45 mg/dL. Diabetics were essentially excluded from this trial. There was a 15% increase in HDL-C and an 18% decrease in TGs at 1 yr of follow-up. However, there was no significant difference in CAD events between the two groups ($p = 0.27$). Although a divergence of the Kaplan-Meier curves occurred at approximately 3 yr, this was not statistically significant (56).

Another recent clinical trial exploring the role of HDL reduction in the secondary prevention of CAD events was the VA-HIT. This study (57) compared the effect of gemfibrozil vs. placebo on CAD endpoints of CHD death or nonfatal MI in men who had low HDL-C (<40 mg/dL) and "normal" or low LDL-C (<140 mg/dL). This lipid profile is felt to comprise approximately one quarter of all CAD patients. Diabetics as well as patients with the constellation of symptoms associated with the metabolic syndrome X. In total, 2531 patients were randomized to gemfibrozil or placebo followed for a mean of 5.1 yr; 25% of patients were diabetic, 57% were hypertensive, and 61 % had prior MI. Baseline TC was 175 mg/dL, HDL-C was 32 mg/dL, LDL-C was 111 mg/dL, and TG was 161 mg/dL. At one year follow-up there was a 7.5% increase in HDL-C and a 22% decrease in the primary endpoint of CHD death or MI, a 22 % reduction in CHD death alone, a 22% reduction in non-fatal MI alone, and a 27% reduction in stroke ($p = 0.05$ for all).

These data provide powerful new evidence that raising low HDL-C in patients with CAD improves outcomes. Importantly these two new clinical trials extend the benefits of lipid modulation to new subsets of patients: those with low HDL and low HDL and diabetics with isolated low HDL and elevated TGs.

GUIDELINES FOR THE MODIFICATION OF LIPIDS

A national consensus panel concluded that the risk of coronary disease could be defined by dividing the population into three relative risk groups according to age and sex specific percentiles. The second report of the NCEP (17) chose to define a similar set of relative risk groups using single-cutoff values for the entire adult population. This algorithm presents both of these options for use in therapeutic decision making. Using the NCEP classification results in more repeat measurements of cholesterol and leads to dietary therapy for a larger proportion of patients, but does not make the use of pharmacological therapy any more likely.

Screening

PATIENTS WITHOUT KNOWN CAD

In patients without a history of CHD or other atherosclerotic disease, TC, and HDL-C should be measured in all adults 20 yr of age or older at least once every 5 yr. These values

Table 4
Major CHD Risk Factors Other Than LDL-C According to NCEP ATP-II

Positive risk factors	Negative risk factor
Age	High HDL-C: ≥60 mg/dL
Male ≥45	
Female ≥55[a]	
Family Hx of CHD: 1st-degree relative with MI or SCD	
Male relative: <age 55	
Female relative: <age 65	
Current cigarette smoking	
Hypertension: BP ≥140/90 mmHg or taking antihypertensive	
medication	
Low HDL-C: <35 mg/dL	
Diabetes mellitus	

[a] Or having premature menopause wihout ERT.
From ref. *14*.

Table 5
Risk Stratification for Primary Prevention in Adults:
Classification Based on Total Cholesterol and HDL-C

Cholesterol level	HDL-C	Follow-up
Desirable blood cholesterol	≥35 mg/dL	Repeat testing within 5 yr
<200 mg/dL	<35 mg/dL	Perform fasting lipoprotein analysis
Borderline-high blood cholesterol	≥35 mg/dL and	Reevaluate risk status in
200–239 mg/dL	<2 other risk factors	1–2 yr
	<35 mg/dL or	Perform fasting lipoprotein
	≥2 other risk factors	analysis
High blood cholesterol		Perform fasting lipoprotein
≥240 mg/dL		analysis

From ref. *14*.

may be determined in nonfasting blood samples. Assessment of other nonlipid risk factors should also be made (Table 4). In individuals without CHD, the following classifications and follow-ups are recommended (Table 5).

1. TC < 200 mg/dL is classified as desirable. If HDL-C is >35 mg/dL, follow-up includes general education materials about dietary modification, physical activity, and other risk-reduction activities. Repeating TC and HDL-C measurements in 5 yr is recommended. If HDL-C is <35 mg/dL, a fasting lipoprotein analysis including LDL-C and TG should be performed due to the increased likelihood of abnormalities of these lipid component in the low-HDL subgroup.
2. TC 200–239 mg/dL is classified as borderline high. If HDL-C is >35 mg/dL, and fewer than two other CHD risk factors are present, instruction on dietary modification, physical activity, and other risk-reduction activities should be provided, and TC and HDL-C measurements should be repeated in 1–2 yr. If HDL-C is <35 mg/dL or two or more other risk factors are present, a fasting lipoprotein analysis should be performed.
3. TC >240 mg/dL is classified as high. A fasting lipoprotein analysis should be performed.

In individuals without CHD or other atherosclerotic disease, an LDL-C concentration <130 mg/dL is classified as desirable (Table 6). Individuals with desirable LDL-C levels

Table 6
Primary Prevention in Adults:
Classification Based on LDL-C

LDL-C level	Classification
<130 mg/dL	Desirable
130–159 mg/dL	Borderline-high
≥160 mg/dL	High

From ref. *14*.

Table 7
Risk Stratification for Secondary Prevention in Adults:
Classification Based on LDL-C[a]

LDL-C concentration	Follow-up
Optimal	Individualize instruction on diet and physical activity
≤100 mg/dL	Repeat lipoprotein analysis annually
Higher than optimal	Conduct full clinical evaluation
>100 mg/dL	Evaluate for causes of secondary dyslipidemia
	Evaluate for familial disorders when indicated
	Consider influences of age, sex, and other CHD risk factors
	Initiate therapy

[a]Average of two measurements, 1–8 wk apart.
From ref. *14*.

do not require further evaluation at this time. They should be instructed about dietary modification, physical activity, and other risk-reduction activities. Information about dietary modification, physical activity, and other risk-reduction activities should be provided. Total cholesterol and HDL-C should be measured after 5 yr.

LDL-C concentration from 130–159 mg/dL is classified as borderline high in primary prevention. If fewer than two other risk factors are present, information about dietary modification, physical activity, and other risk-reduction activities should be provided. In addition, repeat lipoprotein analysis should be performed annually.

Individuals classified as having borderline-high LDL-C and who have two or more other risk factors, or as having high LDL-C (>160 mg/dL) should undergo a full clinical evaluation and begin active cholesterol-lowering diet therapy. NCEP provides LDL-C cut-points for initiating diet therapy and considering drug therapy in patients with and without CHD. In addition, NCEP provides a goal or target for LDL-C concentrations following therapy.

Lifestyle intervention, including dietary therapy, should generally be attempted for 3–6 mo prior to initiation of drug treatment. Need for intervention is based on estimation of overall risk. In patients without CHD, treatment and target cut-points vary based on the presence of other risk factors for CHD. In young people with no additional CHD risk factors, drug therapy may be indicated only if LDL-C exceeds 220 mg/dL. On the other hand, physicians may chose to initiate drug therapy in primary prevention at 130 mg/dL if overall risk is high based on multiple risk factors.

Patients with CHD. In patients with CHD, the optimal LDL-C concentration is <100 mg/dL (Table 7). For these patients, individual instruction on the American Heart Association (AHA) Step II Diet and physical activity should be provided, and lipoprotein analysis should be conducted annually.

Table 8
Step I and Step II Diet Recommendations

	Step I diet (% of total calories)	Step II diet (% of total calories)
Total fat	<30%	<30%
Saturated fat	8–10%	<7%
Polyunsaturated fat	Up to 10%	Up to 10%
Monounsaturated	Up to 15%	Up to 15%
Carbohydrates	50–60%	50–60%
Protein	15%	15%
Cholesterol	<300 mg/d	<200 mg/d

In CHD patients with LDL-C >100 mg/dL, and in high-risk primary prevention patients, clinical evaluation should be carried out and cholesterol-lowering therapy should be initiated based on the recommended cut-points. Clinical evaluation includes medical history, physical examination, and laboratory tests; and assessment for familial disorders (when indicated) and for causes of secondary dyslipidemia. If LDL-C remains at 100–130 mg/dL in secondary prevention despite lifestyle changes, the physician should use clinical judgment of overall risk to determine whether drug therapy should be initiated.

For secondary prevention in adults with evidence of CHD or other atherosclerotic disease, lipoprotein analysis after 12 h fasting should be performed. Definitive lipoprotein analysis should be performed when the patient is not in the recovery phase from an acute event that can alter (lower) the usual LDL-C concentration. Nevertheless, physicians may wish to begin lipid-lowering therapy before a patient is discharged from the hospital in view of risk factor analysis.

Decisions should be based on the average of two LDL-C determinations 1–8 wk apart. If the first two LDL-C determinations differ by >30 mg/dL a third test result should be obtained within 1–8 wk and the average value of the tests used.

The Expert Panel on Detection, Evaluation, and Treatment of High Blood Cholesterol on Adults *(14)* recommends that an optimal LDL-C concentration in the patient with CHD should be <100 mg/dL. In patients who have achieved this level, repeat lipoprotein analysis should be performed annually. In patients with higher than optimal LDL-C (<100 mg/dL) a full clinical examination should be conducted, and a search for secondary causes of dyslipidemia and familial disorders should be initiated in conjunction with a consideration for the influences of age, gender, and other CHD risk factors. Once these factors are fully evaluated, therapy should be initiated.

Treatment of Hyperlipidemia

DIET

NCEP and AHA guidelines promote a diet in which fat composes only 30% or less of the day's total calories. The committee on nutrition from the AHA, based on recommendations from the World Health Organization, suggests that fat calories constitute no less than 15% of total calories. The Step-One and Step-Two AHA diets (Table 8) utilize dietary therapy to reduce the intake of saturated fat and cholesterol in order to lower the LDL-C. The first step in dietary therapy, usually the Step-One diet, parallels NCEP recommendations. A change from the average American diet to the Step-One diet of <10% saturated fatty acids and <300 mg/d of cho-lesterol reduces serum cholesterol levels by approximately 7%, whereas further restriction to <7% saturated fatty acids and <200 mg/d cholesterol (Step-Two Diet) should reduce cholesterol levels by an additional 3–7%.

EXERCISE

Many large epidemiologic investigations have failed to demonstrate consistently a correlation between reported physical activity and lipid values in populations not specifically selected for hyperlipidemia.A paucity of cross-sectional studies have investigated physical activity and hypercholesterolemia. Yet it is generally accepted that exercise improves the spectrum of lipid abnormalities in conjuction with a healthy diet and weight loss.

PHARMACOTHERAPY

The AHA-ACC (American College of Cardiology) guidelines for modifying cholesterol levels in persons without CHD indicate that the goal of therapy is (1) an LDL-C <130 mg/dL and in documented CHD (2) is to lower LDL-C levels to below 100 mg/dL. The guidelines also recommend that an HMG Co A reductase inhibitor or statin be the initial therapy in patients with TG levels lower than 400 mg/dL

The statins' high efficacy in LDL-C lowering and few side effects make them an attractive choice for patients with established CHD. Given the early benefits of cholesterol lowering in patients with CHD and substantial risk of recurrent, often fatal events, it is inappropriate to wait several month before beginning drug therapy. If LDL-C levels are higher than 100 mg/dL at the time of a patient's 4–6-wk follow-up after MI, the patient should be considered a candidate for drug intervention.

The target level of 100 mg/dL or below may be difficult to attain. Consequently combination therapy is often required. The best combination is one of a statin with a bile acid sequestrant, as the sequestrant provides little added toxicity. Moreover, the LDL-C lowering required may not necessitate the a full sequestrant dosage. Combining a statin with niacin may also enhance LDL-C lowering but also increases the risk of drug-induced myopathy. Because patients may have a risk of myopathy as high as 3% when taking this drug combination, all patients should be instructed to report any muscle pain, and to discontinue drug use should this occur until a medical evaluation and creatine kinase (CK) levels are determined. Patients with low HDL-C, high TG, and high LDL-C levels may benefit from the combination of a statin, either with niacin or gemfibrozil. When a statin is used with gemfibrozil, the report of myopathy may be as high as 5%. Occasionally, triple drug therapy is necessary to lower LDL-C levels to less than 100 mg/dL. These patients require careful monitoring for liver and muscular toxicity.

Statins (HMG CoA Reductase Inhibitors)

HMG CoA reductase inhibitors competitively inhibit the rate-limiting enzyme in hepatic cholesterol synthesis, 3-hydroxy-3-methylglutaryl-coenzyme A. This results in a compensatory increase in hepatic LDL receptor activity and appears to have some effect on LDL production rates. The Food and Drug Administration (FDA) has approved Llovastatin (Merck Sharpe & Dohme), pravastatin (Bristol-Myers Squibb), simvastatin (Merck & Co.), fluvastatin (Hoest Marion Roussel), atorvastatin (Parke Davis), and cerivastatin (Bayer) for use in the United States.

INDICATIONS

In patients who have hypercholesterolemia, these compounds can achieve reductions of 30–50%, and, when combined with a resin, reductions of 50–60% are possible. They have a small effect on reducing fasting plasma triglyceride concentrations, but this masks a significant reduction in postprandial triglyceridemia. Like the resins, these agents are useful in treating patients who have elevations in LDL-C but are not the agents of choice for treating hypertriglyceridemia. They appear to have little effect on Lp(a). Recommendations vary on what time of day to take the medication and whether it should be taken in conjunction with meals.

HMG CoA reductase inhibitors are now included by the NCEP ATP II among first-line alternatives for the treatment of hypercholesterolemia. The category includes six drugs: lovastatin, simvastatin, pravastatin, fluvastatin, atorvastatin, and the newest agent cerivastatin. The HMG CoA reductase inhibitors are indicated as an adjunct to diet for reduction of elevated TC in patients with hypercholesterolemia (types IIa and IIb) when nonpharmacologic measures such as diet are inadequate. Although HMG CoA reductase inhibitors may be effective in lowering total and LDL cholesterol in patients with mixed hyperlipidemias (elevated cholesterol and TGs), the agents have not been extensively studied in subjects with lipoprotein lipase functional impairment with severe elevation in TGs (types I), remnant clearance abnormalities due partially to an abnormal apoE isoform, and accompanied by both high TG and cholesterol values (type III), isolated elevations in TGs and reductions in HDL (type IV), and profound increases in TGs predominantly from an intestinal origin (type V).

Efficacy and Safety Profile. HMG CoA reductase inhibitors are extremely effective in reducing LDL-C in most patients with primary hypercholesterolemia. The HMG CoA reductase inhibitors decrease total cholesterol in the range of 15–60%, LDL-C by 20–60%, and increase HDL-C by 5–15%. Declines in apolipoprotein B commensurate with LDL reductions have been also demonstrated. TGs have been reduced by 10–25%. TG lowering parallels LDL lowering, in that higher doses of more potent agents produce TG reductions of over 40%. The HMG CoA reductase inhibitors appear to have minimal effects on apolipoprotein A-I, A-II, and Lp(a).

The first four HMG CoA reductase inhibitors (lovastatin, simvastatin, pravastatin, and fluvastatin) are well tolerated, efficacious, and approximately equivalent with respect to safety profiles during monotherapy within trials. However, the safety and efficacy of cerivastatin and atorvastatin have not been determined in large clinical trials. Given their similar drug class, there is no reason to believe these agents will not perform as effectively and safely as the earlier statins. Fewer than 5% of patients in controlled clinical trials report side effects with HMG CoA reductase inhibitors, the most common of which are mild GI disturbances (nausea, abdominal pain, diarrhea, constipation, flatulence), which rarely warrants therapy discontinuation. Headache, fatigue, pruritis, and myalgia are other minor side effects that seldom prompt treatment termination.

ADVERSE EFFECTS

Liver Function Test Abnormalities. Mild transient elevations in liver enzymes have been reported with all HMG CoA reductase inhibitors. Elevations in serum amino transferases three times the upper limit of normal have occurred in <2% of patients in controlled clinical trials. At the usual midrange dosing, the frequency is <1%. In general, for each doubling of statin dose, there is an 0.6% increase in risk for transaminase elevation.

Therapy should be discontinued when a greater than threefold elevation occurs. Enzyme levels typically return to normal within 2 wk and either lower doses of the same medication can be reinstituted or a different HMG CoA can be utilized. Monitoring of hepatic aminotransferase levels is recommended for those taking HMG CoA reductase inhibitors at 6 wk, 3 mo, and semiannually after drug initiation. Due to the excellent safety profiles of pravastatin and simvastatin, the FDA recommends discontinuing hepatic enzyme monitoring after 3 mo for pravastatin, and after 6 mo of continuous same dose therapy for simvastatin.

Myopathy. Myopathy, a rare but potentially serious side effect of HMG CoA reductase inhibitors, occurs with muscle symptoms and serum CK elevations to more than 10 times the upper limit of normal. CK measurements are not required unless symptoms are present. When statins are used in combination with certain pharmaceutical agents, e.g., erythromycin, gemfibrozil, azole antifungals, cimetidine, methotrexate, and/or cyclosporine, the risk of CK elevation and myositis increases. Pravastatin and fluvastatin combinations are considered relatively safe, as they do not use the P450 3A4 microsomal pathways. These drug combinations should either be avoided, or used judiciously with interval measurements of CK's and liver function tests.

COST EFFECTIVENESS OF STATINS

Cost effectiveness studies in patients with established CHD are consistent in demonstrating that intervention with lipid-lowering drugs is highly cost effective. The incremental cost of intervention may be negative or cost saving in some instances. The cost of cholesterol lowering is less than the cost of doing nothing and allowing the patient to proceed to another event.

Initial data from the 4S study indicate that in patients with established CHD, the addition of simvastatin to the treatment of 100 patients with CHD over 6 yr could be expected to prevent 4 of 9 deaths, 7 of 21 nonfatal MIs, and 6 of 19 bypass procedures. Formal analysis of the cost effectiveness of simvastatin indicated a total cost of hospitalization in the placebo group of 52.8 million Swedish kronor (SEK) compared with 36.0 million SEK in the simvastatin group. This amounted to a 32% reduction per patient.

STATINS IN PATIENTS WITH HYPERTRIGLYCERIDEMIA

Recent clinical trials have proven that statin therapy causes a marked reduction CAD risk in patients with hypercholesterolemia. It remains to be determined whether stain therapy will decrease serum TGs and reduce risk in this population. In patients with normal TG levels, statin therapy decreases TG levels to a lesser percent than LDL levels. In patients with hypertriglyceridemia, percentage reductions in LDL and TG are similar. This implies a common mechanism of action of statins on both LDL and TGs. Whereas the absolute reduction in TG dose is proportional to the statin dose, the percent TG lowering relative to LDL reduction remains constanat across all statins and all doses. Atorvastatin provides the ability to significantly lower both LDL and TGs. It has been shown to decrease TGs by 27–46% across its dosing range.

One approach to the risk reduction in patients with hypertriglyceridemia is to decrease the concentrations of atherogenic TG-rich lipoproteins. This can be achieved through the use of statins, thereby simultaneously decreasing TG and LDL-C. Statins appear to be the first line of therapy in patients with combined elevations of LDL-C and moderate elevations of TGs. No trials have been performed using statins as the primary therapy for hypertriglyceridemia. Clinical efficacy can be xtrapolated from the large body of evidence accumulated across broad populations with different forms of dyslipidemia.

There are insufficient trial data to justify the use of statins as first-line therapy in the treatment of hypertriglyceridemia. However, in selected high-risk patients, TG-lowering medications in combination with a statin may be used. Risk reduction with combination therapy of a TG-lowering agent and statin has not been achieved in a clinical trial.

HMG CoA Reductase Inhibitors and Combination with Other Agents

One third of patients with hypercholesterolemia do not respond adequately to monotherapy alone. In few cases, poor response represents poor absorption of the medicaitons. More often, failures involve subjects with LDL values above 160 mg/dL, and primarily those above 190 mg/dL. The latter cases are often associated with inherited disorders of metabolism, e.g., familial hypercholesterolemia (FH), familial defective apoB, or familial combined hyperlipidemia. If the patient has an LDL >160 mg/dL, a polygenic form of hyperlipidemia should be considered. Prior to the release of atorvastatin and cerivastatin, a majority of CHD subjects required two or three agents to maintain their LDL values less than 100 mg/dL. This may be somewhat easier with the availability of progressively more potent agents. Combination therapy may be required in only the most extreme cases.

STATINS PLUS RESINS

In the isolated forms of LDL elevation, HMG CoA reductase inhibitors and bile acid resins exhibit highly complementary mechanisms of action in combination therapy, and are therefore useful for the treatment of severe hypercholesterolemia. By disrupting the enterohepatic recirculation of bile acids, the sequestrants induce a compensatory rise in conversion of hepatic cholesterol to bile acids, as well as a secondary rise in hepatic cholesterol synthesis. This phenomenon consequently upregulates hepatic LDL receptor expression and thereby decreases LDL serum concentration. Adding an HMG CoA reductase inhibitor blocks the secondary rise in cholesterol synthesis and therefore produces a further increase in hepatic LDL receptors. This combination has been found to be additive in altering LDL levels. Because the HMG CoA reductase inhibitor acts systemically, whereas the resin is nonsystemic, systemic drug interactions are thus minimized.

Combination therapy reduces LDL by 30–55%. This combination was initially administered to familial hypercholesterolemic subjects, using high doses of both statins and resins. More recently, the issues of lower dose preparations using resins and statins have been reviewed, favoring the addition of low dose resins rather than the doubling of ongoing statin agents. Usually, the addition of 4–8 g of a resin to an ongoing statin regimen will result in greater LDL lowering than doubling the statin dose. The marginal value of adding resin to a statin will likely diminish as the potency of available statin agents increases. The angiographic trial Lipoprotein and Coronary Atherosclerosis Study (LCAS) utilized fluvastatin alone, or a combination of fluvastatin and resin when LDL was >160 mg/dL. Similar angiographic benefits were observed in monotherapy and combined cohorts, suggesting that LDL lowering is the relevant parameter, not the means by which it is achieved.

In some patients with combined or mixed hyperlipidemias, resin may not be advocated because of its triglyceride elevating effect, and statin therapy alone may not be adequate to lower LDL-C.

Bile Acid-Binding Resins

Bile acid-binding resins have been used for more than 25 yr. Intestinal binding of bile salts by the resin decreases bile salt resorption through the enterohepatic recirculation route. Hepatic cholesterol, HMG CoA reductase activity, and hepatic cholesterol synthesis are increased. Inhibition of normal bile salt resorption also has been hypothesized as the cause of increased plasma triglyceride concentrations by enhanced activity of phosphatidic acid phosphatase. In type II hyperlipidemia patients, resin therapy can result in LDL-C reductions of approximately 72 mg/dL, or 27%, and an HDL-C increase of 2–3 mg/dL, or 4%. There appears to be little effect on Lp(a).

INDICATIONS

Because of their long history for safety and efficacy, and because of their nonsystemic nature, bile acid-binding resins are the first line drugs of choice for reduction of plasma LDL-C.

Resins are useful for patients who have mild elevation in plasma LDL-C and who do not fall within the classic hyperlipidemia definition (90th percentile) and in whom reduction is warranted because of high-CAD risk from other factors. In this group, it is important to note that low-dose resin therapy can have a significant effect on LDL-C reduction. One-half the recommended full dose of six packets per day can achieve approximately 75% of the full-dose LDL-C reduction. A colestipol dose of 5 g/d (16% full dose) can achieve 50% of the LDL-C reduction as that of a 50% dose. Approximately 50% of moderately hypercholesterolemic subjects can achieve the US NCEP goal of an LDL-C < 130 mg/dL with less than 50% of the full resin dose. It is no longer necessary to dose patients two of three times per day. Once-a-day dosing achieves nearly the same effect as twice-a-day dosing.

COMPLIANCE

Common patient complaints include difficulty in ingesting the resins, GI distress, and constipation. Several tricks are available to enhance compliance. First, for all diet, exercise, weight reduction, and drug therapies, compliance can be enhanced greatly by effective use of a dedicated nurse. Second, the resins can be mixed in various liquid media, including juices and semisolid foods such as applesauce. Third, combining either mineral oil or supplemental fiber can reduce constipation complaints, and some fibers can further reduce LDL-C by approximately 10%. Bowel gas can be reduced by using simethicone.

Nicotinic Acid

Nicotinic acid is a B vitamin that affects the lipoprotein system mediated through nicotinamide adenine dinucleotide (NAD), or NADP, by the inhibition of adenylate cyclase. Only nicotinic acid or its glycine conjugate (nicotinuric acid) has an antilipolytic effect. Nicotinamide is inactive with regard to lipoprotein change. Nicotinic acid inhibits endogenous cholesterol synthesis, increases catabolism, and reduces the plasma concentrations of nonesterified fatty acids by its action at the level of the adipocyte. Rapid release of prostaglandins from platelets is thought to be responsible, in part, for the vasodilation and flush response. Like other medications, nicotinic acid has pharmacologic effects that may benefit atherosclerosis that are not reflected in plasma lipoprotein measurements. These effects include prostaglandin/thromboxane perturbations, platelet aggregation inhibition, and fibrinolysis. A long-acting, once-a-day niacin that is dosed at bedtime was recently approved by the FDA. This niacin has a significant effect in reducing small dense LDL, and in LDL pattern B subjects achieves a mean 40% reduction in LDL-C.

INDICATIONS

Nicotinic acid is useful in patients who have elevated TGs, TG-rich lipoproteins, LDL-C, reductions in HDL-C, and LDL subclass pattern B. Effects on lipids are commonly seen after the renal threshold is exceeded, which generally is around 1500 mg/d. The response of plasma lipoproteins is dose dependent within the range of approximately 1500–6000 mg/d. Unmodified or time-release nicotinic acid can result in 10–25% reductions in daily doses of 1500–3000 mg. Nicotinic acid is one of the few lipid medications that appears to have some effect on Lp(a). Nicotinic acid can suppress expression of LDL subclass pattern B when triglycerides are reduced below approximately 140 mg/dL.

COMPLIANCE

Nicotinic acid is the lipid-altering drug with the most potential for side effects and, consequently, adherence problems. Because of nicotinic acid's great potential benefit, it is worth expending extra effort on achieving compliance. Individual variability exists in the side effects to such an extent that it often can be attributed to differences in formulation. For this reason, obtaining several brands and testing each for individual tolerance can be helpful. Slowly titrating the dose from 100–500 mg three times day (TID) over a 1-mo period can ease the patient into a therapeutic dose range. The prostaglandin-mediated flush can be ameliorated in part by ingesting 2.5 grains of aspirin 15 min before the niacin dose. Avoiding alcohol, monosodium glutamate, hot beverages, and spicy foods also can help ameliorate the flush. Gastrointestinal distress can be reduced by ingesting niacin with food. The most important tool to enhance adherence is a dedicated lipid nurse.

Niaspan® (KOS Pharmaceutical) is a new once-a-night niacin preparation dosed from 500–3000 mg/d. Niaspan has been compared with immediate-release niacin and found to have comparable benefits with fewer side effects. The new formulation of this product as well as the evening dosing reduces the apparent flushing episodes. LDL reductions of 10%, 18%, and 20% are found with 1, 2, and 3 g of Niaspan, respectively. Parallel to these changes, HDL increases by 15%, 25%, and 30%, whereas TGs decrease by 10%, 35%, and 45%. The reduction in Lp(a) was found to be 10%, 25%, and 30% for the 1-, 2-, and 3-g doses. Glucose increases by an average of 6%, uric acid increases by 34%, and some decrease in phosphorus (−16%) was also noted. Overall, an approximate 10% of study participants increased their aspartate transaminase (AST) from baseline, but only 2% went above two times the upper limit of normal, the latter consistent with that found in the placebo group. Long-term 2-yr studies resulted in 2 patients out of 500 discontinuing Niaspan due to liver function elevations (<0.5%), with less than 1% having AST/ALT (alanine transaminase) elevations beyond two times the upper limit of normal. Concomitant statin therapy reduced LDL another 14% on the average, but appeared to modestly reduce the Lp(a) benefit (not significant). Niaspan is a good alternative to regular niacin preparations, with 70% of patients not having reported flushing. Given some of the foregoing trials, niacin or one of its analogs should perhaps be administered more often in "mixed" phenotype patients. It is noted to decrease "dense" LDL particle concentration in such subjects. Statin–niacin outcome trials are clearly needed.

Fibric Acid Derivatives

Fibric acid derivatives enhance lipoprotein lipase activity and hepatic bile secretion and reduce hepatic TG production. TG and LDL-C response to these agents depends on the lipoprotein abnormality and specific fibric acid derivative used. TG reductions between 8% and 72%, LDL-C reductions between 0% and 35%, and HDL-C increases between 0% and 25% have been reported. Generally, the greatest benefit is seen in patients who have elevations in plasma TG, although fenofibrate has been reported to produce significant LDL-C reduction (approximately 1.2 mmol/L) in type IIa patients. In hypertriglyceridemic patients who initially have low or normal LDL-C, gemfibrozil treatment may result in an increase in LDL-C, perhaps because of an increase in LDL production or a decrease in fractional LDL clearance rates. This response suggests the presence of a second lipoprotein abnormality that often requires two-drug therapy.

INDICATIONS

These agents are useful in the treatment of hypertriglyceridemia and in selected patients who have elevated LDL-C in combination with elevated TGs. The HDL-C level often is reported to increase significantly when initial HDL-C is low or when it is associated with reduction of TGs. These agents are the drugs of choice in type III hyperlipidemia. In the Helsinki Heart Study, gemfibrozil (600 mg twice daily [BID]) resulted in an overall 42% reduction in TGs, 10% reduction in LDL-C, and a 10% increase in HDL-C.

COMPLIANCE

These drugs generally are well tolerated. Occasionally mild GI distress (nausea) is experienced in the first week. To reduce this potential side effect, it can be useful to start therapy with one-half the normal dose for several days before increasing to a full dose.

FENOFIBRATE

Fenofibrate is a fibric acid derivative, dosed at 200 or 400 mg/d. It is absorbed and rapidly converted into fenofibric acid, the active metabolite. The vast majority of the drug is protein bound, with a 4-h time to peak plasma levels. Elimination half-life is approximately 20 h. The micronized form of fenofibrate—smaller particles and an absorption rate that is almost twice as fast as regular fenofibrate (200 mg/d)—was used in 1334 subjects with serum triglycerides above 200 mg/dL and total cholesterol >250 mg/dL. LDL was decreased by 27%, triglycerides by approximately 50% and HDL increased overall by 15% (increased by 30% in those subjects whose baseline values were <35 mg/dL). LDL lowering is dependent on the baseline LDL value, with 10% reductions at a baseline of 150 mg/dL, and 25% reduction at a baseline of 190 mg/dL. Combination statin–fenofibrate therapy reduces LDL in an additive fashion. Fenofibrate appears to decrease the density of LDL, and upregulate both lipoprotein lipase and apoCIII, thereby enhancing the cabolism of TG-rich particles. These alterations, including the increase in HDL-associated apoAI and apoAII production, is related to fenofibrate-induced activation of the peroxisome proliferator-activated receptors (PPARs). This superfamily of nuclear hormone receptor genes operate as transcription factors, and can secondarily result in upregulation of several lipoprotein related enzymes and proteins. Furthermore, fenofibrate can produce reductions in both fibrinogen (7–23%) as well as in Lp(a) (>7%).

Fenofibric acid is excreted primarily through the kidney, and therefore needs a dosing modification in renal failure. It is recommended that coumadin be dosed at one-third its standard dose when administered with fenofibrate, with careful follow-up of protimes.

Table 9
Effect of Cholesterol Lowering on Stroke Events: A Meta-Analysis of Statin Trials

Investigators	Statin	% ↓ in LDL-C	Sample size	Event rates[a] placebo/drug
First-degree prevention				
Shepherd et al.	P	26	3302	3.2./2.8
Salonen et al.	P	29	224	6.0/3.0
Mercuri et al.	P	22	151	0.0/0.0
Furberg et al.	L	28	231	1.4/0.0
Second-degree prevention				
PMSGCRP[b]	P	26	530	11.3/0.0
Pitt et al.	P	28	206	3.3/0.0
Crouse et al.	P	28	75	13.2/4.4
Jukema et al.	P	28	450	4.6/2.2
Sacks et al.	P	32	2081	7.5/5.2
Blankenhorn et al.	L	32	134	0.0/0.0
Waters et al.	L	29	165	0.0/6.1
4S[c]	S	38	2221	7.6/5.6

[a] Annual rate per 1000 patients.
[b] Pravastatin Multinational Study Group for Cardiac Risk Patients.
[c] Scandinavian Simvastatin Survival Study Group.
L = lovastatin; P = pravastatain; S = simvastatin.
From ref. 26.

Glucose tolerance is not affected by this agent, and no lithogenic potential has been observed. Creatine phosphokinase (CPK) elevations are noted in 0.6–1.1% of cases, but appear to be usually associated with renal failure. Liver enzymes increase in <2% of cases, whereas GI disturbances (constipation, dyspepsia, and diarrhea) account for well over 50% of side effects and leads to over 3.5% discontinuation rates.

Comparatively, fenofibrate generally reduces LDL by at least 5–10% more than gemfibrozil, with a modest enhanced effect on HDL and TGs. Clinical outcomes data with fenofibrate are scant.

CLINICAL EFFICACY IN SPECIAL POPULATIONS

Statins and Stroke

Although the link between elevated cholesterol and CAD is well established, the link between elevated cholesterol and stroke had been less convincing. Recent clinical trials (26) and meta-analyses (27,28) of HMG CoA reductase inhibitors have demonstrated a significant reduction in ischemic stroke in patients with a history of CAD both with and without elevated cholesterol (Table 9). Both the 4S and CARE studies strongly suggest that statin therapy results in a decrease in the risk for stroke.

In a recent meta-analysis (27) of 16 published trials testing statins from 1985–1995, statins had a clear benefit on stroke and total mortality. In 29,000 subjects considered in the meta-analysis, the average reductions in total and LDL-C achieved were a large −22 to 30%, respectively. A total of 454 strokes and 1175 deaths occurred. Individuals assigned statin drugs had a 29% decrement in stroke (95% [CI] 14–41%) as well as a reduction in total mortality of 22% (95%[CI], 12–31%). Additional data regarding non-CVD mortality and cancer indicate no enhanced risk with the use of statins in these trials.

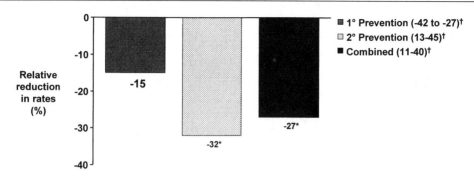

*P=0.001.
†95% confidence interval of percentage of relative reduction.

Fig. 9. Effects of statins on stroke events: a meta-analysis of primary- and secondary-prevention trials. *p = 0.001. †95% confidence interval of percentage of relative reduction. Adapted from ref. 26.

In a meta-analysis (26) by looking at 12 trials of both primary and secondary prevention (n = 7808 primary; n = 11,710 secondary) a 27% risk reduction was seen in the group receiving statins for secondary prevention (p = 0.001) but not in the primary prevention group. In the statin group, 182 strokes were observed, whereas 248 were observed in the placebo group followed for a mean of 4 yr (Fig. 9). In a meta-analysis of 28 trials, Bucher and co-workers (28) noted a 20% risk reduction in stroke with the use of statins. Twenty other trials using alternative cholesterol-lowering approaches were also examined. Resins that reduced death from CHD by 31%, equivalent to that of statins, as well as diet and fibrates, demonstrated no stroke benefits.

The LIPID (12) trial recently reported a significant decrease in stroke mortality with the use of statins. A 23% reduction in stroke was found with a 25% lowering of LDL-C through the use of pravastatin. The basis for this benefit could be the reduction in cardiovascular disease and therefore a reduction in cardiac sources of embolic phenomenon, or perhaps more probable, a direct effect on vasoregulation in the cerebral vasculature. Carotid internal medical thickness (IMT) measurements were reduced in the pravastatin group for the full 4- to 5-yr period of the LIPID trial. Other studies using other statins have reported similar benefits.

Importantly, fewer cerebrovascular events occurred among those patient treated in the 4S, CARE, LIPID, and AFCAPS/TEXCAP studies. These results, and the uniformity in results from the three aforementioned meta-analyses recently reported, provide a clear basis for statin therapy to decrease the incidence of stroke. Even though we await subanalyses of these investigations, this finding may require a rethinking of lipid-lowering therapy in the elderly toward a more aggressive posture.

CARDIAC TRANSPLANT RECIPIENTS

Transplant-associated atherosclerosis is a major cause of cardiac allograft failure after the first year following transplantation (29). Several distinct features are unique for atherosclerosis that develops following transplantation as compared with the commonly occurring disease. The pathological process involves the coronaries in a concentric fashion and often involves the epicardial and intramyocardial branches (29). Although the role of conventional risk factors in the development of transplant-associated atherosclerosis has not yet been defined, it seen logical to control those that are amenable to treatment.

Over 60% of transplant patients are observed to have hypercholesterolemia *(30)*. Because vascular disease is a major cause of ultimate transplantation failure, and cholesterol reduction in CHD patients has been profoundly successful, serious efforts at cholesterol lowering have been made within the transplantation population. At the present time, lovastatin, pravastatin, and simvastatin are the only pharmaceutical agents that have demonstrated a benefit toward reducing rejection after human cardiac transplantation, and decreasing the level of vasculopathy *(31–36)*.

The Kobashigawa study *(36)* included 47 transplant subjects who initiated 20 mg pravastatin 1–2 wk after surgery (increased to 40 mg within 8 wk), and 50 transplant subjects who did not have statin agents administered. Baseline characteristics were generally similar. Cholesterol values at 12 mo were 193 mg/dL vs. 248 mg/dL for pravastatin vs. placebo, respectively. One-year survival was 94% vs. 78% ($p = 0.025$), cardiac rejection with hemodynamic compromise 3% vs. 14% ($p = 0.005$), and intravascular ultrasound (IVUS)-defined maximal intimal thickness was 0.11 vs. 0.23 mm ($p = 0.002$).

In a 4-yr prospective randomized study *(37)* with heart transplant recipients (35 cases, 37 control subjects), the efficacy of simvastatin was assessed. The simvastatin group had significantly lower LDL-C concentrations (115 vs. 156, $p = 0.002$), an improved long-term survival (88.6% vs. 70.3%, $p = 0.05$) and a lower incidence of accelerated graft vessel disease (16.6% vs. 42.3%, $p = 0.045$). The results of this trial show that simvastatin decreased the incidence of transplant atherosclerosis and reduced mortality from graft failure due to acute rejection confirming earlier reports by Kobashigawa.

However, as much as the hypothesis tested was a reasonable one based on clinical trial data related to cholesterol lowering, mechanism of benefit in transplant patients remains unclear. In the Kobashigawa study, LDL lowering did not specifically correlate with vascular benefits, and in the Wenke study *(37)*, no suggestion of this correlation was reported. Thus, some of the immune-related activity of HMG CoA reductase inhibitors, rather than LDL lowering per se, may be relevant to the observed benefits. Wenke notes that a large percentage of cyclosporin is bound to LDL, so that LDL reduction could lead to more free cyclosporin availability to ward off rejection.

Cyclosporine-induced alterations in the metabolism of HMG CoA reductase inhibitor as well as steroid-derived lipoprotein metabolic abnormalities critically impact the treatment and expected benefit of lipid-lowering agents toward vascular disease *(31,38,39)*. Due to the metabolic compromise of statins by cyclosporine, toxicity may be observed at higher statin doses. An increase in serum levels has been documented for all the available HMG CoA reductase inhibitors when coadministered with cyclosporine. Therefore, the use of these agents in cardiac transplantation has been of concern due to the possibility of myositis and potential rhabdomyolsysis. Most of the recent studies in transplanted patients have, therefore, been carried out using relatively low doses of statins. This paradigm may change as more sites begin to use fewer lipid-targeted agents, e.g. tacrolimus. Statins are successful in reducing LDL values, and appear more potent potentially due to the consequences of medication use and/or discontinuation as described. Specifically, these agents include lovastatin, simvastatin, and pravastatin for lowering cholesterol in heart transplant recipients treated with cyclosporine and prednisone. Although mechanisms of action remain to be elucidated, the survival benefit demonstrated suggests the importance of prophylactic statin use in all transplant candidates.

LDL Lowering and Revascularization

The Atorvastatin versus Revascularization Treatment (AVERT) study provides intriguing data on the role of lipid lowering in the management of patients with mild coronary atherosclerosis. It is known that lipid lowering has been effective in the reduction of percutaneous revascularization rates. In the 4S trial, PTCA was reduced by 37% with aggressive lipid lowering ($p = 0.00001$). Studies of PTCA vs. standard therapy have failed to demonstrate a significant reduction in coronary events. It was therefore hypothesized that in a population with mild to moderate CAD under consideration for coronary revascularization via PTCA, that aggressive lipid lowering would provide a significant reduction in clinical events and improved outcomes.

The AVERT Trial randomized 341 patients with CAD (one lesion of greater than or equal to 50% stenosis), LDL-C greater than 115 mg/dL, left ventricular ejection fraction (LVEF) greater than 40% to either PTCA and standard care, or to medical management and aggressive lipid lowering with atrovastatin 80 mg/dL. Patients with left main or its equivalent of three-vessel CAD were excluded.

The AVERT trial showed a trend toward improved outcomes with medical therapy and aggressive lipid lowering compared with PTCA and standard medical care. There was a 13% ischemic event rate in individuals receiving atorvastatin vs. a 21% ischemic event rate in individuals randomized to PTCA. This represented a 36% reduction in events in the group treated with high-dose atorvastatin, although this did not represent a statistically significant difference ($p = 0.048$). In general, high-dose atorvastatin was well-tolerated with only a 2.4% incidence of AST or ALT abnormalities (greater than three times normal). The AVERT trial is a small, underpowered trial with a short follow-up time. It represents a highly selected population that may not have clinical relevance. It does, however, serve as an interesting hypothesis-generating trial that adds insights into the role of lipid lowering in patients undergoing revascularization and points to the potential therapeutic benefits in this subset.

Finally, the ongoing Myocardial Ischemia Reduction with Aggressive Cholesterol Lowering (MIRACL) trial will test the hypothesis that lipid lowering in unstable angina (USA) or non-Q-wave myocardial infarction (NQWMI) will reduce myocardial ischemia and recurrent events. This study will randomize 3000 patients with USA or NQWMI to atorvastatin 80 mg/d or placebo, beginning within 1–4 d of hospitalization and continuing for 16 wk of follow-up. The primary outcome measure is the time to occurrence of an ischemic event, defined as death, nonfatal MI, resuscitated cardiac arrest, or recurrent symptomatic myocardial ischemia with emergency rehospitalization. This study should define whether or not acute cholesterol lowering should play a role in patients with USA and MI and add to our understanding of the use of these agents acutely.

LIPID-LOWERING THERAPY AFTER CORONARY ARTERY BYPASS SURGERY

Atherosclerotic lesions develop at an accelerated rate in saphenous vein grafts (SVGs) compared with native coronary arteries, and thrombosis also contributes to occlusion. In a follow-up study of 82 patients 10 yr after coronary artery bypass surgery, subjects who demonstrated progression or inception of coronary artery narrowing had higher values of VLDL, LDL, and lower values for HDL, even though standard traditional risk factors such as cigarette use, blood pressure, and diabetes were equivalent (40). On multivariate analyses, the HDL value and the LDL-related apoB concentration were the best variables to predict who would progress. Subsequently, in a seminal work by Blankenhorn and colleagues *(41)* beneficial effects of cholesterol lowering on atherosclerosis in saphenous vein grafts in a randomized intervention trial in 162 men younger than 60 yr of age who took niacin and cholestipol or placebo for 2 yr was reported. Both LDL-C and the TG/HDL-C component of the lipid profile were profoundly improved. The post-CABG *(42)* study has furthered the findings of this original work, having been carried out over a longer period of time with more carefully defined measures of quantitative angiography, and a broader range of patients.

A total of 1351 patients were randomized, 92% of them were men with a mean age at entry of 61.5 yr. In addition to a step I diet, patients were randomly assigned to receive one of two different lipid lowering regimens: the "aggressive" treatment arm (targeting an LDL goal of 60–85 mg/dL) included treatment starting with lovastatin 40 mg/d, whereas the "moderate" treatment arm (targeting an LDL goal of 130–140 mg/dL) started with lovastatin 2.5 mg/d. Cholestyramine was added if it was required to meet goal.

The post-CABG study, in which patients were recruited who had undergone CABG 1 to 11 yr prior to randomization, was designed to evaluate whether aggressive lowering of LDL would be more effective than moderate lowering in reducing the progression of atherosclerotic lesions in SVGs. The trial was blinded to intensity of treatment. Male participants had at least two patent SVGs (at least one in women) and LDL levels of 130–175 mg/dL after diet therapy. The primary endpoint was significant worsening of the atherosclerosis (progression of ≥0.6 mm) over a 4.5-yr time period, and secondary endpoints including new occlusions, new lesions, and luminal narrowing.

A mean LDL level of 95 mg/dL was achieved in the aggressive arm and an 135 mg/dL LDL value in the moderate treatment arm. Analyses of the 1192 follow-up angiograms showed less progression of atherosclerosis in the SVGs of patients who underwent aggressive vs. moderate LDL-lowering therapy. A modified ratio estimate (MRE) statistic was used to calculate the mean percentage of grafts per patient showing progression (defined as a decrease in lumen diameter of at least 0.6 mm), which was the primary endpoint. The MRE statistic for the combined endpoint of progression or death was 27% in the aggressive group vs. 39% in the moderate treatment group ($p < 0.001$). New lesions occurred in 10% of the patients in the aggressive group and in 21% of the moderate group. Occlusion occurred in 6% of patients in the aggressive group and in 11% of patients in the moderate group. Low-dose warfarin treatment, one arm of the study, showed no statistically significant benefit over placebo in any of the angiographic or clinical measures.

Although the trial was not powered to detect differences in clinical events, the rate of revascularization procedures (repeat bypass surgery or angioplasty) was 6.5% in the aggressive cholesterol treatment group and 9.2% in the moderate treatment group ($p = 0.03$), a 29% reduction.

These results suggest at least one of two positions: a 35% LDL reduction is more advantageous than simply a 15% reduction, or that it is important to target LDL levels to less than 100 mg/dL. Whether the conclusion is one or both, aggressive cholesterol lowering in patients with SVGs can reduce the progression of atherosclerotic narrowing of grafts, occlusion of grafts, and the need for repeat coronary bypass surgery or balloon angioplasty. The post-CABG and Blankenhorn data strongly suggest use of LDL-lowering agents after these procedures.

CONCLUSION

Treatment of hypercholesterolemia with HMG CoA reductase inhibitors has revolutionized therapy for the prevention of CAD. New provocative trials have greatly expanded the role of statins in the primary and secondary prevention of CAD. Dramatic reductions in cardiovascular morbidity and mortality could be achieved with the implementation of preventive strategies including the aggressive use of statins in the management of patients at risk for CAD. Statins provide the clinician with powerful new agents to prevent and potentially reverse CAD.

A greater understanding of the pathophysiologic mechanisms leading to acute coronary syndromes as well as an elucidation of lipid metabolism has lead to the development of powerful lipid-lowering therapies. These agents have afforded clinicians the opportunity to arrest and potentially reverse CAD. New agents directed at defined metabolic pathways may offer attractive therapies for lipid lowering in select patient populations. Elucidating of the molecular mechanisms involved in lipoprotein metabolism and its relation to acute coronary syndromes will lead to improved therapies and potentially new classes of drugs for the targeted treatment of CAD.

REFERENCES

1. Simon LA. Interrelations of lipids and lipoproteins with coronary artery disease mortality in 19 countries. Am J Cardiol 1986;57:5–10.
2. Kannel WB, Castelli WD, Gordon T, McNamara PM. Serum cholesterol, lipoproteins and risk of coronary artery disease: The Framingham Study. Ann Intern Med 1971;74:1–12.
3. Kannel WB, Castelli WP, Gordon T. Serum cholesterol lipoproteins and risk of coronary heart disease. Ann Intern Med 1971;74:1–12.
4. Kannel WB. Lipids, diabetes, and coronary heart disease: insights from the Framingham Study. Am Heart J 1985;110:110–116.
5. Kannel WB, Neaton JD, Wentworth D, et al. Overall and coronary heart disease mortality rates in relation to major risk factors in 325,348 men screened for MRFIT. Am Heart J 1986;112:825–836.
6. Kannel WB. Cholesterol and risk of coronary heart disease and mortality in men. Clin Chem 1988; 341B:B53–B59.
7. 1997 Heart and Stroke Statistical Update. Dallas: American Heart Association, 1996.
8. Pfeffer M, Sacks F, Lemuel A, et al. Cholesterol and recurrent events: a secondary prevention trial for normolipidemic patients. Am J Cardiol 1995;76:98C–106C.
9. Scandinavian Simvastatin Survival Study Group. Randomised trial of cholesterol lowering in 4444 patients with coronary heart disease: the Scandinavian Simvastatin Survival Study (4S). Lancet 1994; 344:1383–1389.
10. Group SSSS. Baseline serum cholesterol and treatment effect in the Scandinavian Simvastatin Survival Study (4S). Lancet 1995;345:1274–1275.
11. Shepherd J, Cobbe SM, Ford I, et al. Prevention of coronary heart disease with pravastatin in men with hypercholesterolemia. N Engl J Med 1995;333:1301–1307.
12. Tonkin A. Management of the Long-Term Intervention with Pravastatin in Ischaemic Disease (LIPID) study after the Scandinavian Simvastatin Survival Study (4S). Am J Cardiol 1995;107C–112C.
13. Downs J, Beere P, Whitney E, et al. Design and rationale of the Air Force/Texas Coronary Atherosclerosis Prevention Study (AFCAPS/TexCAPS). Am J Cardiol 1997;80:287–293.
14. Expert Panel on Detection, Evaluation, and Treatment of High Blood Cholesterol in Adults. Summary of the second report of the National Cholesterol Education Program (NCEP) expert panel on detection, evaluation, and treatment of high blood cholesterol in adults (Adult Treatment Panel-II). JAMA 1993; 269:3015–3023.
15. Stafford R, Blumenthal D, Pasternak R. Variations in cholesterol management practices of U.S. physicians. J Am Coll Cardiol 1997;29:139–146.
16. MRFIT Research Group. Multiple risk factor changes and mortality results. JAMA 1982;248:1465–1477.

17. National Cholesterol Education Program Expert Panel. Summary of the second report of the National Cholesterol Education Program Expert Panel on detection, evaluation, and treatment of high blood cholesterol in adults (Adult Treatment Panel II). JAMA 1993;269:3015–3023.

18. Superko H. What can we learn about dense low density lipoprotein and lipoprotein particles from clinical trials? Curr Opin Lipidol 1996;7:363–368.

19. Family Study Committee for the Lipid Research Clinics Program. The collaborative Lipid Research Clinics Program Family Study. I. Study design and description of data. Am J Epidemiol 1984;119:931–943.

20. Family Study Committee for the Lipid Research Clinics Program Family Study. The collaborative Lipid Research Clinics Program Family Study. Bivariate path analysis of lipoprotein concentration. Genet Res 1983;42:117–135.

21. Lipid Research Clinics Program. The Lipid Research Clinics Coronary Primary Prevention Trial results. II. The relationship of reduction in incidence of coronary heart disease to cholesterol lowering. JAMA 1984;251:365–374.

22. Frick MH, Elo O, Haapa K, et al. Helsinki Heart Study. Primary-prevention trial with gemfibrozil in middle-age men with dyslipidemia. N Engl J Med 1987;317:1235–1245.

23. Manninen V, Elo MO, Frick MH, et al. Lipid alterations and decline in the incidence of coronary heart disease in the Helsinki Heart Study. JAMA 1988;260:641–651.

24. Pedersen T. Scandinavian Simvastatin Survival Study. AHA Scientific Sessions, 1997.

25. Pedersen TR, Kjekshus J, Pyorala K, et al. Effect of simvastatin on ischemic signs and symptoms in the Scandinavian simvastatin survival study (4S). Am J Cardiol 1998;81:333–335.

26. Crouse JR, Byington RP, Hoen HM, Furberg CD. Reductase inhibitor monotherapy and stroke prevention. Arch Intern Med 1997;157:1305–1310.

27. Hebert PR, Gaziano JM, Chan KS, Hennekens CH. Cholesterol lowering with statin drugs, risk of stroke, and total mortality. An overview of randomized trials. JAMA 1997;278:313–321.

28. Bucher HC, Griffith LE, Guyatt GH. Effect of HMGcoA reductase inhibitors on stroke. A meta-analysis of randomized, controlled trials. Ann Intern Med 1998;128:89–95.

29. Billingham ME. Cardiac transplant atherosclerosis. Transplant Proc 1987;19:19–25.

30. Gamba A, Mamprin F, Fiocchi R, et al. The risk of coronary artery disease after heart transplantation is increased in patients receiving low-dose cyclosporine, regardless of blood cyclosporine levels. Clin Cardiol 1997;20:767–772.

31. Vanhaecke J, Van Cleemput J, Van Lierde J, et al. Safety and efficacy of low dose simvastatin in cardiac transplant recipients treated with cyclosporine. Transplantation 1994;58:42–45.

32. PFCheung AK, De Vault GA Jr, Gregory MC. A prospective study on treatment of hypercholesterolemia with lovastatin in renal transplant patients receiving cyclosporine. J Am Soc Nephrol 1993;3:1884–1891.

33. Kuo PC, Kirshenbaum JM, Gordon J, et al. Lovastatin therapy for hypercholesterolemia in cardiac transplant recipients. Am J Cardiol 1989;64:631–635.

34. Ogawa N, Koyama I, Shibata T, et al. Pravastatin prevents the progression of accelerated coronary artery disease after heart transplantation in a rabbit model. Transplant Int 1996;9:S226–S229.

35. Kobashigawa JA, Murphy FL, Stevenson LW, et al. Low-dose lovastatin safely lowers cholesterol after cardiac transplantation. Circulation 1990;82:IV281–IV283.

36. Kobashigawa JA, Katznelson S, Laks H, et al. Effect of pravastatin on outcomes after cardiac transplantation. N Engl J Med 1995;333:621–627.

37. Wenke K, Meiser B, Thiery J, et al. Simvastatin reduces graft vessel disease and mortality after heart transplantation: a four-year randomized trial. Circulation 1997;96:1398–1402.

38. Vathsala A, Weinberg RB, Schoenberg L, et al. Lipid abnormalities in cyclosporine-prednisone-treated renal transplant recipients. Transplantation 1989;48:37–43.

39. Kasiske B, Tortorice K, Heim-Duthoy K, et al. The adverse impact of cyclosporine on serum lipids in renal transplant recipients. Am J Kidney Dis 1991;17:700–707.

40. Campeau L, Enjalbert M, Lesperance J, et al. The relation of risk factors to the development of atherosclerosis in saphenous-vein bypass grafts and the progression of disease in the native circulation. A study 10 years after aortocoronary bypass surgery. N Engl J Med 1984;311:1329–1332.

41. Blankenhorn DH, Nessim SA, Johnson RL, et al. Beneficial effects of combined colestipol-niacin therapy on coronary atherosclerosis and coronary venous bypass grafts. JAMA 1987;257:3233–3240.

42. The Post Coronary Artery Bypass Graft Trial Investigators. The effect of aggressive lowering of low-density lipoprotein cholesterol levels and low-dose anticoagulation on obstructive changes in saphenous-vein coronary-artery bypass grafts. N Engl J Med 1997;336:153–162.

43. Weekly Pharmacy Reports—"The Green Sheet," 1998;47:1.
44. Castelli WP, Garrison RJ, Wilson WF, et al. Incidence of coronary heart disease and lipoprtein choles-terol levels: the Framingham Study. JAMA 1986;256:2835–2838.
45. Family Study Committee for the Lipid Research Clinics Program. The collaborative Lipid Research Clinics Program Family Study. I. Study design and description of data. Am J Epidemiol 1984;119:931–943.
46. Family Study Committee for the Lipid Research Clinics Program Family Study. The collaborative Lipid Research Clinics Program Family Study. Bivariate path analysis of lipoprotein concentration. Genet Res 1983;42:117–135.
47. Lipid Research Clinics Program. The Lipid Research Clinics Coronary Primary Prevention Trial results. II. The relationship of reduction in incidence of coronary heart disease to cholesterol lowering. JAMA 1984;251:365–374.
48. Namboodiri KK, Green PP, Kaplan EB, et al. Family aggregation of high density lipoprotein choles-terol. Collaborative Lipid Research Clinics Program Family Study. Arteriosclerosis 1983;3:616–626.
49. Assmann G, Schulte H. Role of triglycerides in coronary artery disease: lessons from the Prospective Cardiovascular Muenster Study. Am J Cardiol 1992;70:10H–13H.
50. Assman G, Schulte H. Obesity and hyperlipidemia: results from the Prospective Cardiovascular and Muenster (PROCAM) study. In: Bjorntorp P, Brodoff B, eds. Obesity. JB Lippincott, New York, 1992, pp. 502–511.
50a.Fontbonne A, Charles MA, Thilbult N, et al. Hyperinsulinemia as a predictor of coronary heart disease mortality in a healthy population: The Paris Prospective Study, 15 year follow-up. Diabetologia 1991; 34:356–361.
51. Manninen V, Tenkanen L, Koskinen P, Huttunen JK, et al. Joint effects of serum triglycerides and LDL cholesterol and HDL cholesterol concentrations on coronary heart disease risk in the Helskinki Heart Study—implications for treatment. Circulation 1992;85:37–45.
52. National Center for Health Statistics. National Health and Nutrition Examination Survey (III) (data collected 1991–1994) 1994.
53. Jukema JW, Bruschke AV, van Boven AJ, et al. Effects of lipid lowering by pravastatin on progression and regression of coronary artery disease in symptomatic men with normal to moderately elevated serum cholesterol levels. The Regression Growth Evaluation Statin Study (REGRESS). Circulation 1995;15: 91(10):2528–2540.
54. Grundy S. Lipids, nutrition, and CAD. In: Fuster V, Ross R, Topol EJ, eds. Atherosclerosis and Coro-nary Artery Disease. Lippincott-Raven, Philadelphia, 1996, pp. 2v.
55. Levine GN, Keaney JF Jr, Vita JA. Cholesterol reduction in cardiovascular disease. Clinical benefits and possible mechanisms. N Engl J Med 1995;332(8):512–521.
56. Bezafibrate Infarction Prevention Study. Secondary prevention by rasing HDL cholesterol and reducing triglyceride in patients with coronary artery disease. Circulation 2000, July 4;102:21–27.
57. Rubins HB, Robins SJ, Collins D, et al. Gemfibrozil for the secondary prevention of coronary heart disease in men with low levels of high-density lipoprotein cholesterol. Veterans Affairs High-Density Lipoprotein Cholesterol Intervention Trial Study Group. N Engl J Med 1999;341:410–418.

6

Management of Hypertension
Implications of JNC VI

Donald G. Vidt, MD

CONTENTS

INTRODUCTION

Hypertension awareness, treatment, and control rates have increased progressively over the past three decades. Data from the third National Health and Nutrition Examination Survey conducted from 1988–1991 indicate that the percentage of those aware of hypertension had increased to 73% *(1)*. Of those aware, 55% were being treated, and 29% were controlled to a blood pressure of <140/90 mmHg. This information was considered in the preparation of the fifth report of the Joint National Committee on the Prevention, Detection, Evaluation, and Treatment of High Blood Pressure (JNC V) published in 1993 *(2)*. Unfortunately, these awareness, treatment, and control rates have lessened since publication of the JNC V report (Table 1). Declines in age-adjusted mortality rates for stroke and coronary heart disease appear to be leveling in recent years *(3)*. In fact, the age-adjusted stroke rate actually increased in the United States in 1993 for the first time in more than two decades. The incidence of end-stage renal disease (ESRD), for which high blood pressure is the second most common antecedent, continues to increase, as does the prevalence of congestive heart failure wherein the majority of patients also have antecedent hypertension *(4,5)*.

From: *Contemporary Cardiology: Preventive Cardiology:*
Strategies for the Prevention and Treatment of Coronary Artery Disease
Edited by: J. Foody © Humana Press Inc., Totowa, NJ

Table 1
Trends in the Awareness, Treatment, and Control
of High Blood Pressure in Adults: United States, 1976–1994[a]

	NHANES II (1976–1980) (%)	NHANES III (Phase 1) 1988–1991 (%)	NHANES III (Phase 2) 1991–1994 (%)
Awareness	51.0	73.0	68.4
Treated	31.0	55.0	53.6
Controlled[b]	10.0	29.0	27.4

[a]Adults age 18–74 yr with SBP ≥ 140 mmHg or DBP ≥ 90 mmHg or taking anti-hypertensive medication.

[b]SBP <140 mmHg and DBP < 90 mmHg.

Source: Adapted from Burt V, Cutler JA, Higgins M, et al. Trends in the prevalence, awareness, treatment, and control of hypertension in the adult US population: Data from the health examination surveys, 1960 to 1991. Hypertension 1995;25:305-313. Unpublished data from the National Center for Health Statistics, 1997 (NHANES III, Phase 2).

The sixth JNC report (JNC VI), published in 1997, has undertaken the formulation of clinical policy and therapeutic recommendations based wherever possible on sound, evidence-based data from randomized, controlled clinical trials (6). A large body of clinical studies has also been reviewed and summarized in an effort to provide clinicians and other health care providers with potential advantages and/or cautions regarding selection of anti-hypertensive therapy. It is recognized that a multitude of comorbid conditions will impact the clinician's selection of initial or subsequent agents for the treatment of hypertension.

The current classification of blood pressure (BP) for adults 18 yr and older is seen in Table 2. This classification was first offered in 1993 in the JNC V report. It was modified slightly in the preparation of JNC VI with the deletion of stage 4 hypertension in view of the relatively small numbers of patients in this category, and the belief that all patients with a BP of 180 mmHg systolic and/or 110 mmHg diastolic or greater warrant immediate evaluation and consideration for appropriate therapy.

RISK STRATIFICATION

JNC VI has taken an aggressive approach to the initial assessment of the hypertensive patient together with subsequent recommendations for aggressive treatment not only in patients with sustained systolic and/or diastolic hypertension, but also in selected patients with high–normal BP. The presence or absence of target-organ damage, clinical heart disease, or other cardiovascular risk factors such as smoking, dyslipidemia, and diabetes mellitus, independently modify the risk for subsequent cardiovascular disease in the hypertensive patient (Table 3).

In the course of the initial evaluation, health providers are encouraged to identify and note the presence or absence of any evidence of target-organ damage or other major risk factors. This information is readily available in the course of a thorough history and physical examination together with a few selected laboratory studies suggested for evaluation of new hypertensive patients.

Table 2
Classification of Blood Pressure for Adults Age 18 Years and Older[a]

Category	Systolic (mmHg)		Diastolic (mmHg)
Optimal[b]	<120	and	<80
Normal	<130	and	<85
High-normal	130–139	or	85–89
Hypertension			
Stage 1[c]	140–159	or	90–99
Stage 2[c]	160–179	or	100–109
Stage 3[c]	≥180	or	≥110

[a]Not taking antihypertensive drugs and not acutely ill. When systolic and diastolic blood pressures fall into different categories, the higher category should be selected to classify the individual's blood pressure status. For example, 160/92 mmHg should be classified as stage 2 hypertension, and 174/120 mmHg should be classified as stage 3 hypertension. Isolated systolic hypertension is defined as SBP ≥ 140 mmHg and DBP < 90 mmHg and staged appropriately (e.g., 170/82 mmHg is defined as stage 2 isolated systolic hypertension).

In addition to classifying stages of hypertension on the basis of average blood pressure levels, clinicians should specify presence or absence of target organ disease and additional risk factors. This specificity is important for risk classification and treatment (see Table 4).

[b]Optimal blood pressure with respect to cardiovascular risk is <120/80 mmHg. However, unusually low readings should be evaluated for clinical significance.

[c]Based on the average of two or more readings taken at each of two or more visits after initial screening.

Adapted from ref. 6.

Table 3
Components for Cardiovascular Risk Stratification in Patients with Hypertension[a]

Major risk factors	Target organ damage/clinical cardiovascular disease
Smoking	Heart disease
Dyslipidemia	Left ventricular hypertrophy
Diabetes mellitus	Angina/prior myocardial infarction
Age older than 60 yr	Prior coronary revascularization
Gender (men and postmenopausal women)	Heart failure
Family history of cardiovascular disease:	Stroke or transient ischemic attack
women under age 65 or men under age 55	Nephropathy
	Peripheral arterial disease
	Retinopathy

[a]See Table 4.
From ref. 6.

Based on this assessment of target-organ damage and/or other risk factors, and the level of BP, each patient's risk group can be determined as illustrated in Table 4. Patients with hypertension are stratified into risk groups for subsequent therapeutic decisions. This stratification is similar to those recently recommended by the World Health Organization (WHO) Expert Committee on Hypertension Control (7). Obesity and physical inactivity are also predictors of cardiovascular risk, but are of less significance in the selection of antihypertensive drugs than those considered.

Table 4
Risk Stratification and Treatment[a]

Blood Pressure Stages (mmHg)	Risk group		
	A	B	C
	No risk factors No TOD/CCD[b] (see Table 3)	At least one risk factor, not including diabetes mellitus No TOD/CCD[b] (see Table 3)	TOD/CCD[b] and/or diabetes, with or without other risk factors (see Table 3)
High-normal (130–139/85–89)	Lifestyle modification	Lifestyle modification	Drug therapy[c]
Stage 1 (140–159/90–99)	Lifestyle modification (up to 12 mo)	Lifestyle modification[d] (up to 6 mo)	Drug therapy
Stage 2 and 3 (≥160/≥100)	Drug therapy	Drug therapy	Drug therapy

For example: A patient with diabetes and a BP of 142/94 mmHg plus left ventricular hypertrophy should be classified as having stage 1 hypertension with TOD (LVH) and with another major risk factor (diabetes). This patient would be categorized as stage 1, risk group C, and recommended for immediate initiation of pharmacologic treatment.

[a]Lifestyle modification should be adjunctive therapy for all patients recommended for pharmacologic therapy.
[b]TOD/CCD = target organ disease/clinical cardiovascular disease.
[c]For those with heart failure or renal disease or those with diabetes mellitus
[d]For patients with multiple risk factors, clinicians should consider drugs as initial therapy plus lifestyle modifications.
Adapted from ref. 6.

Risk Groups

A: Patients with high-normal BP or stage 1, 2, or 3 hypertension who exhibit no evidence of clinical cardiovascular disease, target-organ damage, or other risk factors.
B: No clinical cardiovascular disease or target-organ damage, but who have one or more of the risk factors shown in Table 4, but not diabetes mellitus.
C: Patients with clinical manifestations of cardiovascular disease, or target-organ damage, or diabetes mellitus with or without other risk factors.

This classification system should provide a reasonably simple matrix for clinicians to make a determination regarding the early institution of drug therapy, and/or the appropriateness of continued lifestyle modification.

AWARENESS OF THE TOTAL CARDIOVASCULAR RISK PROFILE

In addition to identifying risk strata for individual patients, the current risk stratification can help facilitate an assessment of overall cardiovascular risk for each patient. Tables, formulas, and computer software programs can help calculate total cardiovascular risk by means of data from epidemiologic studies. Aggressive treatment of hypertension, when indicated, could be accomplished as part of the strategy for reducing total cardiovascular risk.

PREVENTION
AND LIFESTYLE MODIFICATIONS

The goal of prevention and management of hypertension is to reduce morbidity and mortality by the least intrusive means possible. Primary prevention provides an opportunity to interrupt and prevent the long-term costs of treating hypertension and its complications. An effective, populationwide strategy to prevent BP rise with age and to reduce BP levels, could have a significant effect on overall cardiovascular morbidity and mortality (8).

A major portion of cardiovascular disease morbidity and mortality occurs in people whose BP is above the optimal level (120/80 mmHg) but not yet in the hypertensive range (≥140/90 mmHg) (9). Aggressive lifestyle modification has been suggested as a means of achieving modest BP reductions in patients with high–normal or stage 1 hypertension in an effort to reduce their overall cardiovascular risk. Unfortunately, most patients with established hypertension do not achieve significant lifestyle changes, do not take medication, or do not take a sufficient amount of medication to achieve control of BP. Even carefully controlled clinical trials of nonpharmacologic therapy have been associated with only modest reductions in BP, despite protocols that would be difficult to achieve in a population-based strategy aimed at prevention (10,11).

Of interest is a newly designed trial of hypertension prevention (TROPHY) to be initiated in 1999. This clinical trial will randomize patients to receive an angiotensin II antagonist (candesartan) or placebo therapy for 24 mo followed by an additional 24 mo of placebo-only treatment and observation to determine if a period of drug therapy in patients with high–normal BP can prevent the progression of BP to hypertensive levels over time. It has been noted from multiple hypertension treatment trials that discontinuation of medication is not necessarily associated with immediate resumption of hypertensive BP levels. Why some patients do not become hypertensive again after a period of pharmacologic therapy is not well understood, but these observations will undoubtedly be the subject of significant future clinical studies.

A Role for Lifestyle Modification

Lifestyle modifications have proven effective in lowering BP in some patients, and can reduce other cardiovascular risk factors at little cost and minimal risk. Patients should be strongly encouraged to initiate and maintain lifestyle modifications because even when not adequate for controlling hypertension, they may still help lower the dosage of antihypertensive medications required.

Wherever possible, JNC VI has used evidence-based data to offer appropriate recommendations for clinicians. Special considerations in the selection of therapy include demographic characteristics, concomitant diseases that may be beneficially or adversely affected by the chosen agent, quality of life, cost, and use of other drugs that may lead to drug interactions.

INITIAL DRUG THERAPY

Joint National Committee reports have traditionally offered a simplified algorithm to assist clinicians in the decision process relative to initial and subsequent antihypertensive therapy. Figure 1 shows the algorithm presented in JNC VI. As with previous reports, lifestyle modifications should be continued because these interventions may have an

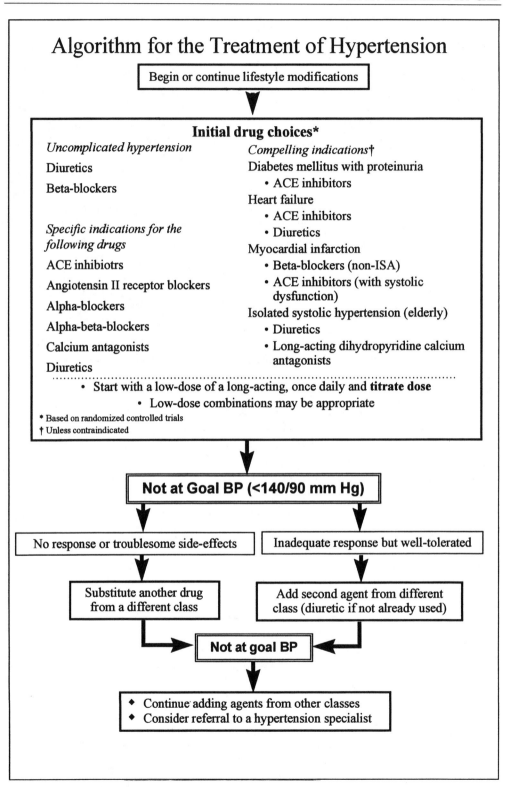

Algorithm for the Treatment of Hypertension

Begin or continue lifestyle modifications

Initial drug choices*

Uncomplicated hypertension

Diuretics

Beta-blockers

Specific indications for the following drugs

ACE inhibiotrs

Angiotensin II receptor blockers

Alpha-blockers

Alpha-beta-blockers

Calcium antagonists

Diuretics

Compelling indications†

Diabetes mellitus with proteinuria
  • ACE inhibitors
Heart failure
  • ACE inhibitors
  • Diuretics
Myocardial infarction
  • Beta-blockers (non-ISA)
  • ACE inhibitors (with systolic dysfunction)
Isolated systolic hypertension (elderly)
  • Diuretics
  • Long-acting dihydropyridine calcium antagonists

  • Start with a low-dose of a long-acting, once daily and **titrate dose**
  • Low-dose combinations may be appropriate

* Based on randomized controlled trials
† Unless contraindicated

Not at Goal BP (<140/90 mm Hg)

No response or troublesome side-effects

Inadequate response but well-tolerated

Substitute another drug from a different class

Add second agent from different class (diuretic if not already used)

Not at goal BP

  ♦ Continue adding agents from other classes
  ♦ Consider referral to a hypertension specialist

Fig. 1. Algorithm for the treatment of hypertension. Adapted from ref. *6*.

additive effect with subsequent pharmacologic therapy in selected patients. Initiation of treatment with one of the newer fixed combinations of antihypertensive drugs may be appropriate for initial therapy, and this topic is addressed later in this section.

As in earlier JNC reports, JNC VI has again recommended diuretics or beta-adrenergic blockers for initial therapy because of proven benefits in the reduction of morbidity and mortality demonstrated in randomized clinical trials *(12–14)*. These classes of agents are preferred for initial drug therapy if there are no contraindications to their use in the individual patient and if there are not special indications for selection of an alternative agent. Alternative drug classes include the calcium antagonists, angiotensin-converting enzyme (ACE) inhibitors, alpha-$_1$ receptor blockers, the alpha–beta blocker labetalol, and the newer angiotensin II receptor antagonists. Extensive clinical trials comparing diuretics and/or beta blockers with the newer classes of agents are currently underway, but except for long-acting dihydropyridine calcium antagonists, results are not yet available to influence treatment recommendations.

For selected patients with high-normal BP, and patients with stage 1 or 2 hypertension, therapy will usually be initiated with a single drug. Therapy should be started with a low dose of long-acting, once-daily agent, and dosage should be titrated with care to minimize the risk of adverse effects. Selected low-dose combinations of long-acting agents may be appropriate for initial as well as subsequent therapy. If there is no response to the initial drug, or if troublesome adverse effects develop, a drug from a different class may be substituted. On the other hand, if a partial response is observed and the agent is well tolerated, the initial drug should be continued with the addition of a second agent from a different class. If a diuretic was not selected as the first drug, it will often be useful as a second step agent because its addition usually enhances the effects of other drugs. If addition of a second agent produces satisfactory BP control, an attempt to withdraw the first agent may be considered, as monotherapy with all classes of available agents can provide adequate BP control for approximately half of patients treated. If BP is not controlled with a combination of agents, the clinician may continue adding agents from other classes or may consider referral to a hypertension specialist.

Combining antihypertensive drugs with different modes of action will often allow smaller doses of individual agents to be used to achieve control and minimize the potential for dose-dependent adverse effects. Prior JNC reports and most clinical treatment recommendations discourage the use of fixed-combination agents, especially for initial therapy. Many of the early fixed-drug combinations were inappropriate from the standpoint of dosages offered or the duration of action of individual drug components. Some of the earliest fixed-combinations included agents with very short duration of action in the same tablet with agents of long duration of action. Newer fixed combinations offer the advantage of more appropriate dosages together with prolonged duration of action for each component to facilitate once-daily dosing. Newer combinations have also taken advantage of clinical data supporting the additive effects of individual components when used together (Table 5).

For all patients with stage 2 or 3 hypertension, pharmacologic therapy is indicated even in the absence of evident target organ damage or other major risk factors. Evidence supports the aggressive treatment for all hypertensive patients. Although the initial goal of achieving BP below 140/90 mmHg remains appropriate, available and emerging data support further reductions in BP with due regard for cardiovascular function, especially in older patients. If a BP of 120/80 mmHg is indeed representative of "normal" BP in our

Table 5
Combination Drugs for Hypertension[a]

Drug	Trade name
Beta-adrenergic blockers and diuretics	
Atenolol 50 or 100 mg/chlorthalidone 25 mg	Tenoretic
Bisoprolol 2.5, 5, or 10 mg/hydrochlorothiazide 6.25 mg	Ziac[b]
Nadolol 40 or 80 mg/bendroflumethiazide 5 mg	Corzide
Propranolol (extended release) 80, 120, or 160 mg/ hydrochlorothiazide 50 mg	Inderide LA
ACE inhibitors and diuretics	
Benazepril 5, 10, or 20 mg/hydrochlorothiazide 6.25, 12.5, or 25 mg	Lotensin HCT
Enalapril 5 or 10 mg/hydrochlorothiazide 12.5 or 25 mg	Vaseretic
Lisinopril 10 or 20 mg/hydrochlorothiazide 12.5 or 25 mg	Prinzide; Zestoretic
Angiotensin II receptor antagonist and diuretic	
Losartan 50 mg/hydrochlorothiazide 12.5 mg	Hyzaar
Valsartan 80 or 100 mg/hydrochlorothiazide 12.5 mg	Diovan HCT
Calcium-channel antagonists and ACE inhibitors	
Amlodipine 2.5 or 5 mg/benazepril 10 or 20 mg	Lotrel
Diltiazem 180 mg/enalapril 5 mg	Teczem
Verapamil (extended release) 180 or 240 mg/trandolapril 1, 2, or 4 mg	Tarka
Felodipine 5 mg/enalapril 5 mg	Lexxel
Other combinations	
Triamterene 37.5, 50, or 75 mg/hydrochlorothiazide 25 or 50 mg	Dyazide, Maxide
Spironolactone 25 or 50 mg/hydrochlorothiazide 25 or 50 mg	Aldactazide
Amiloride 5 mg/hydrochlorothiazide 50 mg	Modiuetic

[a]These agents are appropriate for once-daily adminstration.
[b]Approved for initial therapy.
Adapted from ref. 6.

society, and with the disappointing results to date in control efforts in hypertension, it would seem time to revise BP goals downward. There is now convincing evidence to support a treatment goal of 130/85 mmHg for hypertensive patients with congestive heart failure (CHF), and those with both diabetic and nondiabetic renal disease. In the latter group of patients with renal disease and proteinuria exceeding 1 g/d, there is evidence suggesting that preservation of renal function can be achieved by aggressively lowering BP to levels of 125/75 mmHg.

COMPELLING INDICATIONS FOR SELECTED AGENTS

There are four comorbid conditions for which sound, evidence-based data strongly support treatment with selected classes of agents, if not as initial therapy, then certainly added to the treatment regimen.

Congestive Heart Failure

Data from the Framingham Heart Study continue to implicate hypertension as the major cause of left ventricular failure in the United States (15). Treatment trials have demonstrated that drug therapy of hypertension improves myocardial function and prevents or markedly reduces the incidence of heart failure and cardiovascular mortality (13).

Data from more than 30 controlled clinical trials have shown that ACE inhibitors, when used alone or in conjunction with digitalis and/or diuretics, effectively reduce subsequent hospitalizations and/or mortality by a substantial 35% *(16)*. Unfortunately, many potential heart failure candidates for ACE inhibitors are not receiving these agents and when they are administered, they are often given in insufficient doses to derive the full benefits.

The recent Assessment of Treatment with Lisinopril And Survival (ATLAS) trial has demonstrated that high-dose lisinopril (30–35 mg/d) when compared to low doses (2–2.5 mg/d) reduced mortality and hospitalizations without significantly increasing adverse reactions to the drug *(17)*. From a safety standpoint, the side effect of cough—the leading reason for discontinuing ACE inhibitor therapy—was less common in the high-dose group, and total withdrawals from the study were numerically higher in the low-dose than the high-dose group.

The role of beta-adrenergic blockers in heart failure presents a therapeutic paradox. These agents are well recognized for their negative inotropic properties and have long been considered contraindicated in heart failure despite limited early observations suggesting benefit in congestive cardiomyopathy. More recently, clinical trials with metoprolol and newer vasodilating beta blockers, carvedilol and bisoprolol, have shown these agents to be beneficial in heart failure when added to standard therapy, including ACE inhibitors *(18–20)*.

The rationale for use of beta blockers is related to potentially deleterious effects of overactivation of the sympathetic nervous system in heart failure. Sympathetic nervous support for the failing heart derives in part from direct chronotropic and inotropic stimulation and partly from vasoconstrictor effects on the peripheral circulation *(21)*. However, prolonged and excessive direct effects of noradrenaline stimulation leads to downregulation of cardiac beta receptors, therefore desensitizing the heart to sympathetic stimulation. Excessive vasoconstriction also contributes to increasing afterload, which places an additional burden on an already compromised left ventricle. Beta-adrenergic blockade upregulates myocardial beta receptors, the myocardium becomes more responsive to graded doses of beta agonists such as noradrenaline, thus improving ventricular function and myocardial contractility *(22)*. Beta-adrenergic blockade added to conventional therapy of heart failure, including ACE inhibitors and diuretics, reduces all-cause mortality by about 30–32%. It is likely that newer guidelines will recommend consideration for beta-adrenergic blockers in addition to ACE inhibitors in the management of patients with CHF.

In patients in whom ACE inhibitors are contraindicated or not tolerated, clinical studies would suggest that the newer angiotensin II antagonists may provide an important therapeutic option. The vasodilator combination of hydralazine and isosorbide dinitrate can also be effective in selected patients *(23)*.

Hypertension and Renal Parenchymal Disease

Hypertension can result from any form of renal disease that reduces the number of functioning nephrons, leading to decreased clearance function together with sodium and water retention. Follow-up studies on large numbers of men screened for the Multiple Risk Factor Intervention Trial (MRFIT) and of male veterans have provided conclusive evidence of a relationship between BP and end-stage renal disease (ESRD) *(24,25)*. Hypertensive nephrosclerosis is among the most common causes of renal failure, second only to diabetes, particularly in African-American males.

The most important action to slow progression of renal failure is to lower BP to a goal of 130/85 mmHg or lower. In most patients with significant renal insufficiency, multiple antihypertensive drugs will be required *(26)*. In patients with proteinuria >1 g/24 h, lowering BP to <125/75 mmHg may have special benefit *(27)*. Reducing dietary sodium to levels lower than that recommended for complicated hypertension may provide additive effects to drug therapy selected *(28)*. ACE inhibitors would appear to be of particular benefit in patients with insulin-requiring diabetes mellitus and nephropathy, in those with proteinuria >1 g/24 h, and with renal insufficiency *(29–31)*. In patients with serum creatinine above 2.5 mg/dL, ACE inhibitors must be used with special caution.

Thiazide diuretics tend to be ineffective in patients with serum creatinine above 2.5 mg/ dL where loop diuretics may be required, often in large doses. The combination of a loop diuretic with a long-acting thiazide diuretic such as metolazone may be effective in patients resistant to a loop diuretic alone. Potassium-sparing diuretics should be avoided in patients with renal insufficiency, and must be used with caution in patients receiving ACE inhibitors or angiotensin II receptor blockers. The latter class of agents can be particularly appropriate for patients in whom ACE inhibitor side effects or intolerance have developed.

In patients with insulin-requiring diabetes mellitus and diabetic nephropathy, ACE inhibitors reduce proteinuria and provide substantial renal protection, reducing by 50% the rate of progression of renal insufficiency to ESRD or mortality *(29)*. Similar renoprotective effects of long-term ACE inhibitor therapy has been demonstrated in non-insulin-requiring (type 2) diabetes mellitus *(32)*.

ACE inhibitors, calcium antagonists, alpha blockers, and diuretics in low doses are preferred agents in the hypertensive diabetic because of fewer adverse effects on glucose metabolism, lipid profiles, and renal function *(33,34)*. Although beta-adrenergic blockers have been generally considered inappropriate in patients with diabetes, the major caution relates to insulin-requiring diabetes with a propensity for insulin-induced hypoglycemic attacks. In this situation, beta blockers can impair glycogenolysis and delay blood glucose recovery. Despite the adverse effects of beta blockers on peripheral blood flow, prolonging of hypoglycemia, and the masking of hypoglycemic symptoms, patients treated with beta blockers experience beneficial reductions of coronary heart disease (CHD) and total cardiovascular events *(35)*.

Postmyocardial Infarction

Following myocardial infarction, beta-adrenergic blockers without intrinsic sympathomimetic activity have proven to reduce the risk for subsequent myocardial infarction or sudden cardiac death. As the only class of cardiovascular drugs approved for cardioprotection, they have sadly been underutilized in recent years by clinicians. A recent report on the effect of beta blockade on mortality among high-risk and low-risk patients following myocardial infarction revealed that only 34% of patients received beta blockers *(36)*. The percentage was even lower among the very elderly, African-Americans, and patients with the lowest ejection fractions, heart failure, chronic obstructive pulmonary disease, elevated serum creatinine concentrations, or type I diabetes mellitus *(37)*. In patients with myocardial infarction and no other complications, treatment with beta-adrenergic blockers was associated with a 40% reduction in mortality. Surprisingly, similar benefits were observed in patients with associated diabetes mellitus, asthma, and obstructive pulmonary disease, as well as those with decreased ejection fraction and renal insufficiency.

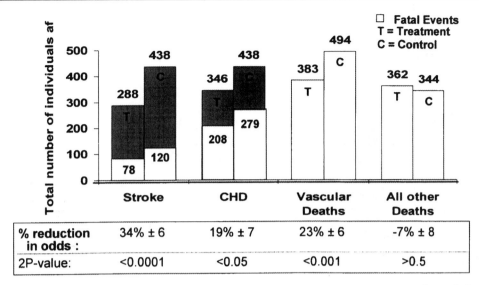

Fig. 2. Five randomized trials of antihypertensive treatment in the elderly; 12,473 patients, follow-up 5 yr.

Isolated Systolic Hypertension

Among older persons, systolic blood pressure (SBP) is a better predictor of events (CHD, cardiovascular disease, heart failure, stroke, end-stage renal disease, and all-cause mortality) than is diastolic blood pressure (DBP) *(38)*. This is particularly relevant to older individuals, in whom the most prevalent form of hypertension is isolated systolic hypertension (ISH) (SBP 140 mmHg or greater, DBP <90 mmHg). Those with stage 1 ISH are at increased cardiovascular risk, but the benefits of treatment in this group have not yet been demonstrated in a controlled clinical trial *(39)*.

Large clinical trials of patients >60 yr have demonstrated the beneficial effects of BP lowering on stroke, CHD, cardiovascular disease, heart failure, and mortality *(16)*. Older patients will often respond to modest salt restriction and weight loss. Keep in mind that the starting dose of antihypertensive drugs in older patients should be about half of that used in younger patients. Thiazide diuretics or beta blockers in combination with thiazide diuretics are recommended because of their established efficacy in reducing mortality and morbidity in older hypertensive patients (Fig. 2) *(14,40)*. These were all diuretic-and/or beta-blocker-based clinical trials, one of which was the Systolic Hypertension in the Elderly (SHEP) trial. As noted from these combined trials, reductions in stroke and CHD events are comparable to those observed in younger patients treated with the same basic regimen.

In 1997, the SYST–EUR trial reported the results of a placebo-controlled trial in 4695 men and women in which the treatment arm was a long-acting dihydropyridine calcium antagonist (nitrendipine). Although designed for a 4-yr follow-up, the study was discontinued after only 2 yr of median follow-up in view of the significance of the results already observed *(41)*. A 42% reduction in total strokes had been observed, together with a marginally significant 26% decline in all cardiac endpoints.

The results of SYST–EUR when compared to those seen in the SHEP trial were strikingly similar except for the apparent benefits on the prevalence of congestive heart failure

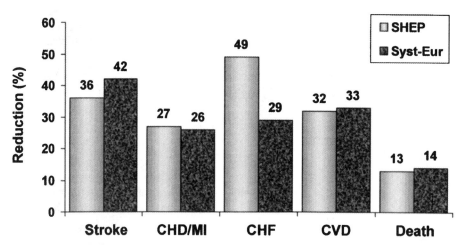

Fig. 3. The results of SYST–EUR when compared to those seen in the SHEP trial were strikingly similar except for the apparent benefits on the prevalence of CHF.

(Fig. 3). However, the duration of follow-up for SYST–EUR was much shorter than for SHEP, which may have had a marked impact on this adverse event. Diuretics and long-acting dihydropyridine calcium antagonists have been considered preferred agents in the initial management of ISH.

The goal of treatment in older patients should be the same as in younger patients, i.e., to achieve a BP <140/90 mmHg. An interim SBP goal of 160 mmHg may be appropriate in older patients with marked systolic elevations in BP. Any reduction in SBP appears to confer benefit, and the closer to normal, the greater the benefit. Additional recommendations regarding hypertension and older patients can be found in the Report by the National High Blood Pressure Education Working Group on Hypertension in the Elderly *(38)*.

OTHER SPECIAL CONSIDERATIONS FOR SELECTED AGENTS

The compelling indications for use of a specific class of agents in the foregoing comorbid conditions are supported by randomized trial data. There are many other comorbid conditions in hypertensive patients that may be beneficially or adversely affected by the antihypertensive agent selected. Practice experience, and/or clinical trials in some cases, and serendipitous observations in others have enabled a compilation of comorbid conditions in which selected antihypertensive agents may prove particularly favorable (Table 6), and others where unfavorable or undesirable effects may be observed (Table 7). It may make particular sense to choose an antihypertensive agent that not only controls or lowers BP but also has a favorable effect on associated comorbid conditions (the "two for one" hypothesis). Similarly, physicians must be alert to those conditions in which the selection of specific agents may beneficially effect BP, but may also have undesirable effects.

Demographics

Age and gender do not appear to be major factors in determining responsiveness to various agents *(42)*. We do know that African-Americans appear to be more responsive to monotherapy with diuretics and calcium antagonists than to beta blockers or ACE inhibitors *(43)*. However, differences in efficacy can usually be overcome by rigid sodium restriction or the addition of a diuretic to the regimen.

Table 6
Considerations for Individualizing Antihypertensive Therapy[a]

Favorable effects on comorbid conditions

Angina	Beta blockers, calcium antagonists
Atrial tachycardia, atrial fibrillation	Beta blockers Calcium antagonists (non-dihydropyridine)
Cyclosporine-induced hypertension	Calcium antagonists
Dyslipidemia	Alpha blockers
Essential tremor	Beta blockers (noncardioselective)
Hyperthyroidism	Beta blockers
Migraine	Beta blockers (noncardioselective), calcium antagonists nondihydropyridine)
Osteoporosis	Thiazide diuretics
Preoperative hypertension	Beta blockers
Prostatism (BPH)	Alpha blockers
Renal insufficiency (caution with renovascular hypertension)	ACE inhibitors, loop diuretics
Type II diabetic nephropathy	ACE inhibitors, calcium antagonists (nondihydropyridine)

[a]Conditions and drugs are listed in alphabetic order.

Table 7
Considerations for Individualizing Antihypertensive Therapy[a]

Unfavorable effects on comorbid conditions

Bronchospastic disease	Beta blockers[b]
Bradycardia, 2° or 3° heart block	Beta blockers[b], calcium antagonists (nondihydropyridine)[b]
Depression	Beta blockers, central alpha-agonists, reserpine[b]
Dyslipidemia	Beta blockers (non-ISA), diuretics (high-dose)
Gout	Diuretics
Heart failure	Beta blockers (except carvedilol), calcium antagonists
Liver disease	Labetalol[b], methyldopa[b]
Peripheral vascular disease	Beta blockers
Pregnancy	ACE inhibitors[b], A-II receptor blockers[b]
Renal insufficiency	Potassium-sparing agents
Renovascular disease	ACE inhibitors, A-II receptor blockers
Type 1 and 2 diabetes mellitus	Beta blockers[b], high-dose diuretics[b]

[a]Conditions and drugs are listed in alphabetic order
[b]May be used with special monitoring, unless contraindicated.

Quality of Life

Although antihypertensive agents are not free of adverse effects, careful selection, and appropriate drug titration can achieve suitable control of BP and maintain or even improve the overall quality of life of the treated hypertensive patient *(12)*.

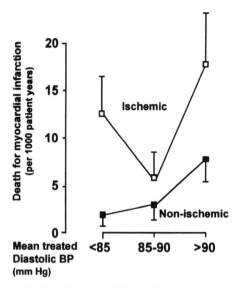

Fig. 4. Mortality rate from MI related to treated BP, 902 points on atenolol for 6.1 yr. In the original report by Cruickshank, a "J-curve" relationship had been observed between DBP and death from myocardial infarction. From Cruiksank et al. Lancet 1987;1:581. © The Lancet Ltd., 1987.

Cost Considerations

The cost of therapy may present a barrier to treatment in selected patients. Among anti-hypertensive agents, generic formulations are generally acceptable. If newer agents prove equally effective to older drugs, cost should be considered in choosing the appropriate agent; if they prove to be more effective, then cost should be a secondary consideration. Remember that the overall cost of medication may be reduced by using fixed-combination tablets, and by using long-acting preparations that can be administered once daily.

TREATING TO LOWER BP GOALS

The issue of how far BP should be lowered to achieve greatest benefit, in terms of reduced cardiovascular morbidity and mortality, has generated significant scientific debate. In the original report by Cruickshank, a "J-curve" relationship was observed between DBP and death from myocardial infarction (MI) (Fig. 4) *(44)*. A number of other studies have also reported similar relationships between the lower BP in response to therapy and increased coronary mortality *(45–47)*. It would appear however, that these relationships with DBP are limited to patients with a clinical history of ischemic CAD. It is also of particular interest that no J-curve relationship was observed in Cruickshank's original observations when SBP was controlled to levels below 130 mmHg. Similarly, neither the SHEP or the SYST–EUR trials demonstrated a J-shaped relationship of SBP reduction to the risk of stroke or all-cause mortality for either the placebo or the treatment groups combined.

Although a J-curve relationship probably does exist in treated subgroups of participants with clinical heart disease, the absolute safe level of DBP reduction is still unclear. Fletcher and Bullpitt have presented a very challenging review in which they summarize studies relating the level of BP during treating of hypertension to the risk of stroke and CHD in an effort to identify the optimal BP levels to be achieved by treatment *(48)*. They concluded that it was reasonable to lower DBP to below 85 mmHg, giving maximal benefit of reducing of stroke and myocardial infarction, as compared to those having DBPs greater than 100 mmHg. They also recommended that SBP be lowered to below 125 mmHg, as there was no indication that doing so had any adverse effects.

The real issue is not whether the relation between achieved BP and cardiovascular events is J-shaped, but rather whether there are additional risks or benefits in lowering BP in hypertensive patients to fully normotensive levels, i.e., below 130/85 mmHg.

An earlier post hoc analysis of the Medical Research Council Mild Hypertension Trial showed that the relation between nontreatment of BP and stroke flattens below SBP values of 135–140 mmHg, and DBP values of 85–90 mmHg, but with no evidence of increased events at lower values (49). Similar results were suggested from a post hoc analysis of the International Prospective Primary Prevention Study in Hypertensives (IPPSH) (50).

JNC VI has also summarized randomized clinical trial data in support of treating BPs to normal levels (below 130/85 mmHg) in hypertensive individuals with selected comorbid conditions including CHF, diabetic nephropathy, and nondiabetic progressive renal failure.

The recently reported, randomized Hypertension Optimal Treatment (HOT) trial was designed to assess the association between target DBP (i.e., ≤ 90 mmHg, ≤ 85 mmHg, or ≤ 80 mmHg) and major cardiovascular events (i.e., nonfatal MI, nonfatal stroke, and cardiovascular death) (51). It was also designed to test the association between major cardiovascular events and DBP achieved during treatment, and to find out whether the addition of low doses of aspirin to antihypertensive treatment further reduced the rate of major cardiovascular events.

This study group consisted of 18,799 patients age 50–80 yr, randomized and followed for an average of 3.8 yr. The lowest incidence of major cardiovascular events occurred at a mean achieved DBP of 82.6 mmHg. The lowest risk of cardiovascular mortality occurred at 86.5 mmHg. Further reductions below these BP levels were safe. In patients with diabetes mellitus there was a 51% reduction in major cardiovascular events in the target group below 80 mmHg, compared with the target group below 90 mmHg ($p = 0.005$). Aspirin reduced major cardiovascular events by 15% and all MIs by 36% with no effect on stroke. There were 7 fatal bleeds in the aspirin group, and 8 in the placebo group, and 126 versus 79 major bleeds in the two groups.

The HOT study showed that intensive lowering of BP in patients with hypertension was associated with a lower rate of cardiovascular events, the benefits shown by lowering the diastolic pressure down to 82.6 mmHg. Lower BPs down to 120 mmHg systolic or 70 mmHg diastolic demonstrated no further benefit, but did not cause any significant additional risk. On the whole, the rate of cardiovascular events observed during treatment initiated with the calcium antagonist, felodipine, was much lower than that seen in previous prospective studies, with diuretic- or beta-blocker-initiated treatment, probably because of the pronounced lowering of BP in this study (52). In fact, 86% of the patients had final DBPs below 90 mmHg, whereas fully 55% of patients randomized to the below 80 mmHg target achieved and maintained this goal BP. Finally, a small dose of aspirin in well-controlled hypertensives reduced the risk of acute MI without exaggerating the risk of cerebral bleeding. The use of aspirin with antihypertensive therapy can, therefore, be recommended, providing that BP is well controlled and the risk of gastrointestinal and nasal bleeding carefully assessed.

The HOT trial was an international trial performed in the outpatient setting. Why is it that 86% of patients in this clinical trial were maintained at a diastolic pressure below 90 mmHg, whereas NHANES III survey data suggest that only 27% of treated hypertensives across the United States are controlled at BPs below 140/90 mmHg? The evidence continues to mount that lower goal BPs are associated with lower risks of cardiovascular morbidity and mortality. As opposed to a forced titration study such as the HOT trial, physicians in the practice setting are far less aggressive in managing the hypertensive population. Despite the fact that only 30–60% of hypertensives will be controlled with any single drug, even at maximal doses, physicians persist in their intentions to control hypertension in patients with single-drug therapy. Surveys have suggested further that in the majority of uncontrolled hypertensives, there is reticence to increase dosages or add agents to the regimen in an effort to achieve lower BP goals (Cardiomonitor Study [unpublished], Taylor Nelson Healthcare, Epson, Surrey, England, 1992–1997). This is particularly true in systolic hypertension. International survey information suggests that there is little inclination to treat SBPs even to levels of <160 mmHg.

SUMMARY

JNC VI took an assertive approach to assessment of the hypertensive patient, together with subsequent recommendations for aggressive treatment not only in patients with sustained systolic and or diastolic hypertension, but also in selected patients identified with high–normal BP. Wherever possible, sound, evidence-based data from randomized, controlled trials was used in making therapeutic recommendations.

The shortfall in hypertension control efforts is a major concern, because only 1 in 4 hypertensive individuals in the United States are currently controlled to below target BPs (140/90 mmHg). Efforts are being made to change physicians' attitudes toward treatment that have led to this significant shortfall in control. We must translate the evidence in support of aggressive treatment to lower BP into an action plan that will encourage all providers to take a more vigorous role in their treatment strategies. Current guidelines for lower treatment goals are soundly grounded in research data. Recently reported clinical trials fully support these treatment recommendations. Treating BP to at least normal levels would seem appropriate for most patients as we enter the new millennium.

REFERENCES

1. Burt VL, Cutler JA, Higgins M, et al. Trends in the prevalence, awareness, treatment, and control of hypertension in the adult US population. Data from the health examination surveys, 1960 to 1991 [published erratum appears in Hypertension 1996 May;27(5):1192]. Hypertension 1995;26:60–69.
2. Joint National Committee. The fifth report of the Joint National Committee on Detection, Evaluation, and Treatment of High Blood Pressure (JNCV). Arch Intern Med 1993;153:154–183.
3. Data calculated for the National Heart, Lung, and Blood Institute staff, J. Cutler, Principal Investigator, January 1997.
4. United States Renal Data System 1997 Annual Data Report. Bethesda, MD: US Department of Health and Human Services, National Institute of Diabetes and Digestive and Kidney Disease.
5. Levy D, Larson MG, Vasan RS, et al. The progression from hypertension to congestive heart failure. JAMA 1996;275:1557–1562.
6. Joint National Committee. The sixth report of the Joint National Committee on the Prevention, Detection, Evaluation and Treatment of High Blood Pressure (JNC VI). Arch Intern Med 1997;157:2413–2446.
7. WHO Expert Committee on Hypertension Control. Hypertension Control: Report of a WHO Expert Committee. WHO Technical Report Series, no. 862, 1996, Geneva, Switzerland, World Health Organization.
8. National High Blood Pressure Education Program (NHBPEP) Working Group. National High Blood Pressure Education Program Working Group report on primary prevention of hypertension. Arch Intern Med 1993;153:186–208.
9. Burt VL, Whelton P, Roccella EJ, et al. Prevalence of hypertension in the US adult population. Results from the Third National Health and Nutrition Examination Survey, 1988-1991. Hypertension 1995;25:305–313.

10. The Trials of Hypertension Prevention Collaborative Research Group. Effects of weight loss and sodium reduction intervention on blood pressure and hypertension incidence in overweight people with high-normal blood pressure. The Trials of Hypertension Prevention, Phase II (TOHP II). Arch Intern Med 1997;157:657–667.

11. Appel LJ, Moore TJ, Obarzanek E, et al. A clinical trial of the effects of dietary patterns on blood pressure. DASH Collaborative Research Group. N Engl J Med 1997;336:1117–1124.

12. Psaty BM, Smith NL, Siscovick DS, et al. Health outcomes associated with antihypertensive therapies used as first-line agents. A systematic review and meta-analysis. JAMA 1997;277:739–745.

13. Moser M, Hebert PR. Prevention of disease progression, left ventricular hypertrophy and congestive heart failure in hypertension treatment trials. J Am Coll Cardiol 1996;27:1214–1218.

14. MacMahon S, Rodgers A. The effects of blood pressure reduction in older patients: An overview of five randomized controlled trials in elderly hypertensives. Clin Exp Hypertens 1993;15:967–978.

15. Vasan RS. The role of hypertension in the pathogenesis of heart failure. A clinical mechanistic overview. Arch Intern Med 1996;156:1789–1796.

16. Garg R, Yusuf S, for the Collaborative Group on ACE Inhibitor Trials. Overview of randomized trials of angiotensin-converting enzyme inhibitors on mortality and morbidity in patients with heart failure. JAMA 1995;273:1450–1456.

17. Massie BM, Cleland JG, Armstrong PW, et al. Regional differences in the characteristics and treatment of patients participating in an international heart failure trial. The Assessment of Treatment with Lisino-pril and Survival (ATLAS) Trial Investigators. J Cardiac Fail 1998;4:3–8.

18. Packer M, Bristow MR, Cohn JN, et al. The effect of carvedilol on morbidity and mortality in patients with chronic heart failure. U.S. Carvedilol Heart Failure Study Group. N Engl J Med 1996;334:1349–1355.

19. Australia/New Zealand Heart Failure Research Collaborative Group. Randomised, placebo-controlled trial of carvedilol in patients with congestive heart failure due to ischaemic heart disease. Lancet 1997; 349:375–380.

20. Hjalmarson A, Waagstein F. The role of beta-blockers in the treatment of cardiomyopathy and ischaemic heart failure. Drugs 1994;47(Suppl 4):31–39.

21. Eichhorn EJ. The paradox of beta-adrenergic blockade for the management of congestive heart failure. Am J Med 1994;92:527–538.

22. van Zwieten PA. The rationale for the use of beta-blockers in the treatment of congestive heart failure. Am J Geriatr Cardiol 1992;(August):57–61.

23. Cohn JN, Archibald DG, Ziesche S, et al. Effect of vasodilator therapy on mortality in chronic congestive heart failure. Results of a Veterans Administration Cooperative Study. N Engl J Med 1986;314:1547–1552.

24. Perry HM Jr, Miller JP, Fornoff JR, et al. Early predictors of 15-year end-stage renal disease in hyper-tensive patients. Hypertension 1995;25(4 Pt 1):587–594.

25. Klag MJ, Whelton PK, Randall BL, et al. Blood pressure and end-stage renal disease in men. N Engl J Med 1996;334:13–18.

26. Klag MJ, Whelton PK, Randall BL, et al. End-stage renal disease in African-American and white men. 16-year MRFIT findings. JAMA 1997;277:1293–1298.

27. Lazarus JM, Bourgoignie JJ, Buckalew VM, et al. Achievement and safety of a low blood pressure goal in chronic renal disease. The Modification of Diet in Renal Disease Study Group. Hypertension 1997;29: 641–650.

28. National High Blood Pressure Education Program (NHBPEP) Working Group. 1995 Update of the Working Group Reports on Chronic Renal Failure and Renovascular Hypertension. Arch Intern Med 1996;156:1938–1947.

29. Lewis EJ, Hunsicker LG, Bain RP, Rohde RD, for the Collaborative Study Group. The effect of angio-tensin-converting-enzyme inhibition on diabetic nephropathy. N Engl J Med 1993;329:1456–1462.

30. Klahr S, Levey AS, Beck GJ, et al. The effects of dietary protein restriction and blood-pressure control on the progression of chronic renal disease. N Engl J Med 1994;330:877–884.

31. Maschio G, Alberti D, Janin G, et al. Effect of the angiotensin-converting-enzyme inhibitor benazepril on the progression of chronic renal insufficiency. The Angiotensin-Converting-Enzyme Inhibition in Progressive Renal Insufficiency Study Group. N Engl J Med 1996;334:939–945.

32. Ravid M, Lang R, Rachmani R, Lishner M. Long-term renoprotective effect of angiotensin-converting enzyme inhibition in non-insulin-dependent diabetes mellitus. A 7-year follow-up study. Arch Intern Med 1996;156:286–289.

33. American Diabetes Association. American Diabetes Association: clinical practice recommendations 1997. Diabetes Care 1997;20(Suppl 1):S1–S70.

34. National High Blood Pressure Education Program (NHBPEP) Working Group. National High Blood Pressure Education Program Working Group report on hypertension in diabetes. Hypertension 1994;23: 145–158.

35. Curb JD, Pressel SL, Cutler JA, et al, for the Systolic Hypertension in the Elderly Program Cooperative Research Group. Effect of diuretic-based antihypertensive treatment on cardiovascular disease risk in older diabetic patients with isolated systolic hypertension. JAMA 1996;276:1886–1892.

36. Hennekens CH, Albert CM, Godfried SL, et al. Adjunctive drug therapy of acute myocardial infarction —evidence from clinical trials. N Engl J Med 1996;335:1660–1667.

37. Gottlieb SS, McCarter RJ, Vogel RA. Effect of beta-blockade on mortality among high-risk and low-risk patients after myocardial infarction. N Engl J Med 1998;339:489–497.

38. National High Blood Pressure Education Program (NHBPEP) Working Group, Roccella EJ, Coordinator. National High Blood Pressure Education Program Working Group Report on hypertension in the elderly. Hypertension 1994;23:275–285.

39. Sagie A, Larson MG, Levy D. The natural history of borderline isolated systolic hypertension. N Engl J Med 1993;329:1912–1917.

40. SHEP Cooperative Research Group. Prevention of stroke by antihypertensive drug treatment in older persons with isolated systolic hypertension: final results of the Systolic Hypertension in the Elderly Program (SHEP). JAMA 1991;265:3255–3264.

41. Staessen J, Fagard R, Thijs LG, et al. Morbidity and mortality in the placebo-controlled European trial on isolated systolic hypertension in the elderly. Lancet 1997;350:757–764.

42. Gueyffier F, Boutitie F, Boissel JP, et al. Effect of antihypertensive drug treatment on cardiovascular outcomes in women and men. A meta-analysis of individual patient data from randomized, controlled trials. The INDANA Investigators. Ann Intern Med 1997;126:761–767.

43. Materson BJ, Reda DJ, Cushman WC, et al. Department of Veterans Affairs Cooperative Study Group on Antihypertensive Agents: Single-drug therapy for hypertension in men: A comparison of six anti-hypertensive agents with placebo [published correction appears in N Engl J Med 1994;330:1689]. N Engl J Med 1993;328:914–921.

44. Cruickshank JM, Thorpe JM, Zacharias FJ. Benefits and potential harm of lowering high blood pressure. Lancet 1987;1:581–584.

45. Cooper SP, Hardy RJ, Labarthe DR, et al. The relation between degree of blood pressure reduction and mortality among hypertensives in the Hypertension Detection and Follow-Up Program. Am J Epidemiol 1988;127:387–403.

46. Waller PC, Isles CG, Lever AF, et al. Does therapeutic reduction of diastolic blood pressure cause death from coronary heart disease? J Hum Hypertens 1988;2:7–10.

47. Fletcher AE, Beevers DG, Bulpitt CJ, et al. The relationship between a low treated blood pressure and IHD mortality: A report from the DHSS Hypertension Care Computing Project (DHCCP). J Hum Hypertens 1988;2:11–15.

48. Fletcher AE, Bulpitt CJ. How far should blood pressure be lowered? N Engl J Med 1992;326:251–254.

49. Medical Research Council Working Party. The MRC Mild Hypertension Trial: Some subgroup results. In: Strasser T, Gauten D, eds. Mild Hypertension: From Drug Trials to Practice. Raven Press, New York, 1987, pp. 9–20.

50. The IPPPSH Collaborative Group. Cardiovascular risk and risk factors in a randomized trial of treatment based on the beta-blocker oxprenolol: the International Prospective Primary Prevention Study in Hypertension (IPPPSH). J Hypertens 1985;3:379–392.

51. Hansson L, Zanchetti A, Carruthers SG, et al. Effects of intensive blood-pressure lowering and low-dose aspirin in patients with hypertension: principal results of the Hypertension Optimal Treatment (HOT) randomised trial. Lancet 1998;351:1755–1762.

52. Vidt DG, Pohl MA. Aggressive blood pressure lowering is safe, but benefit is still hard to prove. Cleve Clin J Med 1999;66:105–111.

7

Diabetes Mellitus, Hyperinsulinemia, and Coronary Artery Disease

Byron J. Hoogwerf, MD

CONTENTS

INTRODUCTION

Diabetes mellitus is associated with an increased risk for coronary heart disease (CHD), less favorable outcomes from intervention procedures, and CHD-related mortality *(1,8,9,31,34,39,47,51,52,65,69–71,75,76,78,91,93,95,99,102,105,115,116,124, 125,127,128,130,140,147,148)* (Table 1). This observation is true for both types 1 and 2 diabetes as well as for secondary forms of diabetes. Hyperglycemia by itself likely contributes to this risk; however, diabetes mellitus—especially type 2—and impaired glucose tolerance are associated with a number of other CHD risk factors, which include dyslipidemia, hypertension, central obesity and a procoagulant state *(26,28,30,33,36,42, 43,75–77,85,106,109,110,116,126,141,145,146,149)*. These risk factors are associated with insulin resistance and have also been described as the "metabolic syndrome" for CHD. There are accumulating data to suggest that these abnormalities may be associated with endothelial cell dysfunction. In addition, the concepts of protein glycation, as well as oxidized lipoproteins as possible mechanisms for CHD have been proposed *(14, 19,92,129)*.

Accumulating intervention trial data to suggest that intervention on these CHD risk factors may reduce the risk for CHD in diabetic patients. CHD risk reduction with lipid lowering has been reported from analysis of diabetic patients in several intervention trials *(32, 44,50,57,66,83,89a,90,94,107,117,118,121,123)*. Observational data and intervention

From: *Contemporary Cardiology: Preventive Cardiology:*
Strategies for the Prevention and Treatment of Coronary Artery Disease
Edited by: J. Foody © Humana Press Inc., Totowa, NJ

Table 1
Summary of Relationships Between DM and CHD Risk

CHD risk in DM
    2–5-fold increased risk for CHD
    2–5-fold increased risk for CHD death
    Increased risk for morbidity and mortality following MI
    Increased risk for adverse outcomes following PTCA/stent/CABG
Clustering of CHD risk factors in DM
    Traditional risk factors
        Dyslipidemia
        Increased TGs
        Decreased HDL-C
        Small dense LDL
        Hypertension
        Central obesity
    Nontraditional risk factors
        Hyperinsulinemia
        Procoagulant profile
           Increased platelet aggregation
           Increased PAI-1
           Increased fibrinogen
        Proteinuria
        Glycation of proteins
        Oxidation of lipoproteins

trials have shown a relationship between the level of hyperglycemia and atherosclerotic disease risk *(39,49,84,89,102,106,134,137,138)*. CHD risk reduction from the management of hypertension *(59,73,132,133)* and use of antiplatelet regimens *(9,21,36)* can be inferred from other studies in diabetic patients. Finally, independent effects of and angiotensin-converting enzyme (ACE) inhibitor therapy and lack of benefit from vitamin E in diabetic patients have been reported *(60–64)*.

This chapter summarizes the observational studies showing the relationship between glucose and CHD risk, the intervention trial data assessing reduction in glucose, lipids and blood pressure on CHD risk, review of treatment strategies for these common risk variables, and a summary of outcomes following myocardial infarction and intervention therapy in diabetic patients.

RELATIONSHIP OF GLUCOSE TOLERANCE AND CHD

Diabetes Mellitus

Diabetes mellitus (DM) is associated with a doubling of CHD risk *(47,75,76,105,128, 140,143a)*. In women the risk may increase as much fivefold. Several prospective observational studies have confirmed these risk relationships. The Framingham Study has demonstrated an overall doubling of CHD risks in men and shown that in women with diabetes, that CHD risk is comparable to that of age-matched male counterparts. Furthermore, this study has shown that in the presence of other CHD risk factors (smoking, hypercholesterolemia, hypertension, left ventricular hypertrophy), diabetes still contributes to CHD risk *(75,76,143a)* (Fig. 1). The Multiple Risk Factor Intervention Trial (MRFIT) has evaluated more than 300,000 screenees. The presence of diabetes in these men tripled

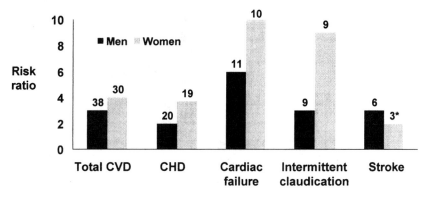

P<0.001 for all values except *P<0.05.

Fig. 1. Framingham Heart Study 30-yr follow-up: Age-adjusted annual risk of vascular disease end points in patients with diabetes (ages 35–64). From Wilson PWF, Kannel WB. In: Hyperglycemia, Diabetes and Vascular Disease. Ruderman N, et al., eds. Oxford, 1992, pp. 21–29 *(143a).*

the risk for subsequent CHD events and CHD deaths *(128).* This relationship held true even when there is adjustment for other CHD risk factors.

Several observational cohort studies have looked at the relationship between baseline glycemic control and atherosclerotic risk. The Wisconsin Epidemiologic Study of Diabetic Retinopathy (WESDR) used baseline hemoglobin A_{1c} as a predictor of subsequent CHD events in the three diabetes subgroups (≤30 yr old on insulin; >30 yr old on insulin; 30 yr old not on insulin). Each of these subgroups carries a progressive increase in CHD events across quartiles of baseline hemoglobin A_{1c} *(102).* More recently, Scandinavian studies have demonstrated that less than glucose values in diabetic patients may predict the risk for stroke or cause mortality *(87,89).*

Therefore, the *presence* of hyperglycemia as well as the *degree* of hyperglycemia and the presence of other CHD risk factors are associated with an increased risk for CHD events in diabetic patients.

Impaired Glucose Tolerance

Impaired glucose tolerance has been defined either in terms of fasting glucose values of ≤126 mg/dL (previously less than 140 mg/dL, greater than 110 mg/dL). Other definitions also included a 30–90 min plasma glucose value greater than 200 with a 2-h blood glucose value of between 140 and 200 mg/dL 2 h following a 75-g glucose challenge. Subjects with impaired glucose tolerance are also at increased risk for CHD. A number of studies have now demonstrated that impaired glucose tolerance is associated with central (or visceral) obesity, hypertension, and dyslipidemia. The dyslipidemia is further characterized as one in which there is an elevation of total triglyceride (TG), reduction in high-density lipoprotein cholesterol (HDL-C), and increased concentrations of small dense low-density lipoprotein cholesterol (LDL-C) *(28,112,126,136,145).* Clustering of such risk factors may be greater in women *(145).*

Normal Glucose Concentration

Recent data to suggest that CHD risk may be associated with increasing glucose concentrations *(12,24,49,127),* even in the normal range (≤110 mg/dL). These studies have

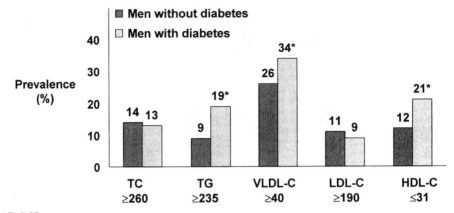

*P<0.05.
LRC approximate 90th percentile age- and sex-matched values, except for
HDL-C (10th percentile).

Fig. 2. Abnormal lipid levels in men with type 2 diabetes. Adapted from Garg A, Grundy SM. Diabetes Care 1990;13:153–169.

not uniformly adjusted for the other more traditional CHD risk factors, although some data suggest that there is an increased risk for clustering of other CHD risk factors with high/normal glucose concentrations.

CORONARY HEART DISEASE RISK FACTORS ASSOCIATED WITH GLUCOSE INTOLERANCE

Traditional

DYSLIPIDEMIA

The dyslipidemia of diabetes has been characterized in a number of studies. Typically, diabetic patients have higher mean TG concentrations, lower HDL-C concentrations, and LDL-C concentrations that are comparable to a nondiabetic population (Figs. 2 and 3). However, LDL composition is altered with higher concentrations of small dense LDL. This is the more atherogenic moiety and may be more susceptible to oxidation (*see* subheading "Glycation and Glycoxidation of Proteins," p. 122). Increased TG concentrations may be the result of increased production of very-low-density lipoprotein (VLDL) (perhaps related to the hyperglycemia) as well as diminished clearance of TG concentrations. Hydrolysis of TGs via capillary lipoprotein lipase (LPL) may be impaired. LPL is an insulin-sensitive enzyme. Therefore, either insulinopenia or insulin resistance contribute to diminished clearance of TGs.

HYPERTENSION

Both type 1 and type 2 diabetic patients have an increased risk for hypertension. In type 1 diabetes, this is almost always associated with evidence of diabetic nephropathy (in the early stages with evidence of microalbuminuria). Hypertension in type 2 diabetes occurs independently of clinical evidence of diabetic nephropathy. The mechanism for hypertension is not entirely established. Some evidence suggests that hyperinsulinemia may be associated with salt retention or increased sympathetic tone. Both mechanisms have been invoked as contributors to hypertension associated with diabetes.

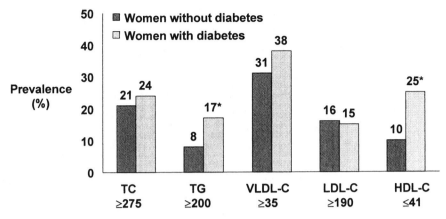

*P<0.05.
LRC approximate 90th percentile age- and sex-matched values, except for
HDL-C (10th percentile).

Fig. 3. Abnormal lipid levels in women with type 2 diabetes. Adapted from Garg A, Grundy SM. Diabetes Care 1990;13:153–169.

OBESITY

Increased body weight is associated with diabetes. Several observational studies have demonstrated that central obesity or an increased waist-to-hip ratio (more recently, simply a waist circumference) is associated with an increased risk for diabetes as well as associated CHD risk factors. Central obesity is associated with hyperinsulinemia and insulin resistance. Visceral fat (more than abdominal subcutaneous fat) is associated with diabetes, hyperinsulinemia, and the other risk factors for CHD. The mechanism by which obesity may contribute to CHD risk is uncertain. Visceral fat may increase delivery of free fatty acids to the liver. Visceral fat may be associated with cytokine production, which contributes to endothelial cell dysfunction.

SMOKING

Smoking has long been known to be a risk for CAD. There are now data to suggest smoking increases the risk for insulin resistance in type 2 diabetes and impaired glucose tolerance. The mechanism by which this occurs is not yet established.

Nontraditional CHD Risk Factors

There are other risk factors that may be associated with diabetes and impaired glucose tolerance that, in turn, may be associated with an increased risk of CAD.

HYPERINSULINEMIA

Hyperinsulinemia, especially when associated with central obesity, is associated with increased CHD risk in several observational studies *(3,13,33,34,42,43,55,77,87,106,109, 110,112,114,116,119,126,131,136,141,149)*. In many of these studies, hyperinsulinemia is associated with traditional risk factors. Hyperinsulinemia appeared to be additive to risks associated with lipid abnormalities including increased LDL-C and lipoprotein B. Hyperinsulinemia is associated with increased plasminogen activator inhibitor 1 (PAI-1). Insulin is also associated with tissue growth, suggesting that it may contribute to such things as smooth muscle proliferation that may be important in the atherosclerotic process. However, it is not yet clear whether insulin (or perhaps proinsulin) is itself atherogenic or whether this increased risk for CHD is a result of the other factors.

EXOGENOUS HYPERINSULINEMIA

Diabetic patients who are taking insulin are also at increased risk for CHD events. Insulin has been in proposed as the culprit. These studies cannot consistently take into account the duration of diabetes, however. Since one third to one half of people in the United States who have diabetes are unaware of the diagnosis, adjusting for the duration of the disease is difficult. Furthermore, the accumulating evidence that type 2 diabetes is characterized not only by insulin resistance but by declining beta cell function suggests that all patients with type 2 diabetes have had the disease long enough to exhibit beta cell failure.

PROTEINURIA

There is increased in attention to proteinuria, renal failure, and associated dyslipidemia as risk factors for CAD in patients with diabetes *(58,79,97,135)*. Whether proteinuria again simply marks for duration of diabetes or reflects loss of vascular integrity in general (both microvascular and macrovascular disease) is not that clear. In the face of proteinuria, the rate of progression to end-stage renal disease can be slowed by aggressive blood pressure management, especially with the use of ACE inhibitors, as well as improved glycemic control. Since both of these interventions may have beneficial effect on CHD risks, whether reduction in proteinuria has independent benefit on CHD risk is not yet established.

INCREASED PROCOAGULANT STATE

Diabetes mellitus is associated with an increased risk for atherothrombosis, probably as a result of increased platelet aggregation, increased fibrinogen, and elevated PAI-1 levels *(26,75,85,98,146)*. How much these variables affect the risk for initial CHD events, the increased risk for recurrent myocardial infarction (following first MI), and worse outcomes following revascularization procedures is not yet established.

GLYCATION AND GLYCOXIDATION OF PROTEINS (*SEE* CHAPTER 3)

Oxidized lipoproteins *(15,20,92,129)* have several features that suggest that they may increase the risk for the development of atherosclerotic plaque including increased foam-cell formation, cytotoxicity to endothelial cells, and increased smooth muscle formation. Two features of diabetes may increase the risk for oxidation. Glycated lipoproteins appear to have increased susceptibility to oxidation leading to the term "glycoxidation." In addition, small dense LDL is also more susceptible to oxidation. Therefore, both hyperglycemia and presence of increased concentrations of small dense LDL suggest that if lipoprotein oxidation is important in the atherosclerotic process, it may contribute to the increased risks seen in diabetic patients.

INTERVENTION TRIALS OF CHD
RISK REDUCTION IN DIABETES MELLITUS

Glycemic Control

Five major randomized trials looking glycemic control and complications in type 2 diabetes mellitus have been reported. The Japanese study of Ohkkubo and colleagues was designed to look at microvascular complications *(103)*. The four of intervention trials that have addressed relationships between glycemic control and CHD risk reduction deserve comment. The University Group Diabetes Program (UGDP) was the first major, randomized clinical trial designed to compare the effects of placebo and four different treatment rooms (tolbutamide, phenformin, insulin with variable dose strategy, and insulin with standard or "fixed" dose strategy) on CHD risk reduction *(81)*. In retrospect, the UGDP probably was underpowered to test the hypothesis. Furthermore, the well-known results were confounded by the observation that the tolbutamide group had an increased number of coronary events and mortality. The trial could not demonstrate any reduction in CHD risks with the insulin therapies. Conversely, it did not show any adverse effect of insulin therapy. The VA trial was a pilot study that assessed intensive glucose control in 75 diabetic men compared to conventional control in a similar group (control). Although an incremental difference in hemoglobin A_{1c} of 2% was met (this was the intent of the pilot), the trial could not show clear differences between treatment groups for coronary events *(2,4)*. Although a greater number of events were reported in the intensively controlled group, when this was adjusted for pre-existing coronary disease, there were no statistically significant differences. The DIGAMI Study (Diabetic Patients with Acute Myocardial Infarction) studied patients with diabetes who had a myocardial infarction. Patients were randomized to intensified glucose control both in the immediate postinfarction state as well as for a period of time after the infarction (compared to a conventional post-MI approach). The risk for subsequent MIs was reduced in the more intensively treated group *(96)*. Whether this is the result of more intensive follow-up or whether the postinfarct period will actually predict a reduction in CHD risk as a result of glucose lowering again, cannot be addressed by this study. Finally, the United Kingdom Prospective Diabetic Study (UKPDS) reported a 16% reduction in risk for atherosclerotic events in patients who were more intensively treated *(134,137–139)*. This did not quite achieve statistical significance ($p = 0.052$). There were no clear differences among the oral agent and insulin treatment arms.

Lipid Lowering (Tables 2 and 3)

Nine large ($n \geq 1350$ subjects) randomized trials of cholesterol lowering demonstrate benefits of cholesterol lowering *(17,32,44,50,57,66,83,89a,90,94,107,111,117,118,123)*. Seven of these trials included diabetic patients in their design *(32,44,90,107,117,118, 121)*. Four of the trials have reported the results in the diabetic patients separately from the main trial *(17,50,57,66,83,111)*. Benefits of LDL-C reduction in diabetic patients can be determined from the main results report in two of the studies *(32,94)*. Each study has demonstrated reductions in CHD events as a result of interventions that resulted in reductions of LDL-C/non-HDL-C and/or increases of HDL-C. In these studies, diabetic subjects have usually had higher risk for events in both the placebo and treatment (gemfibrozil or statin ± bile acid sequestrant) arms. However, the incremental reduction in risk is the same or greater in the diabetic subjects. Details of studies that reported on diabetic patients are provided as follows.

In the Helsinki Heart Study *(44,83)* data on 135 diabetic subjects were reported. Diabetic subjects on placebo had a higher 5-yr incidence of CHD death and MI (10.5%) than for the other subjects in the placebo group (7.4%). On gemfibrozil the incidence of CHD and MI in diabetic subjects was 3.4%, which was comparable to other subjects on gemfibrozil (3.3%). The net result was that there was a greater reduction in the risk for CHD

Table 2
Major Lipid-Lowering Trials and Diabetic Subsets

Trial name	Abbreviation	Refs.	Medication(s)	N	Median or mean follow-up (yr)	Lipid changes	Endpoints	% Reduction in events	Diabetic subjects—n
Primary prevention									
Lipid Research Clinics Primary Prevention Trial	LRC-CPPT	89a	Questran	3906	7.4	LDL-C decr. 12%	Nonfatal MI, death from CHD	19	None
Helsinki Heart Study	HHS	44,83	Gemfibrozil	4081	5	non-HDL-C decr. 14% LDL-C decr. 11% TG decr. 35% HDL-C incr. 11%	CHD events	34	135
West of Scotland Coronary Prevention Trial	WOSCOPS	123	Pravastatin	6595	4.9	LDL-C decr. 26%	Nonfatal MI, death from CHD	31	76
Air Force/Texas Coronary Atherosclerosis Prevention Study	AFSCAPS/TexCAPS	32	Lovastatin	6505	5.2	LDL-C decr. 25%, HDL-C incr. 6%	Fatal or nonfatal MI, unstable angina, sudden cardiac death	37	155/239[a]
Secondary prevention									
Scandinavian Study of Simvistatin	4S	57,111,121	Simvistatin	4444	5.4	LDL-C decr. 34% HDL-C incr. 8% TG decr. 9%	All-cause mortality Fatal or nonfatal, definite or probable MI	30	202[b] 483[b]
Post Coronary Artery Bypass Graft Trial	Post-CABG	17,66,107	Lovastatin (and questran)	1351	4.3	Two LDL-C targets	Composite[c]		116
Cholesterol and Recurrent Events	CARE	50,118	Pravastatin	4159	5	LDL-C decr. 28% HDL-C incr. 5% TG decr. 14%	Nonfatal MI, death from CHD	24	586
Long-Term Intevention with Pravastatin in Ischaemic Disease	LIPID	90	Pravastatin	9014	6.1	LDL-C decr. 27% apoB decr. 19% TG decr. 13% HDL-C incr. 4%	CHD death	24	777
Veterans Affairs Cooperative Studies Program High-Density Lipoprotein Cholesterol Intervention Trial	VA-HIT	117	Gemfibrozil	2531	5.1	HDL-C Incr. 6% TG Decr. 31%	CHD death, nonfatal MI	22	627

[a] In AFSCAPS/TexCAPS there were 155 patients with clinically diagnosed diabetes and 239 with clinically diagnosed diabetes plus elevated fasting glucose.
[b] In 4S there were 202 patients with clinically diagnosed DM and 486 with clinically diagnosed diabetes plus elevated fasting glucose.
[c] Primary endpoint(s) in the post-CABG trial were angiographic changes in saphenous vein grafts; the composite clinical endpoints were MI, CHD death, and stroke. Decr. = decrement; incr. = increment.

Table 3
CHD Risk Reduction in Diabetic Patients Based on Intervention Trial Data

Variable	Study	Refs.	Intervention	Outcome[a]
Glycemic control	UKPDS	134,137,138	Oral glucose-lowering agents and insulin	2% Absolute reduction in HgbA1c with 16% reduction in CHD
Lipid lowering				
Primary Prevention	HHS	44	Gemfibrozil	Greater incremental reduction in CHD endpoints in diabetic patients
	AFSCAPS/TexCAPS	32	Lovastatin	Greater incremental reduction in CHD endpoints in diabetic patients
Secondary Prevention	4S	57,110,111	Simvastatin	Greater incremental reduction in CHD endpoints in diabetic patients
	Post-CABG	17,66,107	Lovastatin (+ bile acid resins)	Comparable incremental reduction in composite endpoints in diabetic patients
	CARE	50,118	Pravastatin	Comparable incremental reduction in CHD endpoints in diabetic patients
	LIPID	94	Pravastatin	Comparable incremental reduction in CHD endpoints in diabetic patients
	VAHIT	117	Gemfobrozil	Comparable incremental reduction in CHD endpoints in diabetic patients
Hypertension	UKPDS	139	Atenolol Captopril, nisoldipine	Comparable reduction in endpoints with atenolol and captopril, nisoldipine
	ABCD	35	Enalapril, nisoldipine	Fatal, nonfatal MI and stroke higher with nisoldipine in diabetic patients
	FACET	132	Fosinopril Amlodipine	Cardiovascular events lower with fosinopril than with amlodipine
	HOT	59	Multiple agents (three diastolic BP goals)	Decreased major atherosclerotic events with lowest diastolic BP target
	Syst-Eur	133	Nitrendipine	Decreased mortality, CHD events, and stroke with decreased BP
Aspirin	ETDRS	36	ASA[b] 650 mg/d	Reduction in CHD risk
	HOT	59	Low-dose ASA	Decreased major atherosclerotic events
ACE inhibitors	HOPE	61,64	Ramipril 10 mg/day	Reduction in CHD and stroke comparable in diabetic patients to nondiabetic patients

[a]Not all outcomes reached statistical significance.
[b]ASA = acetylsalicylic acid.

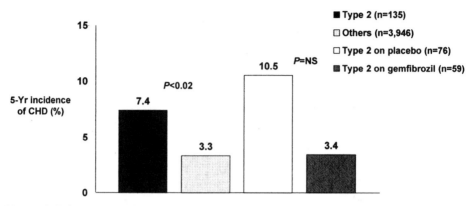

*Myocardial infarction or cardiac death.
NS=not significant.

Fig. 4. Primary CHD* prevention in patients with type 2 diabetes: The Helsinki Heart Study. From Koskinen P, et al. Diabetes Care 1992;15:820–825.

in the diabetic subjects than in the nondiabetic subjects in this trial (Fig. 4). This incremental reduction in risk did not reach statistical significance ($p = 0.19$). In the Scandinavian Simvastatin Survival Study (4S) trial *(57, 111,121)*, the diabetic subjects in the placebo group had a higher incidence of CHD events (CHD-related death or nonfatal MI) compared to subjects without diabetes mellitus (45% vs. 27%). With lipid-lowering therapy the incidence of CHD events was still greater in diabetic subjects (24%) than in nondiabetic subjects (19%). This represented a greater incremental reduction in CHD events for diabetic subjects (55% risk reduction), however, than in nondiabetic subjects (32% risk reduction) (Fig.5). Mortality rates in this trial were also higher in diabetic vs. nondiabetic subjects in both the placebo (25% vs. 11% mortality) and simvastatin groups (14% vs. 8% mortality). There was a greater percent reduction in all cause mortality in diabetic subjects treated with simvastatin compared to those without diabetes mellitus (43% vs. 29%) (Fig. 6). In a subgroup analysis of these same patients *(57)* that included diabetic patients diagnosed clinically (elevated fasting plasma glucose [$n = 483$]) as well as patients with impaired fasting glucose ($n = 678$), there was a progressive increase in the percent of patients (placebo group) with CHD events as a function of increasing glucose category. The LDL-C reduction was comparable among simvastatin-treated groups. The reduction in risk for each of the 4S end points was comparable or greater in the hyperglycemic patients compared to patients with normal fasting glucose concentrations. In a study looking at the effect of pravastatin on coronary events after myocardial infarction in subjects with average cholesterol levels (Cholesterol and Recurrent Events [CARE] study), diabetic subjects had a 25% reduction in nonfatal MI or CHD death when they were treated with pravastatin compared to placebo *(50,118)* (Fig. 7). The effect was similar in the nondiabetic subjects who had a 23% reduction in these events. Summary data from the results of the Air Force/Texas Coronary Atherosclerosis Prevention Study (AFCAPS/TexCAPS) *(32)* primary prevention trial that included 155 type 2 diabetic subjects also suggest higher event rates in the diabetic patients in both the lovastatin- and placebo-treatment arms of the trial when compared with the nondiabetic patients. Although the numbers were too small to show statistically significant differences in event rates with lovastatin therapy, the incremental difference (reduction) in event rates between lova-

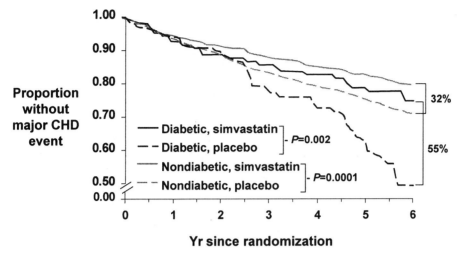

Fig. 5. Major CHD event reduction in a subgroup of patients with diabetes. From Pyörälä K, et al. Diabetes Care 1997;20:614–620.

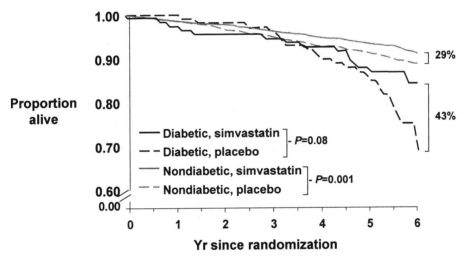

Fig. 6. Total mortality reduction in a subgroup of patients with diabetes. From Pyörälä K, et al. Diabetes Care 1997;20:614–620.

statin and placebo was greater in diabetic patients than in nondiabetic patients in this trial. The risk reduction for CHD events in the Long-Term Intervention with Pravastatin in Ischemic Disease (LIPID) trial was slightly less in the diabetic subjects compared with the nondiabetic subjects. Finally, in the Post-Coronary Artery Bypass Grafting (CABG) trial the reduction in the occurrence of angiographic outcomes and clinical events with treatment in the Post-CABG trial was not statistically significant between diabetic ($n = 116$) and nondiabetic ($n = 1235$) patients, the consistency in risk reduction (as determined by risk ratio) was the same (or perhaps even greater) in the diabetic patients *(17,66)*.

The Veterans Affairs High-Density Lipoprotein Cholesterol Intervention Trial (VAHIT) reported a mean HDL-C, which was 6% higher, and mean TG was 31% lower in the gemfibrozil group compared with the placebo group; no differences in LDL-C were reported. The reduction in non-fatal MI and CHD death was reported to be comparable in diabetic subjects and the group as a whole *(117)*.

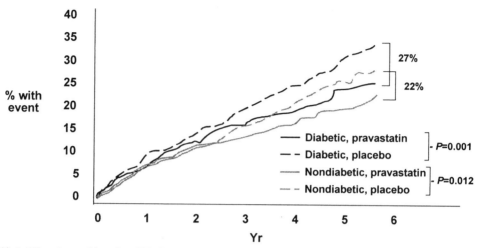

N=4,159 males and females; 976 diabetics.

Fig. 7. CARE: reduction of coronary events in patients with diabetes. From Goldberg R, et al. Circulation 1998;98:2513–2519.

These trials support the concept that a reduction in LDL-C accrues benefit to reduce CHD risk. Reductions in non-HDL-C and increased HDL-C also confer benefit. Aggressive LDL-C reduction may attenuate or eliminate some of the risk associated with TG and HDL-C abnormalities, but this concept currently derives from post-hoc analysis of data. No large randomized trial has tested this concept in prospective fashion.

Hypertension (Table 3; see Chapter 6)

Several trials of blood pressure lowering *(5,5a,9,14,25,26a,35,59,73,74,99,108,122, 132,133)* have shown a reduction in CHD events in patients with and without DM. Most of the studies on coronary vascular disease (CVD) as well as stroke have been carried out in type 2 diabetic patients. This section discusses selected studies showing general effects of blood pressure (BP) lowering on atherosclerotic disease events as well as the observations with selected classes of antihypertensive agents. There appears to be accumulating data that short-acting calcium channel blockers should be avoided in both patients with and without DM. This subject will not be further discussed in this chapter.

The largest body of reported data in diabetic patients is on the use of angiotensin-converting enzyme (ACE) inhibitors, long-acting calcium channel blockers and diuretics. Unfortunately, there are few comparisons with single agents in each class within a single trial. Blood pressure levels at entry have also been somewhat variable for both systolic and diastolic blood pressure. Most of the trials use a reduction of 20 mmHg for either systolic or diastolic blood pressure or both. There are also widely varying endpoints including combined or individual endpoints that include all-cause mortality, fatal or nonfatal MI, and strokes. Selected trials have used other endpoints including hospitalization for angina. In some of the trials, cardiovascular endpoints were secondary endpoints and the analyses in diabetic patients were often done after trial completion. Nevertheless, the following general conclusions can be drawn. There is atherosclerotic risk reduction in the range of 20–55% with BP lowering in diabetic patients. (These risk reductions are comparable to what can be achieved with aggressive lipid lowering.)

Several studies have looked at ACE inhibitor therapy in diabetic subjects. The Appropriate Blood Pressure in Diabetes (ABCD) trial had a change in creatinine clearance as its primary endpoint with fatal and nonfatal MI as a secondary endpoint *(35)*. It compared 235 diabetic subjects taking enalapril to 235 diabetic subjects taking nisoldipine. There were both normotensive and hypertensive patients in this study. In the report of 470 hypertensive, type 2 diabetic patients, there was comparable BP lowering in the two treatment groups. There was an increased risk for fatal and nonfatal MI with nisoldipine (adjusted risk ratio of 7 with a 95% confidence interval of 2.3–21.4) as well as nonfatal MIs (adjusted risk ratio [RR]: 5.9) and cerebrovascular accidents. (Adjusted RR 2.2 with a confidence interval that bounded unity of 0.7–7.1). The fact that other BP treatment was not controlled may also be a confounding variable, as there was a high discontinuation rate in both groups. Furthermore, the authors acknowledged that they could not "distinguish among a deleterious effect of nisoldipine, protective effect of enalapril and a combination of both as the reason for the difference...." The FACET trial (Fosinopril vs. Amlodipine Cardiovascular Events Randomized Trial in Patients with Hypertension and NIDDM) looked at 380 hypertensive patients *(132)*. The primary outcome was to look at the changes in lipid levels. Cardiovascular events were a secondary outcome. Target BPs were 140/90 (or greater than 20 mm of mercury BP drop if initial BPs are greater than 160/110). This trial demonstrated that a greater number of patients in both groups achieved diastolic BP targets than achieve systolic BP targets. Furthermore, amlodipine was added to more than 30% of the fosinopril group. Fosinopril was added to more than 26% of the amlodipine group. Overall event rates were less with fosinopril than with amlodipine.

The Heart Outcomes Prevention Evaluation Study (HOPE) demonstrated that use of the ACE inhibitor, ramipril 10 mg daily, was associated with a 22% reduction in myocardial infarction and 37% reduction in cardiac death in diabetic patients *(64)*. These results were similar to the reduction in risk reported in the whole HOPE study population *(61)*. The Antihypertensive and Lipid Lowering Treatment to Prevent Heart Attack Trial (ALLHAT) will look at more than 40,000 greater than 55 yr, in whom more than one third will have diabetes, to compare amlodipine, lisinopril, doxazosin, and chlorthalidone on atherosclerotic event rates *(26a)*.

A beneficial effect of other agents including calcium channel blockers is available from other hypertensive trials. Most notable is the Hypertension Optimal Treatment Trial (HOT) with 18,790 patients aged 50–80 yr *(59)*. Target BPs include diastolic pressures of <90 in one group, to ≤85 in a second group, and to ≤80 in a third group. There were approximately 500 type 2 diabetic patients in each arm (total of 1501). The diabetic patients with a BP target of less than 80 compared to the BP target group of less than 90, had a 51% decrease in major cardiovascular events. (Aspirin use in this trial also demonstrated a reduction in atherosclerotic vascular events.) The Systolic Hypertension in Europe (Syst-Eur) *(133)* trial used nitrendipine to lower BP. It included 492 patients with diabetes (4203 patients did not have diabetes). The BP target was at 20 mmHg reduction of systolic BP. There was a reduction in mortality by 55% and decreased cardiovascular events of 26% and strokes of 38% in the diabetic patients with BP reduction.

Finally, it should be noted that the potential beneficial effects of low-dose thiazides have been demonstrated in a number of studies. The Systolic Hypertension in the Elderly Program (SHEP) trial *(122)* was really the first to show significant benefit in diabetic patients. The SHEP trial did not demonstrate statistically significant reduction in mortality; however, the reported reduction was 26%. There was a reduction in cardiovascular

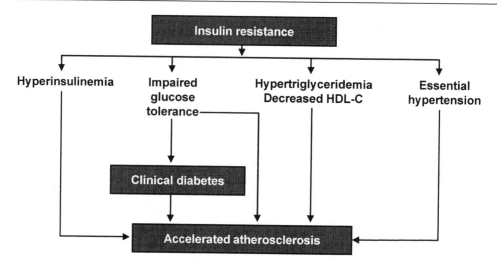

Fig. 8. Insulin resistance and atherosclerosis: posited relationships.

events of 34% and in coronary events of 56%. Stroke reduction was also not statistically significant at 22%.

The use of beta blockers has been incorporated in a number of trials. The beneficial effects of both ACE inhibitor and beta blockers were demonstrated in the UKPDS *(139)*. Furthermore, there appears to be additive effects of BP lowering to hemoglobin A_{1c} reduction in this trial. Greater incremental effects of BP on risk reduction may be seen in patients with higher hemoglobin A_{1c} levels and similarly greater effects of hemoglobin A_{1c} reduction may be seen in patients with higher BP.

Other Atherosclerotic Risk Factors Related to DM

HYPERINSULINEMIA

Hyperinsulinemia *(3,13,33,34,42,43,55,77,87,106,109,110,112,113,116,126,131, 136,141,149)*, and the commonly associated insulin resistance, has been associated with increased risk for CHD. Hyperinsulinemia is often associated with known or suspected risk factors for atherosclerotic vascular disease such as central obesity, DM, dyslipidemia (high TG, low HDL-C, and a small dense LDL-C), hypertension, and increased PAI-1 activity (Fig. 8). This association had been demonstrated in studies of clinical CHD as well as angiographic studies of the carotid arteries. It is not yet clear whether insulin, or perhaps proinsulin, is atherogenic, or whether the risk for atherosclerosis is because hyperinsulinemia is associated with the well-established risk factors noted earlier.

The role by which hyperinsulinemia or "hyperproinsulinemia" may increase the risk for CHD is not yet established. Furthermore, whether it contributes to the risk in similarly in various arterial systems (coronary, cerebral, peripheral) is also not yet established. Many studies have looked at clinical outcomes, and more recently angiographic outcomes have been investigated using such methodologies as angiography of native vessels, saphenous vein graft conduits, and ultrasound of the carotid arteries.

Several observational studies have looked at insulin concentration as a predictor of CHD risk. As early as 1968 Tzargournis and co-workers reported an association of hyperinsulinemia and hypertriglyceridemia in young men with CHD *(136)*. This observation has been confirmed in several subsequent studies that also show an association of hyperinsulinemia with one or more of the following: central obesity, low HDL-C, hypertension, and impaired glucose tolerance. Prospective observational studies have also shown that increased insulin concentrations were associated with an increased risk for future CHD events and CHD-related mortality. Insulin levels obtained 1 h post-oral glucose challenge were associated with increased CHD incidence and mortality in the 3390 participants of the Busselton (Australia) study *(141)*. Relative risk for the top quintile of insulin concentrations (compared to the bottom four quintiles) was 1.67 for CHD events at 6 yr and 1.66 for CHD death at 12 yr. In the Paris Prospective Study, the highest quintiles of fasting insulin and insulin concentrations 2 h after a 75-g oral glucose challenge ($n = 7029$) were associated with a more than twofold increase in CHD risk compared to the lower quintiles *(34)*. In the Quebec Cardiovascular Study *(30)* of 2103 men, insulin concentration predicted CHD events (along with several lipid abnormalities including apo B, LDL-C, HDL-C); insulin concentration amplified the adverse effects of low HDL-C, elevated TGs, and elevated apo B levels.

In the past decade several studies have looked at the relationship between insulin concentrations and other measures of vascular disease. The Atherosclerosis Risk in Communities (ARIC) Study *(42)* used several measures of arterial stiffness in carotid arteries and reported that insulin concentrations were associated with measures reflecting increased stiffness in univariate analyses performed in nondiabetic subjects. In multivariate analyses, serum insulin remained a significant predictor in white men and women, but not in black examinees. In addition, insulin showed a synergistic effect with glucose and TGs in this study. Kekälänen and associates could not show a relationship between insulin concentration or insulin sensitivity in the progression of atherosclerosis as measured by serial ultrasounds in femoral arteries in 118 subjects *(80)*. Agewall and colleagues used carotid ultrasound to look at intima media thickness and plaque status in 25 men with cardiovascular risk factors and 23 matched controls without such risk factors *(3)*. Insulin sensitivity was determined by hyperinsulinemic, euglycemic clamp techniques. Lower insulin sensitivity was associated with intima media thickness (even when adjusted for body weight). However, these authors reported no relationship of insulin sensitivity to plaque status. Laakso and co-workers reported that men with either femoral or carotid (or both) atherosclerosis as determined by ultrasonography had lower glucose disposal rates (insulin resistance) during hyperinsulinemic clamp studies compared to controls without ultrasound evidence of disease *(87)*. However, mean fasting insulin and C-peptide concentrations were similar.

Dysfibrinolysis and Atherosclerosis

There are several lines of evidence to suggest that diabetic patients may be at increased risks for atherothrombosis as a result of increased platelet aggregation, elevated PAI levels and perhaps altered endothelial cell function *(26,85,98,146)*. Nevertheless, there are few randomized controlled trials that assess the benefits of interventions to reduce the risk for thrombogenesis in diabetic patients. One such study was the Early Treatment Diabetic Retinopathy Study (ETDRS *[36]*). The purpose of this study was to assess whether aspirin (650 mg daily) vs. placebo would reduce the risk for progression of diabetic retinopathy. Although there was no benefit in this primary endpoint, there was a reduction in life-table cumulative event rates for fatal or nonfatal MI (relative risk, RR = 0.83; CI 0.66–1.04; $p = 0.04$) in diabetic patients. This study was an important consideration in

Table 4
Glycemic Control for People with Diabetes

Biochemical index	Nondiabetic	Diabetic goal	Action suggested
Preprandial glucose (mg/dL)	<110	80–120	<80 >140
Bedtime glucose (mg/dL)	<120	100–140	<100 >160
Hemoglobin A_{1c} (%)	<6	<7	>8

These values are for nonpregnant individuals. "Action suggested" depends on individual patient circumstances.

Hemoglobin A1c is referenced to a nondiabetic range of 4.0–6.0% (mean 5.0%, standard deviation 0.5%).

From ADA. Diabetes Care 2000;23(Suppl 1):S32–S42 (6a).

the position statement from the American Diabetes Association in recommending aspirin for patients with DM (9,21).

Glucose-Lowering Agents

OVERVIEW

In type 1 DM, insulin use is necessary for adequate glycemic control. Similarly, with increasing duration of type 2 DM, the use of insulin is often necessary for adequate glycemic control. It is beyond the scope of this chapter to discuss the spectrum of insulins and insulin regimens in diabetes. ADA suggested standards for glycemic control are included in Table 4. The oral agents to lower glucose deserve summary comments, however. These agents fall into several general mechanistic classes: insulin secretagogues (sulfonylureas, meglitinides); reduction in hepatic glucose production (metformin); insulin sensitizers (thiazolidinediones); gut-related delay in glucose absorption (carbohydrase inhibitors) (19,22,23,27,29,41,46,48,68,72,88,114,120,142). The mechanisms that increase glucose in type 2 diabetes include abnormalities of insulin production, increased hepatic glucose production, and insulin resistances as well as exaggerated postprandial hyperglycemia. As such, agents that work by different mechanism have additive effects on glucose control. However, the limited ability to characterize the main biochemical abnormality in any single patient limits the ability to select a single agent that will have the greatest efficacy in a single patient. The general efficacy, contraindications, and side effects of each class of agents are discussed briefly.

SULFONYLUREAS

At maximal doses, mean glucose-lowering effects are in the range of 30–60 mg/dL (hemoglobin A_{1c} change of 1–2%). The incremental reduction may be greater with more marked hyperglycemia. In addition, to glucose-lowering effects, there are data for these agents (as well as other sulfonylureas) to indicate that they may have a beneficial effect on the dyslipidemia associated with diabetes by lowering TGs. In some cases, this may be associated by an increase in HDL-C concentrations.

Hypoglycemia may occur with any of the sulfonylureas; however, severe hypoglycemia is infrequent. Weight gain is common with sulfonylureas. Sulfonylureas are cleared by both hepatic and renal routes (depending on the agent). In patients with elevated serum creatinine concentrations, sulfonylurea-dosing schedules should be reduced and increased attention given to increased risk for hypoglycemia.

MEGLITINIDE (REPAGLINIDE)

This oral glucose-lowering agent reduces postprandial glucose. It is rapidly absorbed and has a short metabolic half-life; therefore, it must be taken with meals. The overall efficacy is modest with reduction in hemoglobin A_{1c} in the range of ½–1½%. Among the insulin secretagogue medications, it does have the advantage of use in patients who have renal compromise. It also has relatively little risk for hypoglycemia. Extensive data on beneficial effects on lipid profiles are not available.

METFORMIN

The efficacy of metformin is comparable to that of the sulfonylureas and comparison data with glyburide have been reported. Mean reduction in hemoglobin A_{1c} is between 1 and 2% in many studies. In addition, there is a reduction in total cholesterol (TC), total TGs, and LDL-C. Several studies also report weight reduction in conjunction with metformin use.

A small percentage of people develop a metallic taste with metformin use. This is usually transient. Starting with a low dose can ameliorate it and increasing doses as tolerated. Approximately 5% of patients may develop diarrhea of sufficient degree to preclude metformin use. Finally, with selected patients who have risk for hypoxemia (e.g., with congestive heart failure [CHF]), liver disease or renal compromise, there may be an increased risk for lactic acidosis. Some clinicians also suggest that metformin should not be used in the elderly.

THIAZOLIDINEDIONES

Thiazolidinediones are insulin sensitizers, which require insulin (endogenous or exogenous) to work effectively. As monotherapy they are slightly less efficacious than sulfonylureas and metformin, with hemoglobin A_{1c} reductions in the approx 0.5–1.5% range. Greater efficacy may be achieved with patients who have greater residual beta cell function (presumably shorter duration of disease) or when used in conjunction with sulfonylureas or exogenous insulin administration.

There are some data that suggest use of thiazolidinediones may be associated with improved insulin secretory capacity (even though they are not primarily an insulin secretagogue). These data suggest that with improved insulin sensitivity there is improved beta cell response with entraining of endogenous insulin to nutrient stimulation.

There is an evolving understanding of the potential benefits of thiazolidinediones on lipid profiles. These include changes in LDL-C size from a small dense LDC to a larger LDL that may be less atherogenic and less susceptible to oxidation.

Finally, there is some data to suggest that because of the interaction with a peroxisome proliferator-activated receptor (PPAR), there may be a beneficial affect on CHD risk factor reduction. Some of this may be mediated through macrophage function in which there may be reduced uptake of lipid into macrophages. This, in turn, may reduce the risk for foam-cell formation. Any reduction in lipid oxidation may also decrease the risk for endothelial cell damage and smooth muscle proliferation.

The most serious concern regarding thiazolidinediones is the risk for serious hepatoxicity. Current data suggest that this risk is acceptable with appropriate monitoring of liver enzymes. Weight gain is a common side effect of thiazolidinedione use in some patients. Whether it is associated with increased risk for atherosclerotic disease is unknown. Furthermore, fluid retention is common. Thiazolidinedione use in the face of a history of CHF needs to take fluid retention into consideration.

Table 5
ADA Recommendations: Goals of Lipid Regulation for Adults with Diabetes[a]

Risk	TC	HDL-C	LDL-C	TG
Acceptable	<200	>45	<100	<200
Borderline	200–239	35–45	100–129	200–399
High	≥240	<35	≥130	≥400
Therapy goals				
Macrovascular disease (+)	—	—	≤100	<200
Macrovascular disease (–)[b]	<200	—	≤100	<200

[a] Values represent mg/dL.
[b] With multiple CHD risk factors: HDL <35 mg/dL, smoking, hypertension, family history of premature CHD, or microalbuminuria or proteinuria.
From ADA. Diabetes Care 2000;23(Suppl 1):S57–S60 (9).

CARBOHYDRASE INHIBITORS

The efficacy of the carbohydrate inhibitors (acarbose, miglitol) is modest in mean glycemic reduction. In many trials the reduction in hemoglobin A_{1c} is approximately ½–1%. However, postmarketing data suggest that with marked hyperglycemia the actual reduction in hemoglobin A_{1c} may be somewhat greater than that reported from phase 3 trials. There is a beneficial effect on lipid profiles. The agents do not predispose to weight gain and may ameliorate some of the weight gain associated with sulfonylurea use.

The gastrointestinal side effects of the carbohydrase inhibitors are significant in both frequency and intensity. This has limited their use in the clinical arena in the United States.

Lipid Management in Diabetic Patients

Diabetes is a significant risk factor in risk assessment strategies. Consequently, aggressive lipid-lowering strategies have been recommended for diabetic patients (6a,7,37,38,45, 53,54,56,79,82) (Table 5). Intervention trial and general clinical experience indicate use of statins and fibric acid derivatives in diabetic patients are efficacious and safe. Furthermore, these agents have no known adverse effect on glucose tolerance. Bile acid sequestrants may be somewhat more difficult to use in diabetic patients who are more likely to be hypertensive or require oral agents to manage glucose levels. This "poly-pharmacy" and the effect of the bile acid sequestrants to potentially interfere with absorption of other agents limit their use in some diabetic patients. Furthermore, increased TG levels with bile acid sequestrant use are also a problem in some diabetic patients. Niacin may increase insulin resistance and adversely affect glycemic control. Its use is generally limited to diabetic patients with satisfactory glycemic control (Fig. 9).

Management of Hypertension in Diabetic Patients

The beneficial effects of BP lowering are now well established in both non-diabetic and diabetic patients. Studies show that reduction in systolic BP will result in substantial reduction in atherosclerotic risk. Furthermore, beneficial effects have been shown in diabetic patients with ACE-inhibitors, long acting calcium channel blockers, beta-blocker and diuretics. The absence of extensive head to head comparisons limits the capability to determine which class of agents may have the greatest benefit. Because of the accumulating data that ACE inhibitors may have some advantage in protecting renal function in diabetic patients, this class of agents should generally be consider as the first line agent(s).

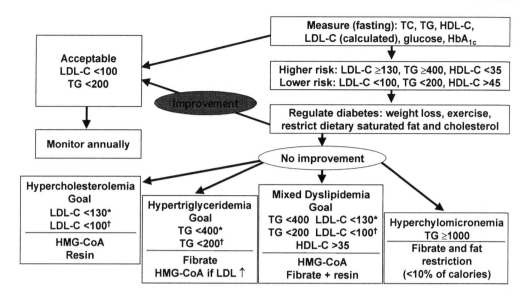

Fig. 9. Approach to patients with diabetes and hyperlipidemia. Adapted from NLEC. (*, Without vascular disease; †, with vascular disease or without vascular disease but with other CHD risk factors).

Potential adverse effects of beta-blockers and diuretics on glycemic control and dyslipidemia need to be balanced by their indications in the face of CHD risk management. Such considerations usually favor their use with usual clinical indications.

Smoking Risk in Diabetic Patients (See Chapter 10)

Smoking clearly increases the risk for CHD risk in diabetic patients. The ADA has formally endorsed the importance of smoking cessation in diabetic patients (8).

Acute Coronary Syndromes in Diabetic Patients

In addition to an increased risk for CHD, many studies have shown that diabetic patients have a worse outcome following a myocardial infarction both in terms of morbidity and mortality (1,10,11,31,39,65,69,78,99,100,104,130,147). Many of these studies report that women with diabetes are a much greater risk for an adverse outcome than their non-diabetic counter parts. Furthermore, the increased number of CHD risk factors in diabetic patients and more diffuse disease appear to be contributing risk factors. Acute management of an acute coronary syndrome is similar in diabetic and non-diabetic patients. The outcomes of thrombolytic therapy may be less favorable in diabetic patients (52,70,95, 148). Limited data suggest that intensive glycemic control in the period surrounding the myocardial infarction may improve outcomes (96).

Vascular Interventions in Diabetic Patients

The results of surgical intervention such as coronary artery bypass procedures also generally have less favorable long term outcomes in diabetic patients (18,40,71,93,101, 107,115) with evidence of earlier graft closure and increased mortality compared to non-diabetic patients. Angioplasty also has a less favorable outcome in such patients (18,51, 97,124,125). The mechanisms for more these adverse outcomes may be related to the increased number of CHD risk factors, including an increased procoagulant risk. Limited data on the effects of aggressive risk factor management suggest that aggressive cholesterol lowering may slow the rate of progression of disease in saphenous vein graft conduits *(66)*. The BARI trial was designed to compare CABG vs. PTCA *(18)*. The subgroup with diabetes had a more favorable outcome with CABG. However, the changing intervention technologies for both CABG and PTCA/Stent procedures, and more aggressive use of antiplatelet therapy limit the ability to apply the BARI results to current clinical practice.

SUMMARY

Diabetic patients are at increased risk for CHD and experience increased morbidity and mortality from CHD compared to their non-diabetic counterparts. Diabetic patients often have a greater number of traditional risk factors such as hypertension, dyslipidemia, obesity as well as a relatively higher procoagulant state (increased fibrinogen, increased PAI-I, increased platelet aggregation. Aggressive risk factor management has comparable or greater benefit in diabetic patients compared to patients without diabetes mellitus (Table 3). Management of acute coronary syndromes and indications for surgical interventions are essentially the same in diabetic and non-diabetic patients, although long-term outcomes are worse in diabetic patients.

REFERENCES

1. Abbott RD, Donahue RP, Kannel WB, Wilson PW. The impact of diabetes on survival following myocardial infarction in men vs. women. The Framingham Study JAMA 1988;260:3456–3460.
2. Abraira C, Colwell J, Nuttall F. Veterans Affairs cooperative study on glycemic control and complications in type II diabetes (VACSDM): results of the feasibility trial. Diabetes Care 1995;18:1113–1123.
3. Agewall S, Fagerberg B, Atvall S, et al. Carotid artery wall intima-media thickness is associated with insulin-mediated glucose disposal in men at high and low coronary risk. Stroke 1995;26:956–960.
4. Abraira C, Emanuele N, Colwell J, et al. Glycemic control and complications in type II diabetes: design of the feasibility trial. Diabetes Care 1995;15:1560–1571.
5. Alderman MH, Cohen H, Roque R, Madhavan S. Effect of long-acting and short-acting calcium antagonists on cardiovascular outcomes in hypertensive patients. Lancet 1997;349:594–598.
5a. Officers and Coordinators for the ALLHAT Collaborative Research Group. Major cardiovascular events in hypertensive patients randomized to doxozosin vs chlorthalidone: The Antihypertensive and Lipid-Lowering Treatment to Prevent Heart Attack Trial (ALLHAT). JAMA 2000;283:1967–1975.
6. Anderson, KM, Wilson PWF, Odell PM, Kannel WB. An updated coronary risk profile: a statement for health professionals. Circulation 1991;83:356–362.
6a. American Diabetes Association Standards of Medical Care for Patients with Diabetes Mellitus. Diabetes Care 2000;23(Suppl 1):S32–S42.
7. American Diabetes Association. Management of dyslipidemia in adults with diabetes. Diabetes Care 2000;23(Suppl 1):557–560.
8. American Diabetes Association. Smoking and diabetes. American Diabetes Association: Clinical Practice Recommendations. Diabetes Care 2000;23(Suppl 1):563–564.
9. American Diabetes Association. Aspirin therapy in diabetes. American Diabetes Association: Clinical Practice Recommendations. Diabetes Care 2000;23(Suppl 1):561–562.
10. Aronson D, Rayfield EJ, Chesebro JH. Mechanisms determining course and outcome of diabetic patients who have had acute myocardial infarction. [Review] Ann Intern Med. 1997;126:296–306.
11. Behar S, Boyko V, Reicher-Reiss H, Goldbourt U. Ten-year survival after acute myocardial infarction: comparison of patients with and without diabetes. SPRINT Study Group. Secondary Prevention Reinfarction Israeli Nifedipine Trial. Am Heart J 1997;133:290–296.
12. Bjornholt JV, Erikssen G, Aaser E, et al. Fasting blood glucose: an underestimated risk factor for cardiovascular death: results from a 22-year follow-up of healthy nondiabetic men. Diabetes Care 1999;22:45–49.

13. Bonora E, Targier G, Zenere MB, et al. Relationship between fasting insulin and cardiovascular risk factors in already present in young men: the Verona Young Men Atherosclerosis Risk Factors Study. Eur J Clin Invest 1997;27:248–254.

14. Borhani NO, Mercuri M, Borhani PA, et al. Final outcome results of the multicenter isradipine diuretic atherosclerosis study. JAMA 1996;276:785–791.

15. Brownlee M, Cerami A, Vlassara H. Advanced glycosylation end products in tissue and the biochemical basis of diabetic complications. N Engl J Med 1988;318:1315–1321.

16. Buse J, Hart K, Minasi L, on behalf of the PROTECT Study Group. The PROTECT Study: final results of a large multicenter post marketing study in patients with type 2 diabetes. Clin Ther 1998;20:257–269.

17. Campeau L, Hunninghake DB, Knatterud G, et al., for the Post CABG Study. Aggressive cholesterol lowering delays saphenous vein graft atherosclerosis in women, in the Elderly and in Patients with Associated Risk Factors: NHLBI Post CABG Clinical Trial. Circulation 1999;99:3241–3247.

18. Chaitman BR, Rosen AD, Williams DO, et al. Myocardial infarction and cardiac mortality in the Bypass Angioplasty Revascularization Investigation (BARI) randomized trial. Circulation 1997;96: 2162–2170.

19. Chiasson JL, Josse RG, Hunt JA, et al. The efficacy of acarbose in the treatment of patients with non-insulin-dependent diabetes mellitus. Ann Int Med 1994;121:928–935.

20. Chisolm GM, Irwin KC, Penn MC. Lipoprotein oxidation and lipoprotein-induced cell injury in diabetes. Diabetes 1992;41(Suppl 2):61–66.

21. Colwell JA. Aspirin therapy in diabetes (Technical Review). Diabetes Care 1997;20:1767–1771.

22. Coniff RJ, Shapiro JA, Seaton TB, et al. A double-blind placebo-controlled trial evaluating the safety and efficacy of acarbose for the treatment of patients with insulin-requiring type II diabetes. Diabetes Care 1995;18:928–932.

23. Coniff R, Shapiro JA, Seaton TB, Bray GA. Multicenter, placebo-controlled trial comparing acarbose (BAY g 5421) with placebo, tolbutamide and tolbutamide-plus-acarbose in non-insulin-dependent diabetes mellitus Am J Med 1995;98:443–451.

24. Coutinho M, Gerstein HC, Wang Y, Yusuf, S. The relationship between glucose and incident cardiovascular events: a metaregression analysis of published data from 20 studies in 95,783 individuals followed for 12.4 years. Diabetes Care 1999;22:233–240.

25. Curb JD, Pressel SL, Cutler JA, et al. Effect of diuretic-based antihypertensive treatment on cardiovascular disease risk in older diabetic patients with isolated systolic hypertension. JAMA 1996;276: 1886–1892.

26. Davi G, Violi F, Giammarresi C, et al. Increased plasminogen activator inhibitor antigen levels in diabetic patients with stable angina. Blood Coag Fibrinolysis 1991;2:41–45.

26a. Davis BR, Cutler JA, Gordon D, et al. for the ALLHAT Research Group. Rationale and design of the Antihypertensive and Lipid-Lowering Treatment to Prevent Heart Attack Trial (ALLHAT). Am J Hypertens 1996;9:342–360.

27. DeFronzo RA, Barzilai N, Simonson DC. Mechanism of metformin action in obese and lean non-insulin-dependent diabetic subjects. J Clin Endocrinol Metab 1991;73:1294–1301.

28. DeFronzo RA, Ferrannini E. A multifaceted syndrome responsible for NIDDM obesity, hypertension, dyslipidemia, and atherosclerotic cardiovascular disease. Insulin resistance. [Review] [307 refs.] Diabetes Care 1991;14:173–194.

29. DeFronzo RA, Goodman AM. Multicenter Metformin Study Group. Efficacy of metformin in patients with non-insulin dependent diabetes mellitus. N Engl J Med. 1995;333:541–545.

30. Deprès J-P, Lamarche B, Mauriège P, et al. Hyperinsulinaemia as an independent risk factor for ischaemic heart disease. N Engl J Med 1996;334:952–957.

31. Donahue RP, Goldberg RJ, Chen Z, et al. The influence of sex and diabetes mellitus on survival following acute myocardial infarction: a community-wide perspective. J Clin Epidemiol 1993;46:245–252.

32. Downs JR, Clearfield M, Weis S, et al. Primary prevention of acute coronary events with lovastatin in men and women with average cholesterol levels: results of AFCAPS/TexCAPS.Air Force/Texas Coronary Atherosclerosis Prevention Study. JAMA 1998;279:1615–1622.

33. Ducimetière P, Eschwège E, Papoz L, et al. Relationship of plasma insulin levels to the incidence of myocardial infarction and coronary heart disease mortality in a middle-aged population. Diabetologia 1980;19:205–210.

34. Eschwège E, Richard JL, Thibult N, et al. Coronary heart disease mortality in relation with diabetes, blood glucose and plasma insulin levels: The Paris Prospective Study, ten years later. Horm Metab Res 1985;15(Suppl):41–46.

35. Estacio RO, Jeffers BW, Hiatt WR, et al. The effect of nisoldipine as compared with enalapril on cardiovascular outcomes in patients with non-insulin-dependent diabetes and hypertension. N Engl J Med 1998;338:645–652.
36. ETDRS Study Group. Aspirin effects on mortality and morbidity in patients with diabetes mellitus—Early Treatment Diabetic Retinopathy Study Report—14. JAMA 1992;268:1292–1300.
37. Expert Panel of Detection, Evaluation, and Treatment of High Blood Cholesterol in Adults. National Cholesterol Education Program. Second report of the expert panel on detection, evaluation and treatment of high blood cholesterol in adults (Adult Treatment Panel II). Circulation 1994;89:1333–1345.
38. Expert Panel of Detection, Evaluation, and Treatment of High Blood Cholesterol in Adults. National Cholesterol Education Program. Summary of the second report of the National Cholesterol Education Program expert panel on detection, evaluation and treatment of high blood cholesterol in adults (Adult Treatment Panel II). JAMA 1993;269:3002–3009.
39. Fava S, Aquilina O, Azzopardi J, et al.The prognostic value of blood glucose in diabetic patients with acute myocardial infarction. Diabetic Med 1996;13:80–83.
40. Fietsam R, Bassett J, Glover JL. Comparisons of coronary artery surgery in diabetic patients. Am Surg 1991;57:551–557.
41. Feinglos MN, Bethol MA. Oral agent therapy in the treatment of type 2 diabetes. Diabetes Care 1999; 22:C61–C64.
42. Folsom AR, Szklo M, Stevens J, et al. A prospective study of coronary heart disease in relation to fasting insulin, glucose, and diabetes. The Atherosclerosis Risk in Communities (ARIC) Study. Diabetes Care 1997;20:935–942.
43. Fontbonne A, Charles MA, Thilbult N, et al. Hyperinsulinemia as a predictor of coronary heart disease mortality in a healthy population: The Paris Prospective Study, 15 year follow-up. Diabetologia 1991; 34:356–361.
44. Frick MH, Elo O, Haapa K, et al. Helsinki Heart Study: primary-prevention trial with gemfibrozil in middle-aged men with dyslipidemia. Safety of treatment, changes in risk factors, and incidence of coronary heart disease. N Engl J Med 1987; 317:1237–1245.
45. Friedrich CA, Rader DJ. Management of lipid disorders. Rheum Clin N Am 1999;25:507–520.
46. Garber AJ, Duncan TG, Goodman AM, et al. Efficacy of metformin in type II diabetes: results of a double-blind, placebo-controlled, dose-response trial. Am J Med 1997;103:491–497.
47. Garcia MJ, McNamara PM, Gordon T, Kannell WB. Morbidity and mortality in diabetics in the Framingham population. Sixteen year follow-up study. Diabetes 1974;23:105–111.
48. Gerich JE. Drug therapy-oral hypoglycemic agents. N Engl J Med 1989;321:1231–1245.
49. Gerstein HC, Pais P, Pogue J, Yusuf S. Relationship of glucose and insulin levels to the risk of myocardial infarction: a case-control study. J Am Coll Cardiol 1999;33:612–619.
50. Goldberg RB, Mellies MJ, Sacks FM, et al. The Care Investigators. Cardiovascular events and their reduction with pravastatin in diabetic and glucose intolerant myocardial infarction survivors with average cholesterol levels: subgroup analyses in the cholesterol and recurrent events (CARE) trial. Circulation 1998;98:2513–2519.
51. Gowda MS, Vacek JL, Hallas D. One-year outcomes of diabetic versus nondiabetic patients with non-Q-wave acute myocardial infarction treated with percutaneous transluminal coronary angioplasty. Am J Cardiol 1998;81(9):1067–1071.
52. Granger CB, Califf RM, Young S. et al. Outcome of patients with diabetes mellitus and acute myocardial infarction treated with thrombolytic agents. The Thrombolysis and Angioplasty in Myocardial Infarction (TAMI) Study Group. J Am Coll Cardiol 1993;21:920–925.
53. Grundy SM, Balady GJ, Criqui MH, et al. Primary prevention of coronary heart disease: guidelines from Framingham. A statement for healthcare professionals from the American Heart Association's Task Force on Risk Reduction. Circulation 1998;97:1876–1887.
54. Grundy SM. Integrating risk assessment with intervention. Primary prevention of coronary heart disease. Circulation 1999;100:988–998.
55. Haffner SM, Mykkänen L, Stern MP, et al. Relationship of proinsulin and insulin to cardiovascular risk factors in nondiabetic subjects. Diabetes 1993;42:1297–1302.
56. Haffner SM. Management of dyslipidemia in adults with diabetes: technical review. Diabetes Care 1998;21:160–178.
57. Haffner SM, Alexander CM, Cook TJ, et al., for the Scandinavian Simvastatin Survival Study Group. Reduced coronary events in simvistatin-treated patients with coronary heart disease and diabetes or impaired glucose levels: Subgroup analyses in the Scandinavian Simvastatin Survival Study. Arch Intern Med 1999;159:2661–2667.

58. Hanninen J, Takala J, Keinanen-Kiukaanniemi S. Albuminuria and other risk factors for moratlity in patients with non-insulin-dependent diabetes mellitus aged under 65 years: a population-based prospective 5-year study. Diabetes Res Clin Pract 1999;43:121–126.

59. Hansson L, Znachetti A, Carruthers SG, et al. Effect of intensive blood-pressure lowering and low-dose aspirin in patients with hypertension: principal results of the Hypertension Optimal Treatment (HOT) randomized trial. Lancet 1998;351:1755–1762.

60. The HOPE Study Investigators. The HOPE (Heart Outcomes Prevention Evaluation) Study: the design of a large, simple randomized trial of an angiotensin-converting enzyme inhibitor (ramipril) and vitamin E in patients at high risk of cardiovascular events. Can J Cardiol 1996;12:127–137.

61. The Heart Outcomes Prevention Evaluation Study Investigators. Effects of an angiotensin-converting-enzyme inhibitor, ramipril, on death from cardiovascular causes, myocardial infarction, and stroke in high-risk patients. N Engl J Med 2000;342:145–153.

62. The Heart Outcomes Prevention Evaluation Study Investigators. Vitamin E supplementation and cardiovascular events in high-risk patients. N Engl J Med 2000;342:154–160.

63. The Heart Outcomes Prevention Evaluation Study Investigators. The MICRO-HOPE Study: rationale and design of a large study to evaluate the renal and cardiovascular effects of an ACE inhibitor and vitamin E in high-risk patients with diabetes. Diabetes Care 1996:19:1225–1228.

64. The Heart Outcomes Prevention Evaluation Study Investigators. Effects of ramipril on cardiovascular and microvascular outcomes in people with diabetes mellitus: results of the HOPE and MICRO-HOPE study. Lancet 2000;355:253–259.

65. Herlitz J, Bang A, Karlson BW. Mortality, place and mode of death and reinfarction during a period of 5 years after acute myocardial infarction in diabetic and non-diabetic patients. Cardiology 1996;87:423–428.

66. Hoogwerf BJ, Waness A, Cressman M, et al., for the Post CABG Trial Investigators. Effects of aggressive cholesterol lowering on clinical and angiographic outcomes in patients with diabetes mellitus: post CABG Trial. Diabetes 1999;48:1289–1294.

67. Horton ES, Whitehouse F, Ghazzi MN, et al. Troglitazone in combination with sulfonylurea restores glycemic control in patients with type 2 diabetes mellitus. The Troglitazone Study Group. Diabetes Care 1998;21:1462–1469.

68. Inzucchi SE, Maggs DG, Spollett GR, et al. Efficacy and metabolic effects of metformin and troglitazone in type II diabetes mellitus. N Engl J Med 1998;338:867–872.

69. Jacoby RM, Nesto RW. Acute myocardial infarction in the diabetic patient: pathophysiology, clinical course and prognosis. [Review] [113 refs] J Am Coll Cardiol 1992;20:736–744.

70. Jelesoff NE, Feinglos M, Granger CB, Califf RM. Outcomes of diabetic patients following acute myocardial infarction: a review of the major thrombolytic trials. [Review] Coron Artery Dis 1996;7:732–743.

71. Johnson WE, Pedraza PM, Kayser KL. Coronary artery surgery in diabetics: 281 consecutive patients followed four to seven years. Am Heart J 1982;104:824–829.

72. Johnston PS, Coniff RF, Hoogwerf BJ, et al. Effects of the carbohydrase inhibitor miglitol in sulfonylure-treated NIDDM patients. Diabetes Care 1994;17:20–29.

73. Jonas M, Reicher-Reiss H, Boyko V, et al. Usefulness of beta-blocker therapy in patients with non-insulin-dependent diabetes mellitus and coronary artery disease. Bezafibrate Infarction Prevention (BIP) Study Group. Am J Cardiol 1996;77:1273–1277.

74. Joint National Committee (JNC-VI). The sixth report of the Joint National Committee on prevention, detection, evaluation and treatment of high blood pressure. Arch Intern Med 1997;157:2413–2446.

75. Kannel WB, D'Agostino RB, Wilson PW, et al. Diabetes, fibrinogen, and risk of cardiovascular disease: the Framingham experience. Am Heart J 1990;120:672–676.

76. Kannel WB. Lipids, diabetes, and coronary artery disease: insights from the Framingham Study. Am Heart J 1985;110:1100–1107.

77. Kaplan NM. Upper-body obesity, glucose intolerance, hypertriglyceridemia, and hypertension. The deadly quartet. [Review][76 refs]. Arch Intern Med 1989;149:1514–1520.

78. Karlson BW, Herlitz J, Hjalmarson A. Prognosis of acute myocardial infarction in diabetic and non-diabetic patients. Diabetic Med 1993;10:449–454.

79. Kasiske B. Hyperlipidemia in patients with chronic renal disease. Am J Kidney Dis 1998;32:S142–S156.

80. Kekäläinen P, Sarlund H, Farin P, et al. Femoral atherosclerosis in middle-aged subjects: association with cardiovascular risk factors and insulin resistance. Am J Epidemiol 1996;144:742–748.

81. Knatterud GL, Klimt CR, Goldner MG, et al. The University Group Diabetes Program: effects of hypoglycemic agents on vascular complications in patients with adult-onset diabetes, VIII. Evaluation of insulin therapy: final report. Diabetes 1982;31(Suppl.15):1–79.

82. Knopp RH. Drug Treatment of lipid disorders. N Engl J Med 1999;341:498–511.
83. Koskinen P, Manttari M, Manninen V, et al. Coronary heart disease incidence in NIDDM patients in the Helsinki Heart Study. Diabetes Care 1992;15:820–825.
84. Kuusisto J, Mykkänen L, Pyörälä K, Laakso M. NIDDM and its metabolic control predict coronary heart disease in elderly subjects. Diabetes 1994;43:960–967.
85. Kwaan HC. Changes in blood coagulation, platelet function, and plasminogen-plasmin system in diabetes (review). Diabetes 1992;41(Suppl 2):32–35.
86. Laakso M, Barrett-Connor E. Asymptomatic hyperglycemia is associated with lipid and lipoprotein changes favoring atherosclerosis. Arteriosclerosis 1989;9:665–672.
87. Laakso M, Sarlund H, Salonen R, et al. Asymptomatic atherosclerosis and insulin resistance. Arterioscler Thromb 1991;11:1068–1076.
88. Lebovitz HE. Effects of oral antihyperglycemic agents in modifying macrovascular risk factors in type 2 diabetes. Diabetes Care 1999;22:C41–C44.
89. Lehto S, Ronnemaa T, Haffner SM, et al. Dyslipidemia and hyperglycemia predict coronary heart disease events in middle-aged patients with NIDDM. Diabetes 1997;46:1354–1359.
89a. Lipid Research Clinics Program. The Lipid Research Clinics and Coronary Primary Prevention Trial results I: Reduction in incidence of coronary disease. JAMA 1984;251:351–364.
90. LIPID Research Study Group. The relationship of reduction in incidence of coronary heart disease to cholesterol lowering. The Lipid Research Clinics Coronary Primary Prevention Trial results. II. JAMA 1984;251:365–374.
91. Lundberg V, Stegmayr B, Asplund K, et al. Diabetes as a risk factor for myocardial infarction: population and gender perspectives. J Intern Med 1997;241:485–492.
92. Lyons TJ. Lipoprotein glycation and its metabolic consequences. Diabetes 1992;41(Suppl 2):67–73.
93. Lytle B, Loop FD, Cosgrove DM, et al. Long-term (5–12 years) serial studies of internal mammary artery and saphenous vein coronary bypass grafts. J Thorac Cardiovasc Surg 1985;80:258–278.
94. The Long-Term Intervention with Pravastatin in Ischaemic Disease (LIPID) Study Group. Prevention of cardiovascular events and death with pravastatin in patients with coronary heart disease and a broad range of initial cholesterol levels. N Engl J Med 1998;339:1349–1357.
95. Mak KH, Moliterno DJ, Granger CB, et al. Influence of diabetes mellitus on clinical outcome in the thrombolytic era of acute myocardial infarction. GUSTO-I Investigators. Global Utilization of Streptokinase and Tissue Plasminogen Activator for Occluded Coronary Arteries. J Am Coll Cardiol 1997: 30:171–179.
96. Malmberg K, Ryden L, Efendic S, et al. Randomized trial of insulin-glucose infusion followed by subcutaneous insulin treatment in diabetic patients with acute myocardial infarction (DIGAMI study): effects on mortality at 1 year. J Am Coll Cardiol 1995;26:57–65.
97. Marso SP, Ellis SG, Tuzcu M, et al. The importance of proteinuria as a determinant of mortality following percutaneous coronary revascularization in diabetics. J Am Coll Cardiol 1999;33:1269–1277.
98. Matsuda T, Morishita E, Jokaji H, et al. Mechanism on disorders of coagulation and fibinolysis in diabetes. Diabetes 1996;45(Suppl 3):S109–S110.
99. Melchior T, Kober L, Madsen CR, et al. Accelerating impact of diabetes mellitus on mortality in the years following an acute myocardial infarction. TRACE Study Group. Trandolapril Cardiac Evaluation. Eur Heart J 1999;20:973–978.
100. Miettinen H, Lehto S, Salomaa V, et al. Impact of diabetes on mortality after the first myocardial infarction. The FINMONICA Myocardial Infarction Register Study Group. Diabetes Care 1998;21:69–75.
101. Morris JJ, Smith LR, Jones RH, et al. Influence of diabetes and mammary artery grafting on survival after coronary bypass. Circulation 1991;84(Suppl. III):III-275–III-284.
102. Moss, SE, Klein, R, Klein BE, Meuer, SM. The association of glycemia and cause-specific mortality in a diabetic population. Arch Intern Med 1994;154:2473–2479.
103. Ohkkubo Y, Kishikawa H, Araki E, et al. Intensive insulin therapy prevents the progression of diabetic microvascular complications in Japanese patients with non-insulin-dependent diabetes mellitus: a randomized prospective 6-year study. Diabetes Res Clin Pract 1995;28:103–117.
104. O'Sullivan JJ, Conroy RM, Robinson K, et al. In-hospital prognosis of patients with fasting hyperglycemia after first myocardial infarction. Diabetes Care 1991;14:758–760.
105. Panzram G. Mortality and survival in type 2 (non-insulin dependent) diabetes mellitus. Diabetologia 1987;30:123–131.
106. Perry IJ, Wannamethee SG, Whincup PH, et al. Serum insulin and incident coronary heart disease in middle-aged British men. Am J Epidemiol 1996;144:224–234.

107. The Post Coronary Artery Bypass Graft Trial Investigators. The effect of aggressive lowering of low density lipoprotein cholesterol levels and low dose anticoagulation on obstructive changes in saphenous-vein coronary-artery bypass grafts. [published erratum appears in N Engl J Med 1997 Dec 18; 337(25): 1859]. N Engl J Med 1997;336:153–162.
108. Psaty BM, Heckbert SR, Koepsell TD, et al. The risk of myocardial infarction associated with anti-hypertensive drug therapies. JAMA 1995;274:620–625.
109. Pyörälä K. Relationship of glucose intolerance and plasma insulin to the incidence of coronary heart disease: results from 2 population studies in Finland. Diabetes Care 1972;2:131–141.
110. Pyörälä K, Savolainen E, Kaukola S, Haapakoski J. Plasma insulin as coronary heart disease risk factor: relationship to other risk factors and predictive value during 9-year follow-up of the Helsinki Policemen Study population. Acta Med Scand 1985;701(Suppl):38–52.
111. Pyörälä K, Pedersen TR, Kjekshus J, et al. Cholesterol lowering with simvastatin improves prognosis of diabetic patients with coronary heart disease. A subgroup analysis of the Scandinavian Simvastatin Survival Study (4S) [published erratum appears in Diabetes Care 1997 June;20(6):1048]. Diabetes Care 1997;20:614–620.
112. Rantala AO, Paivansalo M, Kauma H, et al. Hyperinsulinemia and carotid atherosclerosis in hypertensive and control subjects. Diabetes Care 1998;21:1188–1193.
113. Reaven GM. Role of insulin resistance in human disease. Diabetes 1988;37:1495–1507.
114. Riddle MC. Overview of current therapeutic options: session summary. Diabetes Care 1999;22:C76–C78.
115. Risum FL, Abdelnoor M, Svennevig JL, et al. Diabetes mellitus and morbidity and mortality risks after coronary artery bypass surgery. Scand J Thor Cardiovasc Surg 1996;30:71–75.
116. Rönnemaa T, Laakso L, Pyörälä K, et al. High fasting plasma insulin is an indicator of coronary heart disease in non-insulin-dependent diabetic patients and nondiabetic subjects. Arterioscler Thromb 1991;11:80–90.
117. Rubins HB, Robins SJ, Collins D, et al., for the Veterans Affairs High-Density Lipoprotein Cholesterol Intervention Trial Study Group. Gemfibrozil for the secondary prevention of coronary heart disease in men with low levels of high-density lipoprotein cholesterol. N Engl J Med 1999;341:410–418.
118. Sacks FM, Pfeffer MA, Moye LA, et al. The effect of pravastatin on coronary events after myocardial infarction in patients with average cholesterol levels. Cholesterol and Recurrent Events Trial Investigators. N Engl J Med 1996;335:1001–1009.
119. Saloma V, Riley W, Kark JD, et al. Non-insulin dependent diabetes mellitus and fasting glucose and insulin concentrations are associated with arterial stiffness indexes: the Atherosclerosis Risk in Communities (ARIC) Study. Circulation 1995;91:1432–1443.
120. Saltiel AR, Olefsky JM. Thiazolidinediones in the treatment of insulin resistance and type II diabetes mellitus. Diabetes1996;45:1661–1669.
121. Scandinavian Simvastatin Survival Study (4S). Randomized trial of cholesterol lowering in 4444 patients with coronary heart disease: the Scandinavian Simvastatin Survival Study (4S). Lancet 1994;344:1383–1389.
122. SHEP Cooperative Research Group. Prevention of stroke by antihypertensive drug treatment in older persons with isolated systolic hypertension: final results of the Systolic Hypertension in the Elderly Program (SHEP). JAMA 1991;265:3255–3264.
123. Shepherd J, Cobbe M, Ford I, et al., for the West of Scotland Coronary Prevention Study Group. Prevention of coronary heart disease with pravastatin in men with hypercholesterolemia. N Engl J Med 1995;333:1301–1307.
124. Silva JA, Nunez E, White CJ, et al. Predictors of stent thrombosis after primary stenting for acute myocardial infarction. Cathet Cardiovasc Intervent 1999;47:415–422.
125. Silva JA, Ramee SR, White CJ, et al. Primary stenting in acute myocardial infarction: influence of diabetes mellitus in angiographic results and clinical outcome. Am Heart J 1999;138:446–455.
126. Sowers JR. Insulin resistance, hyperinsulinemia, dyslipidemia, hypertension, and accelerated atherosclerosis. [Review] [97 refs]. J Clin Pharmacol 1992;32:529–535.
127. Stamler R, Stamler J. Asymptomatic hyperglycemia and coronary heart disease. J Chron Dis 1979;32:683–691.
128. Stamler J, Vaccaro I, Neaton JD, Wentworth D. Diabetes, other risk factors, and 12-yr cardiovascular mortality for men screened in the Multiple Risk Factor Intervention Trial. Diabetes Care 1993;16:434–444.
129. Steinberg D, Parthasarathy S, Carew TE, et al. Beyond cholesterol: modifications of low-density lipoprotein that increase its atherogenicity (Review) N Engl J Med 1989;320:915–924.

130. Stone PH, Muller JE, Hartwell T, et al. The effect of diabetes mellitus on prognosis and serial left ventricular function after acute myocardial infarction: contribution of both coronary disease and diastolic left ventricular dysfunction to the adverse prognosis. The MILIS Study Group. J Am Coll Cardiol 1989;14:49–57.
131. Stout RA. Insulin and atheroma: 20-yr perspective. Diabetes Care 1990;13;631–654.
132. Tatti P, Pahor M, Byrington RP, et al. Outcome results of the fosinopril versus amlodipine cardiovascular events randomized trial (FACET) in patients with hypertension and NIDDM. Diabetes Care 1998; 21:597–603.
133. Tuomilehto J, Rastenyte D, Birkenhager WH, et al. Effects of calcium-channel blockade in older patients with diabetes and systolic hypertension. Systolic Hypertension in Europe Trial Investigators. N Engl J Med 1999;340:677–684.
134. Turner R, Cull C, Holman R, for the United Kingdom Prospective Diabetes Study Group. United Kingdom Prospective Diabetes Study 17: a 9-year update of a randomized controlled trial on the effect of improved metabolic control on complications in non-insulin-dependent diabetes mellitus. Ann Intern Med 1996;124:136–145.
135. Tuttle KR, Phulman ME, Cooney SK, Short R. Urinary albumin and insulin as predictors of coronary artery disease: an angiographic study. Am J Kidney Dis 1999;34:918–925.
136. Tzargournis M, Chiles JM, Ryan JM, Skillman TG. Interrelationships of hyperinsulinism and hypertriglyceridemia in young patients with coronary heart disease. Circulation 1968;38:1156–1163.
137. UK Prospective Diabetes Study (UKPDS) Group. Intensive blood-glucose control with suphonylureas or insulin compared with conventional treatment and risk of complications in patients with type 2 diabetes (UKPDS 33). Lancet 1998;352:837–853.
138. UK Prospective Diabetes Study (UKPDS) Group. Effect of intensive blood-glucose control with metformin on complications in overweight patients with type 2 diabetes (UKPDS 34). Lancet 1998;352: 854–865.
139. UK Prospective Diabetes Study (UKPDS) Group. Tight blood pressure control and risk of macrovascular and microvascular complications in type 2 diabetes: (UKPDS 38). BMJ 1998;317(7160):703–713.
140. Walter DP, Gatling W, Houston AC, et al. Mortality in diabetic subjects: an eleven-year follow-up of a community-based population. Diabet Med 1994;11:968–973.
141. Welborn TA, Wearne K. Coronary heart disease incidence and cardiovascular mortality in Busselton with reference to glucose and insulin concentrations. Diabetes Care 1979;2:154–160.
142. Whitcomb RW, Saltiel AR. Thiazolidinediones. Exp Opin Invest Drugs 1995;4:1299–1309.
143. Wick G, Schett G, Amberger A, et al. Is atherosclerosis an immunologically mediated disease? Immunol Today 1995;16(1):27–33.
143a. Wilson PWF, Kannel WB. Epidemiology of hyperglycemia and atherosclerosis. In: Ruderman et al., eds. Hyperglycemia, Diabetes and Vascular Disease. Oxford, 1992, pp. 21–29.
144. Wilson PWF, D'Agostino RB, Levy D, et al. Prediction of coronary heart disease using risk factor categories. Circulation 1998;97:1837–1847.
145. Winegard DL, Barrett-Connor E, Crigui M, Suarez L. Clustering of heart disease risk factors in diabetic compared to non-diabetic adults. Am J Epidemiol 1983;117:19–26.
146. Winocour PD. Platelet abnormalities in diabetes mellitus. Diabetes 1992;41(Suppl 2):26–32.
147. Wong ND, Cupples LA, Ostfeld AM, et al. Risk factors for long-term coronary prognosis after initial myocardial infarction: the Framingham Study. Am J Epidemiol 1989;130:469–480.
148. Woodfield SL, Lundergan CF, Reiner JS, et al. Angiographic findings and outcome in diabetic patients treated with thrombolytic therapy for acute myocardial infarction: the GUSTO-I experience. J Am Coll Cardiol 1996;28:1661–1669.
149. Yudkin JS, Denver AE, Mohamed AV, et al. The relationships of concentrations of insulin and proinsulin-like molecules with coronary heart disease prevalence and incidence: a study of two ethnic groups. Diabetes Care 1997;20:1093–1100.

8

Exercise in the Prevention of Coronary Artery Disease

Gordon G. Blackburn, PHD

INTRODUCTION

Coronary artery disease (CAD) is a chronic, multifactor disease that has powerful contributing genetic components as well as strong lifestyle components that increase the risk for the development and progression of the disease. Risk factors for CAD have been historically divided into Nonmodifiable, Primary Modifiable, and Secondary Modifiable. The primary focus of medicine has been on the treatment of established CAD and preventive efforts have more aggressively addressed areas where direct pharmacological intervention is available *(1)* *(see* Table 1). This is especially evident with respect to hypertension, hyperlipidemia and anti-platelet aggregation therapy.

For centuries the medical community has supported the role of regular, moderate exercise as means of maintaining health and preventing disease. Scientific data, collected extensively in the last half of the twentieth century, has repeatedly validated this concept. Most studies have been underpowered and no one randomized clinical trial has definitively demonstrated the benefits of exercise in the prevention of CAD. However, the data supporting the benefits of exercise in reducing the risk of development and progression of CAD are so striking that multiple national health care agencies and organizations have issued recent position statements regarding the benefits and recommendations for regular physical activity as a strategy to reduce the risk of CAD. These have included the Centers for Disease Control and Prevention (CDC) *(2)*, American Heart Association (AHA) *(3)*, National Institutes of Health (NIH) *(4)*, Surgeon General *(5)*, and the American College of Sports Medicine *(6)*. So strong is the evidence of the association between sedentary living and the development of heart disease that the American Heart Association moved

From: *Contemporary Cardiology: Preventive Cardiology:*
Strategies for the Prevention and Treatment of Coronary Artery Disease
Edited by: J. Foody © Humana Press Inc., Totowa, NJ

Table 1
Estimates of Levels of Utilization
of Risk Reduction Measures Patients
Surviving an MI in the United States in 1996

Exercise (cardiac rehabilitation)	<10%
Smoking cessation	20%
Estrogen replacement (women)	20%
Cholesterol-lowering diet	20%
Cholesterol-lowering drug	30%
Beta blocker therapy	40%
ACE inhibitor therapy	60%
Aspirin therapy	70%

"sedentary lifestyle" into the Primary Modifiable risk category in 1992, stating that "inactivity increases the risk of CAD" and regular exercise can help to control blood lipid abnormalities, control obesity, independently but modestly lower blood pressure in the hypertensive patient, and lower coronary mortality (7). However, despite half a century of recurrent scientific findings outlining the benefits of exercise both for primary and secondary prevention, our society remains remarkably sedentary and the utilization of cardiac rehabilitation programs abysmally low. It has been estimated that 20% of the North American population is totally sedentary and 60% have no regular exercise. It has also been estimated that only 20–25% of the North American population exercise appropriately to achieve the desired benefits attributed to an active lifestyle.

EXERCISE AND PRIMARY PREVENTION

Modern epidemiological studies investigating the relationship between activity and the development of CAD began with the report by Morris and colleagues (8) looking at a large population of civil servants from England. The authors compared CAD rates between sedentary bus drivers and the more active conductors, who at that time walked throughout the double-decker buses collecting fares. Comparisons were also made between active postal workers, who walked, delivering letters, and the more sedentary clerks. In both groups, the active cohort had half the age-adjusted incidence for myocardial infarction (MI) and the sedentary cohort was at twice the risk for sudden or early death following an MI. Although these studies were later revealed to have significant design flaws, that may have accounted for a higher risk population being hired for the sedentary jobs, it suggested the positive relationship between regular activity and decreased risk of developing heart disease. However, as stated by Oberman (9), "The observed association between inactivity and CAD in the prospective studies could represent several possible hypotheses: (1) exercise protects against CAD, (2) exercise indirectly reduces the risk of CAD through changes in other risk factors, (3) subclinical disease prevents people from exercising vigorously at work or during leisure, (4) people predisposed to CAD prefer sedentary activities, or (5) social, cultural, and other factors determine both activity levels and likelihood of CAD." Although epidemiological studies cannot definitively determine a cause-and-effect relationship, if the first hypothesis is not true, one would expect to see variation in the benefits of exercise on the prevention of CAD between studies, the impact of exercise should disappear if other risk factors are not effected by exercise, changes in physical activity levels should not effect CAD risk, there should not be a dose-response effect of exercise on reduction of CAD and the relationship between physical activity and CAD should vary between cultures and job types.

A homogeneous lifestyle and standard of living with varying levels of occupational activity was studied in men and women living on kibbutzim (collective settlements) in Israel. Over 5000 men and 5000 women were studied to determine the relationship between activity and CAD risk. The population was divided into those who spent <80% of their work time seated and those who spent >80% of their work time seated. Although the active population had a higher caloric intake of food, there was no difference between cholesterol levels of the groups. The risk of MI was 2.5 times greater for the sedentary male and 1.8 times greater for the sedentary female. The sedentary kibbutz member was also at greater risk for death from CAD (2.0 times increase for males and 3.0 times increase for females). Controlling for life-style and select risk factors, the protective benefit of physical activity was supported (10).

The protective role of exercise was also supported in a large cohort of longshoremen, in the United States. This longitudinal study objectively measured energy requirements of various job tasks and tracked job assignments for four aged cohorts (35–44, 45–54, 55–64, and 65–74 yr of age at entry into the study in 1951). Tasks were classified into three categories: high (5.2–7.5 kcal/min), intermediate (2.4–5.0 kcal/min), and light (1.5–2.0 kcal/min). Subjects were contacted annually to evaluate job energy requirements and underwent repeated multiphase screening for cigarette smoking, hypertension, history of MI, obesity, abnormal glucose metabolism, and higher cholesterol level over a 21-yr time period. All subjects were followed for 22 yr or until age 75, or death. Over the follow-up period, less than 1% of participants were lost to follow-up.

The age-adjusted coronary death rates were 26.9, 46.3 and 49.0/10,000 work-years for those in the heavy, moderate, and light caloric output jobs, respectively. Cigarette smoking, hypertension, and history of a prior MI all added to the risk of a fatal heart attack. However, differences in mortality rates persisted after correction for risk factors for CAD by multiple logistic analysis. To account for a drop in activity level secondary to subclinical disease, men with job transfers within 6 mo of death were excluded from the analysis without effecting the relationship between higher activity level and lower CAD rates (11–13).

If a genetic predisposition exists, which excludes individuals prone to CAD from exercise, it could be argued that athletes should be at lower risk for CAD than nonathletes. However, if it is habitual activity that offers a protective effect, then regular daily activity, carried on throughout life should be a key factor in reducing CAD risk. Paffenbarger and colleagues (14) studied the relationship between college athleticism and postcollege physical exercise in 16,936 Harvard alumni. The physical exam records of students who entered Harvard between 1916 and 1950 were analyzed along with a questionnaire regarding postcollege physical activity. Physical activity was standardized based on specific activities and estimated weekly caloric expenditures were calculated. During the follow-up period from 1962–1972 there were 572 first-time heart attacks and from 1962–1978, 1413 total deaths. Student athletic participation did not predict low CAD risk, although habitual postcollege exercise did. A strong, inverse, dose-related correlation was observed between exercise level and death from all causes, cardiovascular disease (CVD) and respiratory disease, with individuals expending >2000 kcal/wk at the lowest risk. In addition, the exercise benefit was independent of other risk factors (smoking, obesity, weight gain, hypertension, and family history). Sedentary alumni (<2000 kcal/wk expended in activity) were at 49% greater risk for heart attack as compared to the most active alumni.

Summary papers, outlining the risk of sedentary lifestyle and increased risk of developing CAD were published in 1987 and 1990. The article by Powell and colleagues *(15)* reviewed 43 prospective studies that investigated the relationship between the primary risk for CAD and sedentary lifestyles. The quality of the study designs were evaluated and rated. The authors reported that for studies with good scientific design a strong inverse relationship between physical activity and CAD mortality was consistently observed, with the sedentary population being at twice the risk of the active population. In addition, they found the risk of a sedentary lifestyle to be similar to that of other risk factors, such as elevated cholesterol, cigarette smoking, and hypertension. The studies reported in Powell *(15)* were re-evaluated along with eight more recent studies using meta-analysis *(16)* and revealed similar findings regardless of whether activity was performed on the job or during leisure time.

Not only has daily activity been associated with a reduction in CAD risk, but fitness level has also been correlated with lower mortality levels from CAD. Ekelund and colleagues *(17)* reported on data from the Lipid Research Clinics in which 4276 men between the ages of 30 and 69 yr of age were followed for an average of 8.5 yr. For patients without clinical evidence of CAD and who were not taking cardiovascular drugs there was approximately a three-times greater risk of both cardiovascular and CAD death in the lower-fit group, even after adjustment for age and cardiovascular risk factors.

Most studies have focused on the benefits of exercise and fitness in reducing CAD risk in the male population. Blair and colleagues *(18)* evaluated the impact of fitness on both all-cause death, CAD death, and cancer death in 10,224 men and 3120 women. All individuals were relatively healthy, with no known CVD at entry into the study. Each individual underwent a physical exam, blood work, and a maximal treadmill exercise test. Based on the results of the exercise test, subjects were assigned to a fitness level, adjusted for age, and based on gender and treadmill time. Subjects were followed for an average of 8 yr, during which time there were 283 deaths in the group. Age-adjusted rates of death were calculated with a strong inverse relationship observed between fitness level and mortality. In comparison to the highest-fit group of men, the least-fit group had 3.4 times greater risk of all-cause death and for women the relationship was 4.7 times greater for the least-fit group. Lower mortality rates from CVD and cancer were also observed for both highest-fit men and women and the trends remained significant after adjustment for age, smoking, cholesterol, systolic blood pressure, fasting blood glucose level, family history of CAD, and follow-up interval. It was also observed that decline in death rates associated with higher fitness levels was more pronounced in the older individuals.

The benefit of regular activity for the elderly to reduce the risk of primary CVD was further supported by the recent findings from a follow-up study to the Honolulu Heart Program *(19)*, in which 707 nonsmoking retired men between the ages of 61 and 81 yr of age at entry into the study were evaluated for walking habits. The gentlemen were followed for 12 yr and the primary endpoint evaluated for this study was mortality. At the end of the study period, there were 208 deaths with a strong inverse relationship observed between distance walked and all-cause death, coronary heart disease (CHD) deaths as well as cancer deaths. Individuals who walked less than one mile per day had 1.8 times greater risk for all-cause death, 2.6 times greater risk for CHD death, and 2.4 times greater risk for cancer death as compared to those who walked greater than 2 miles per day. The inverse relationship between distance walked and mortality remained significant even after adjustment for age, overall activity levels, and other risk factors. These findings suggest that the benefits on activity is dose related and can be beneficial for older men.

Although point estimates of physical fitness have repeatedly demonstrated and increased risk associated with a low fitness level *(17,20–23)*, it can always be argued that genetic factors or subclinical disease limit fitness level and it is that relationship rather that fitness itself that accounts for the relationship with mortality. If changes in fitness over time were associated with changes in CAD risk, the cause-and-effect association between fitness and CAD would be strengthened. To test this hypothesis, Blair and colleagues *(24)* studied 9777 men who were initially seen for preventive physical exams that included an exercise test. The participants in the study ranged from 20–82 yr at intake. All subjects returned for a second exam and exercise test approximately 4.9 yr after the first visit and were followed an average of 5.1 yr after the second exam. Of the 9777 men, 6819 were classified as healthy and 2958 were classified as unhealthy because of prior MI, hypertension, diabetes, cancer, abnormal resting electrocardiogram, or abnormal exercise electrocardiogram. All subjects were followed throughout the study and the relationship between fitness change and mortality was evaluated.

Subjects who maintained a fit level at both exams had the lowest risk of mortality and those who were classified as least fit at both exams had the highest risk of mortality. This was true for all-cause as well as cardiovascular mortality. However, of greater significance is the fact that those who went from the unfit to fit category from the first exam to the second exam had a 44% reduction in all-cause mortality and a 52% reduction in cardiovascular mortality. The improvement in fitness was associated with a reduction in death rates even after adjusting for health status, age, and risk factors.

Longitudinal studies demonstrating an inverse relationship between fitness levels or activity patterns and coronary mortality strengthen the concept of a cause-and-effect relationship, but underlying genetic or early environmental biases cannot be controlled for. However, evaluation of activity and mortality in twin pairs can control for both of these issues. Such a study was conducted by Kujala and colleagues *(25)*. In this study same-sex twin pairs (7925 male and 7977 female) between the ages of 25–64 yr were followed for mortality from 1977–1994. Leisure-time physical activity level was evaluated by questionnaire in 1975 and again in 1981. Subjects were free of clinical disease at entry into the study and all subjects were able to exercise. Individuals were classified into one of three categories based on reported intensity and total volume of activity. Sedentary individuals reported no leisure time activity, whereas individuals who reported participating in activities at least as strenuous as vigorous walking, for at least 30 min on average per session and at least six times per month, were placed in the Conditioning category. All others were placed in the Occasional Exercise category.

Over the 17-year follow-up period, 1253 subjects died. After adjusting for age and sex, the conditioning exercisers had a 43% reduction in mortality compared to the sedentary group, which is similar to previous non-twin-pair study findings. However, a more detailed analysis of 434 discordant twin deaths (only one of the twin pair died during follow-up), there was a 56% reduction in all cause death favoring the conditioning exercisers over the sedentary individual and 34% reduction for the occasional exercisers. The benefits of physical exercise persisted after controlling for age, sex, and other predictors of mortality. Even when genetic and early life familial factors are controlled, a reduction in mortality is associated with chronically higher levels of activity.

EXERCISE AND SECONDARY PREVENTION

The role of exercise in individuals with documented CAD has been investigated extensively since the early 1970s with consistent findings with respect to safety, improved functional ability, and the relative reduction of both all-cause and cardiac mortality. However, all of the studies have been statistically underpowered with respect to mortality outcomes, limiting the statistical significance and clinical impact of exercise for individuals with CAD. It is estimated that only 11–38% of qualifying patients participate in cardiac rehabilitation programs (26).

Functional Capacity Improvement

An excellent summary of exercise trials in CAD patients is presented in the Clinical Practice Guidelines for Cardiac Rehabilitation (26). Fourteen randomized trials from the United States and 21 foreign trials were reviewed. Exercise training was found to improve functional level in patients with catheterization documented CAD, as well as following myocardial infarction, coronary artery bypass grafting and percutaneous transluminal coronary angioplasty. The extent of the improvement varied based on the frequency, intensity, and duration of exercise, as well as the time interval over which training was conducted. It is also important to note that no deterioration in exercise tolerance occurred in any patient who underwent exercise training.

Physical Training and Mortality

Numerous trials have been conducted in the United States and internationally, designed to look at exercise and mortality in a CAD population. However, only one trial focusing on activity had more than 1000 patients entering the exercise arm (27). This pales to the 3837 patients randomized to B-blocker or placebo in the Beta Blocker Heart Attack Trial (27a). Low patient numbers and few endpoints have limited the statistical significance of studies looking at exercise and CAD mortality.

Kentala reported one of the first randomized, controlled studies looking at exercise and mortality following myocardial infarction (28). One hundred and fifty-two patients, in a 6–8 wk event, were randomized to either exercise three times per week for 20 min per session or consultation once per week. In a 12-mo follow-up period there were 11 deaths in each of the groups.

Kallio and colleagues (29) reported on the results of a multifactorial intervention program of education, antismoking and dietary advice, discussions on psychosocial problems, and a supervised cycle activity program as compared to the usual care in 375 post-MI patients. The patients were randomized to the intervention group or usual care and followed for 3 yr. The cumulative mortality in the intervention group was 18.6% as compared with 29.4% in the usual care group ($p < 0.02$). This represented a 37% reduction in mortality for the treatment group.

The National Exercise and Heart Disease Project (30) was a multi-center study conducted in the United States. A total of 651 post-MI patients (2–36 mo postevent) were randomized to either usual care or exercise. The exercise prescription was set to 85% of the peak heart rate achieved on the entry exercise test. Exercising patients were monitored by electrocardiography for the first 8 wk and then were allowed to exercise in a supervised gym setting for the next 34 mo. The patients performed interval exercise in the lab for 24 min total and 15 min of steady-state aerobic activity in the gym, followed by 25 min of games. Patients were encouraged to exercise three times per week. At the end of the study period, the cumulative mortality rate for the exercise group was 4.6% vs. 7.3% for the control group. These differences were not statistically significant, but the exercise group had a 37% reduction in mortality.

A recent report on the 19-yr follow-up of long-term survival of patients in the National Exercise and Heart Disease Project revealed a steady decline in all-cause mortality risk estimates for the exercise group compared with the control subjects. The authors concluded that protective mechanisms associated with exercise may be short lived and suggested that to maintain the benefits of exercise it must be performed on a continuous, regular basis. Of note is the finding that for individuals who increased their functional capacity, regardless of study group, there was a consistent 8–14% reduction (per metabolic equivalent (MET) increase in all-cause mortality at every follow-up period *(31)*.

At the end of the 1980s, two meta-analyses were reported, each analyzing 21 randomized, controlled studies of cardiac rehabilitation and the impact on mortality. The findings of both studies were similar, revealing approximately a 20–25% relative reduction in mortality, both all-cause and cardiovascular, for the exercise group as compared to the control group after a 3-yr follow-up period *(32,33)*. The benefits in mortality were realized when exercise was started early after the event as well as late, but the benefit improved the longer the activity was maintained. No difference was observed between the exercise group and the control group for nonfatal infarcts at any follow-up period. The consistent, reproducible finding of reduced cardiac and all-cause mortality strongly argues for the increased use of regular activity as a component of any comprehensive risk reduction program.

Safety of Exercise

The benefits of regular, aerobic exercise has been repeatedly documented in both the primary and secondary preventive population. However, any truly effective therapeutic intervention must provide benefit without increasing morbidity or mortality. The most frequently voiced concerns regarding regular aerobic exercise is that it will precipitate or aggravate an orthopedic complication or trigger sudden death.

In a study reported by Panush and colleagues *(34)* 17 recreational runners, mean age 56 yr, were compared to age-matched, sedentary controls. There was no significant difference reported for problems with degenerative joint disease, osteoarthritis, joint pain, or joint swelling. For individuals with known osteoarthritis, regular, moderate intensity activity, such as walking, increased functional ability and, at the same time, decreased the amount of joint pain in the active participants as compared to sedentary subjects *(35)*. Overall, the incidence of injury in individuals involved in recreational activity, requiring medical care, has been estimated as low as 5% annually *(36)*.

Regular moderate intensity exercise is associated with decreased risk of cardiac mortality, and the incidence of sudden death associated with even vigorous exercise is low at one death/396,000 jogging-hours *(37)* or one sudden coronary death/25,000 marathoners/yr *(38)*. However, it is important to note that vigorous, high-intensity exercise does increase the risk of MI. Siscovick and colleagues studied 133 men with no known prior history of CAD, who experienced a primary cardiac arrest during vigorous activity *(39)*. For men with low levels of habitual physical activity, the relative risk of a cardiac arrest during vigorous exercise was 56 times greater than at other times. Even for men who were routinely active, the risk of cardiac arrest was increased 5 times during vigorous activity. However, the overall risk of cardiac risk (at rest and during vigorous exercise) was reduced by 40% for the routinely active male over the sedentary male, thus supporting the overall benefit of routine exercise and the underlying risk of vigorous physical activity. Similar findings were reported by Mittleman and colleagues (40), who found that there was a 5.9 times greater likelihood of experiencing a myocardial infarction after vigorous exercise (>6 METS), as compared to the likelihood of experiencing a myocardial infarction following less vigorous activity or no activity. In addition they found an inverse dose response relationship in risk with respect to routine frequency of exercise, ranging from 107 times increased relative risk for individuals who exercised less than once per week, to 2.4 times increased risk for individuals who exercised five or more times per week.

The relative safety of individualized, moderate intensity exercise has also been documented in individuals with known CAD. Based on a survey of 167 cardiac rehabilitation programs, covering 51,303 patients during the first half of the 1980s, VanCamp and Peterson reported only three deaths, 21 cardiac arrests, and eight nonfatal MIs (41). This equates to one cardiac arrest per 111,996 patient-hours, one MI per 293,990 patient-hours, and an amazingly infrequent one death per 783,972 patient-hours—the latter incidence being lower than that reported for sudden cardiac death associated with jogging for men with no known prior CAD (37). It is also important to note that there was no significant difference in the rates of events between patients who received continuous electrocardiogram monitoring or those who received intermittent monitoring. This suggests that it is the supervision of patients during individualized, moderate activity, rather than the extent of monitoring, that provides the safety during cardiac rehabilitation classes.

Initiating an Activity Program

The benefits of regular exercise are well documented and although the risk associated with exercise is relatively small, it is real. The risk of cardiovascular and orthopedic complications increase both as individual risk of CAD increases and as the intensity of exercise increases. Therefore, it is appropriate that individuals about to embark on a regular activity program undergo some form of screening to minimize exercise-related complications. The extent of the evaluation should be dependent on the age of the individuals, their health status and the intensity of the exercise they will engage in. The American College of Sports Medicine (ACSM) provides recommendations regarding screening evaluations and testing to guide health care providers involved in the development and administration of exercise prescriptions, outlined in Table 2 (42). It is important to note that for apparently healthy and asymptomatic at risk populations embarking on a moderate-intensity exercise program a medical examination or exercise testing is not recommended, thus removing a significant barrier for many individuals and not placing a major burden on the health care system.

With respect to exercise prescriptions, the graded-exercise test is conducted to provide far more information than simply the presence or absence of significant ST segment changes on the electrocardiogram or exertional angina. The MET level and rate-pressure product at onset of ST changes or symptoms, coupled with the heart rate and blood pressure response to exertion as well as an accurate determination of peak METS or onset/exacerbation of arrhythmias are all key variables to be considered and factored into the exercise prescription. It is also important to consider the impact of medications on the exercise response. Although it may be desirable to have beta blockers and nitrates held prior to

Table 2
ACSM Recommendations for Medical Examination
and Exercise Testing Prior to Participation and Physician Supervision of Exercise Tests

	Medical examination and clinical exercise test recommended prior to:				
	Apparently healthy		Increased risk[a]	Known disease[b]	
	Younger[c]	Older	no symptoms	symptoms	
Moderate exercise (40–60% $VO_{2\,max}$)	No	No	No	Yes	Yes
Vigorous exercise (>60% $VO_{2\,max}$)	No	Yes	Yes	Yes	Yes
	Physician supervision recommended during exercise test:				
	Apparently healthy		Increased risk	Known disease	
	Younger[c]	Older	no symptoms	symptoms	
Submaximal testing	No	No	No	Yes	Yes
Maximal testing	No	Yes	Yes	Yes	Yes

[a] Persons with 2 or more risk factors for CAD.
[b] Persons with known cardiac, pulmonary or metabolic disease
[c] <40 yr for men, <50 yr for women.

diagnostic exercise tests to improve sensitivity, to evaluate typical hemodynamic and chronotropic responses during exertion, it is desirable to have patients take all medications as normally prescribed prior to the graded exercise test.

Mode of exercise testing and conduct of exercise testing are also key factors to consider if the exercise test is to be used to designing activity guidelines. For most individuals, walking-type activity yields the highest functional capacity and peak heart rate. The same person who undergoes a maximal cycle test is likely to achieve approximately 85% of that recorded for the treadmill, with a peak heart rate of 95% that observed during the maximal walking test. For arm-crank exercise tests, the peak functional capacity falls even further, reaching only 50–70% of that measured on the treadmill. Peak heart rate also tends to be lower for arm exercise, as compared to treadmill exercise, reaching only 90% of the latter value (43). These changes in chronotropic response and functional level between modes should be factored in when designing exercise prescriptions to avoid excessive or ineffective intensities. Because of the differences in response between modalities, it is recommended that the primary exercise mode be employed as the exercise test modality whenever possible.

Test technique and patient population can also have a significant impact on the estimated functional capacity. Most standard nomograms used to estimate peak functional capacity from time and workload are based on young, healthy individuals who exercised without holding onto the treadmill bars (44). Although these nomograms have been shown to be accurate for healthy, young- to middle-aged populations without orthopedic limitations and not taking cardiac medications (45), a significant overprediction of functional capacity can occur for the senior, clinical population on medication (46,47). These overestimations can be exaggerated even more if patients are allowed to hold onto the handrails of the treadmill during exercise tests. Peak functional capacity can be overestimated by up to 31% if patients are allowed to pull or even hold onto the front handrail. To achieve the most accurate estimation of functional capacity and minimize patient risk, it is recommended that patients walk, lightly touching the side handrail for balance during the treadmill exercise test *(48,49)*.

Once the patient has been cleared to begin an exercise the specific components of the program can be addressed. Every activity session should be composed of a Warm-Up, Conditioning, and Cool-Down period *(42)*.

The Warm-Up period initiates the exercise session and includes static and range-of-motion stretches as well as low-level aerobic activity at 25–40% of the individual's functional ability. These activities are designed to avoid musculoskeletal injury and allow for gradual hemodynamic and physiologic adaptation to activity. The Warm-Up period should last between 5–15 min depending on the orthopedic, metabolic, or cardiovascular restrictions of the exercising population.

The focus of the exercise prescription is the Conditioning period. The Conditioning period must address six key factors, with the emphasis on each area effected by the overall goal of the activity program: frequency, intensity, mode, duration, rate of progression, and compliance.

FREQUENCY

Recent guidelines regarding activity recommend that for both cardiovascular benefit, overall risk reduction, and weight management, that exercise be conducted on most days of the week. However, the frequency can vary from only three times per week to multiple sessions per day. The goal of the program, the schedule of the individual, and their current level of fitness all impact on frequency. In general, activity must be performed at least three times per week to gain the desired benefit, no matter what the goal. At lower levels of fitness, it may be necessary to increase the frequency of activity to 5–7 d/wk to achieve a desirable caloric expenditure per week. For individuals with musculoskeletal or pulmonary limitations to activity or limited flexibility in their schedule, multiple sessions per day may be advisable. As a general rule exercise, for health purposes should be performed between a basal threshold of three times per week out to five times per week.

INTENSITY

Intensity of exercise is perhaps the hardest area to prescribe and monitor. It is also the most poorly understood component of the exercise prescription. It has been recommended that the exercise be performed at a "moderate" intensity. Based on the ACSM criteria, this would correspond to activities equivalent to 40–60% of peak oxygen uptake, with 40% appearing to be the threshold level below which no improvement in functional ability occurs. However, few individuals know their peak oxygen uptake and in apparently healthy, asymptomatic patients, the need for an exercise test is not indicated *(42)*.

Exercise intensity can be determined in several ways. One of the most common methods is based on a standard, linear, age dependent chronotropic response to exercise. This assumes a standard age dependent peak heart rate and a linear relationship between oxygen uptake and heart rate. When both heart rate response and functional capacity are expressed as percentage of maximal ability, assuming rest levels to be baseline (i.e., resting heart rate equates to 0% and peak heart rate equates to 100%), the linear relationship can be assumed to be a 1:1 relationship, with the intercept passing through the origin. Therefore, when an individual is exercising at 60% of the heart rate reserve [(peak heart rate-resting heart rate) × 0.6) + resting heart rate] they are exercise at approximately 60% of their functional reserve *(50)*. For healthy individuals not taking cardiac medications this method can be helpful in determining the appropriate intensity of aerobic activity. Accuracy of pulse palpation is critical to the utility of this method and individuals unfamiliar with this skill are likely to require brief training. For those not interested in, or capable of, palpating their pulse, the development of accurate heart rate monitors that easily provide constant pulse monitoring provides and alternative method to monitor exercise heart rate responses.

For individuals with documented coronary disease or symptoms in whom an exercise test is recommended prior to initiating an exercise program, the individual heart rate response to activity and actual peak heart rate can be determined. This provides the health care provider developing the exercise prescription with the information necessary to individualize the target heart rate range for exercise. The prescription is more specific to the patient's responses to activity, especially if the patient took all medications as normally prescribed, prior to the exercise test.

Intensity can also be determined based on a more subjective, quantified approach, related to the individual's perception of exercise effort. The Rating of Perceived Exertion (RPE) scales were developed by Borg *(51,52)*. The scales provide numeric values with word anchors that the patient uses to rate the level of exertion they perceive for any given activity. The scales include the older, linear 6–20-point scale, based on the relationship between heart rate and perceived exertion and the newer logarithmic scale ranging from 0–10. Both scales are widely used and correlate well with the relative level of exertion. At an exercise intensity of 50–85% of oxygen uptake, most subjects rate the activity between 12 and 16 ("LIGHT" to "HARD"). On the 10-point scale a similar level of exertion would correspond to 3–6 ("MODERATE" to "HARD").

The RPE method of guiding exercise intensity can be quickly introduced to an individual and can be easily applied during any type of activity. Although there are certain populations who rate activity disproportionately low or high as compared to the actual relative cost *(53)*, for most individuals the RPE can effectively guide exercise intensity across a variety of exercise modalities *(54)*.

For individuals undergoing a graded exercise test, the exercise intensity can be set based on the functional capacity or METS predicted or measured. The relative exercise intensity range should be at least the threshold level of 40% and can range up to 85% of functional reserve, based on the goal of the program, the interest of the patient, and the patient's ability. The majority of individuals receiving optimal return on their effort at intensities between 60 and 75% of functional ability.

To prescribe activities based on METS requires a good understanding of exercise and work physiology so that comparable work levels can be calculated or identified for a variety of modalities. Tables outlining the MET cost of a variety of activities have been published to aid the clinician or exercising individual to identify the cost of activities. One such table is displayed here, dividing activities into three categories based on MET ranges (*see* Table 3).

MODE

For both primary and secondary preventive care the mode of activity recommended is one that is aerobic or rhythmical and repetitive in nature and uses large muscle groups and satisfies the necessary intensity requirement. There is no one mode of activity that is 'best', other than the best activities are the ones that satisfy the components of the exercise prescription for the individual and are engaged in routinely. Common exercise modalities are included in Table 3.

Table 3
Physical Activities Grouped by MET Ranges

A 3–4 METS	B 5–6 METS	C 7–8 METS
Cycling <8 mph	Cycling 8–10 mph	Cycling 11–12 mph
Cycling, stationary— very light effort	Cycling, stationary— light effort	Cycling, stationary— moderate effort
Dancing, slow pace (aerobic, ballroom)	Dance, moderate pace (folk, square, ballet)	Dancing, quick pace
Rowing, stationary 10 mph	Rowing, stationary 15 mph	Rowing, stationary 20 mph
Tennis, table	Tennis, doubles	Tennis, singles
Walking, level 2–3.5 mph	Walking 3.6–4.5 mph	Walk/jog intervals
Water aerobics/walking	Swimming, leisure	Walking upstairs/stair stepper
Bowling	Baseball/softball, nongame	Swimming, laps
Billiards	Basketball, nongame	Baseball/softball game
Croquet	Cross-country skiing <3 mph	Basketball game
Golf, driving range, riding cart	Golf, carrying, pulling clubs	Canoeing, 2–5 mph
Horseback riding, walk	Sailing, small boat	Cross-country skiing, 3–4 mph
Horseshoe pitching	Skiing, downhill, beginner, moderate effort	Hiking
Shuffleboard	Volleyball	Horseback riding, trot
Gardening, light (hand tools, planting)	Gardening, moderate (power tools, dig, rake, hoe)	Hockey, ice and/or field
Grass cutting, riding mower	Grass cutting, push power mower	In-line skating, slow
Housework, general cleaning woodwork	Hunting, small-game, light effort	Racquetball/paddleball, Car washing
		Grass cutting, push handmower
		Hunting, big game (no carcass dragging)
		Wood chopping

DURATION

A minimum of 30 min of aerobic activity per day is recommended. Again the goal of the program and the individual's exercise history, functional ability and schedule will all effect the daily duration. One of the goals of most exercise programs, from a preventive standpoint, is to increase the weekly caloric expenditure, targeting ≥2000 kcal/wk. It will likely be necessary for sedentary individuals to gradually ramp up to this level, which can be accomplished by starting at the 30-min/session level and gradually increasing the duration until the target is accomplished. The frequency of activity will also impact weekly caloric expenditure. Assuming a fixed intensity, more frequent exercise can be conducted for a shorter time period at each session and still achieve the same weekly caloric expenditure.

Recently, emphasis has been directed at the potential benefits of multiple, shorter sessions per day. For some individuals, three 20-min sessions/d may be easier to accomplish than one 60-min session. Certainly, multiple shorter sessions can provide benefit, but the threshold duration for each interval is unclear. Divided intervals of no shorter than 15 min each is recommended.

RATE OF PROGRESSION

As individuals embark on exercise programs, it is important to avoid overly aggressive progression of the exercise program. The rate of progression will depend on the individual's past exercise history, level of conditioning, comorbid conditions, and age. In general the sedentary, deconditioned, elderly patient with multiple comorbid conditions, will require longer to adapt to the activity and progression, in absolute terms, will be slower. Ratings of Perceived Exertion and target heart rate ranges can be helpful in determining individual adaptation and targeting progression.

For the first several months in a program, progression will be somewhat rapid. However, after the first 4–6 mo of exercise, progression will slow as the individual enters a maintenance phase *(42)*.

COMPLIANCE

The benefits of appropriate, regular aerobic exercise, both in primary and secondary prevention patients, have been documented previously in this chapter. The key is that the activity be performed long term, however. Compliance with cardiac rehabilitation programs, a population that could be expected to be more highly motivated than those without known disease, has a compliance rate of 50–75% after 6 mo. To optimize compliance it is necessary to develop activity plans that mesh with the individual's lifestyle and have a minimum number of barriers. In addition to education regarding the benefits of regular exercise, Oldridge recommends that compliance enhancing strategies should include reinforcement control, stimulus control and cognitive/self control procedures *(55)*.

Each activity session should conclude with the Cool-Down period. This is essentially the opposite of the Warm-Up period, allowing the body to gradually transition from the more vigorous Conditioning period to rest. During the Cool-Down activity should be gradually tapered down, rather than abruptly terminated. This prevents venous pooling, hypotension, and an abrupt, relative catecholamine surge that can cause arrhythmias. The Cool-Down period usually lasts from 3–10 min.

SUMMARY

Although no single large, prospective trial has been conducted to decisively demonstrated the benefits of exercise in both the primary and secondary preventive population, the preponderance of the research supports the benefit in reducing future cardiovascular risk. The mechanism or mechanisms through which physical activity reduces this risk of either developing or dying form CAD are unclear. Regardless of the mechanism, it is apparent that regular, aerobic activity should be addressed and optimized in all CAD preventive strategies. Development of an effective exercise program is likely to require more than a casual recommendation. Patients should be appropriately screened, based on their individual risk of complications associated with exercise and individualized programs addressing frequency, intensity, mode, duration and progression should be provided. In addition, as with all lifestyle and risk reduction strategies, strategies to optimize long-term compliance should be incorporated into the management plan.

REFERENCES

1. Pearson TA, Peters TD. The treatment gap in coronary artery disease and heart failure: community standards and the post-discharge patient. Am J Cardiol 1997;80:45H–52H.
2. Pate RR, Pratt M, Blair SM, et al. Physical activity and public health: a recommendation from the Centers for Disease Control and Prevention and the American College of Sports Medicine. JAMA 1995; 273:402–407.
3. Fletcher GF, Balady G, Blair SN, et al. Statement on exercise: benefits and recommendations for physical activity programs for all Americans. A statement for health professionals by the committee on exercise and cardiac rehabilitation of the council on clinical cardiology, American Heart Association. Circulation 1996;94:857–862.
4. NIH Consensus Conference. Physical activity and cardiovascular health. JAMA 1996;276:241–246.
5. Department of Health and Human Services. Physical Activity and Health: a Report for the Surgeon General: U.S. Department of Health and Human Services, Centers for Disease Control and Prevention, National Center for Chronic Disease Prevention and Health Promotion, 1996.
6. Pollock ML, Gaesser GA, Butcher JD, et al. The recommended quantity and quality of exercise for developing and maintaining cardiorespiratory and muscular fitness, and flexibility in health adults. Med Sci Sports Exere 1998;30:975–991.
7. Fletcher AF, Blair SN, Blumenthal J, et al. Statement on exercise: benefits and recommendations for physical activity programs for all Americans. Circulation 1992;86:340–344.
8. Morris JN, Heady JA, Raffle PAB, et al. Coronary heart disease and physical activity of work. Lancet 1953;2:1053–1057, 1111–1120.
9. Oberman A. Exercise and the primary prevention of cardiovascular disease. Am J Cardiol 1985;55: 10D–20D.
10. Brunner D, Manelis G, Modan M, Levin S. Physical activity at work and the incidence of myocardial infarction, angina pectoris and death due to ischemic heart diasease: an epidemiologiical study in Israeli collective settlements (kibbutzim). J Chronic Dis 1974;27:217–233.
11. Paffenbarger RS, Hale WE. Work activity and coronary heart mortality. N Engl J Med 1975;292: 545–550.
12. Paffenbarger RS, Hale WE, Brand RJ, Hyde RT. Work-energy level, personal characteristics and fatal heart attack: a birth-cohort effect. Am J Epidemiol 1977;105:200–213.
13. Brand RJ, Paffenbarger RS, Sholtz RI, Kampert JB. Work activity and fatal heart attack studied by multiple logistic risk analysis. Am J Epidemiol 1979;110:52–62.
14. Paffenbarger RS, Hyde RT, Wing AL, Steinmetz CH. A natural history of athleticism and cardiovascular health. JAMA 1984;252:491–405.
15. Powell KE, Thompson PD, Caspersen CJ, Kendrick JS. Physical activity and the incidence of coronary heart disease. Ann Rev Public Health 1987;8:253–287.
16. Berlin JA, Colditz GA. A meta-analysis of physical activity in the prevention of coronary heart disease. Am J Epidemiol 1990;132:612–628.
17. Ekelund LG, Haskell WL, Johnson JL, et al. Physical fitness as a predictor of cardiovascular mortality in asymptomatic North American men. The Lipid Research Clinics Mortality Follow-up Study. N Engl J Med 1988;319:1379–1384.
18. Blair SN, Hohl HW, Paffenbarger RS, et al. Physical fitness and all-cause mortality: a prospective study of healthy men and women. JAMA 1989;262:2395–2401.
19. Hakim AA, Petrovitch H, Burchfiel CM, et al. Effects of walking on mortality among nonsmoking retired med. N Engl J Med 1998;338:94–99.
20. Bruce RA, Hossack KF, DeRouen TA, Hofer V. Enhanced risk assessment for primary coronary heart disease events by maximal exercise testing: 10 years' experience of Seattle Heart Watch. J Am Coll Cardiol 1983;2:565–573.
21. Erikssen J. Physical fitness and coronary heart disease morbidity and mortality: a prospective study in apparently healthy, middle-aged men. Acta Med Scand Suppl 1986;711:189–192.
22. Lie H, Mundal R, Erikssen J. Coronary risk factors and incidence of coronary death in relation to physical fitness: seven year follow-up study of middle-aged and elderly men. Eur Heart J 1985;6:147–157.
23. Sandvik L, Erikssen J, Thaulow E, et al. Physical fitness as a predictor of mortality among healthy, middle-aged Norwegian men. N Engl J Med 1993;328:533–537.
24. Blair SN, Kohl HW, Barlow CE, et al. Changes in physical fitness and all-cause mortality: a prospective study of healthy and unhealthy men. JAMA 1995;273:1093–1098.

25. Kujala UM, Kaprio J, Sarna S, Koskenvuo M. Relationship of liesure-time physical activity and mortality: the Finnish twin cohort. JAMA 1998;279:440–444.
26. Wenger NK, Froelicher ES, Smith LK, et al. Cardiac Rehabilitation. Clinical Practice Guideline No. 17. Rockville, MD: US Department of Health and Human Services, Public Health Service, Agency for Health Care Policy and Research, National Heart, Lung, and Blood Institute, 1995.
27. Lamm G, Denolin H, Dorossiev D, Pisa Z. Rehabilitation and secondary prevention of patients after acute myocardial infarction. Adv Cardiol 1982;31:107–111.
27a. Beta Blocker Heart Attack Trial. A randomized trial of propranolol in patients with acute myocardial infarction. I. Mortality results. JAMA 1982;26:247(12):1707–1714.
28. Kentala E. Physical fitness and feasibility of physical rehabilitation after myocardial infarction in men of working age. Ann Clin Res 1972;4(Suppl 9):1–84.
29. Kallio V, Hamalainen H, Hakkila J, Luurila OJ. Reduction in sudden deaths by a multifactorial intervention programme after acute myocardial infarction. Lancet 1979;2:1091–1094.
30. Shaw LW. Effects of a prescribed supervised exercise program on mortality and cardiovascular morbidity in patients after a myocardial infarction. The National Exercise and Heart Disease Project. Am J Cardiol 1981;48:39–46.
31. Dorn J, Naughton J, Imamura D, Trevisan M. Results of a multicenter randomized clinical trial of exercise and long-term survival in myocardial infarction patients. The National Exercise and Heart Disease Project (NEHDP). Circulation 1999;100:1764–1769.
32. Oldridge NB, Guyatt GH, Fischer ME, Rimm AA. Cardiac rehabilitation after myocardial infarction: combined experience of randomized clinical trials. JAMA 1988;260:945–950.
33. O'Connor GT, Burnig JE, Yusuf S, et al. An overview of randomized trials of rehabilitation with exercise after myocardial infarction. Circulation 1989;80:234–244.
34. Panush RS, Schmidt C, Caldwell JR, et al. Is running associated with degenerative joint disease? JAMA 1986;255:1152–1154.
35. Kovar PA, Allegrante JP, MacKenzie CR, et al. Supervised fitness walking in patients with osteoarthritis of the knee. Ann Intern Med 1992;116:529–534.
36. Blair S, Kohl H, Goodyear N. Rates and risks for running and exercise injuries: studies in three populations. Res Q Exer Sports 1987;58:221–228.
37. Thompson PD, Funk EJ, Carleton RA, Sturner WQ. Incidence of death during jogging in Rhode Island from 1975 through 1980. JAMA 1982;247:2535–2538.
38. Noakes TD. Heart disease in marathon runners: a review. Med Sci Sports Exer 1987;19:187–194.
39. Siskovick DS, Weiss NS, Fletcher, RH, Lasky T. The incidence of primary cardiac arrest during vigorous exercise. N Engl J Med 1994;311:874–877.
40. Mittleman MA, Maclure M, Tofler GH, et al. Triggering of acute myocardial infarction by heavy physical exertion: protection against triggering by regular exertion. N Engl J Med 1993;329:1677–1683.
41. VanCamp SP, Peterson RA. Cardiovascular complications of outpatient cardiac rehabilitation programs. JAMA 1986;256:1160–1163.
42. American College of Sports Medicine. ACSM's Guidelines for Exercise Testing and Prescription 5th ed. Williams & Wilkins, Baltimore, MD, 1995, p. 373.
43. Blackburn GG. Cardiorespiratory responses to six-week limb-specific exercise conditioning programs: The Pennsylvania State University, 1984.
44. Bruce RA, Kusumi F, Hosmer D. Maximal oxygen intake and nomographic assessment of functional aerobic impairment on cardiovascular disease. Am Heart J 1973;85:546–562.
45. Blackburn G, Harvey S, Wilkoff B. A chronotropic assessment exercise protocol to assess the nedd and efficacy of rate responsive pacing. Med Sci Sports Exer 1988;20:S21.
46. Sullivan M, McKirnan MD. Errors in predicting functional capacity for postmyocardial infarction patients using a modified Bruce protocol. Am Heart J 1984;107:486–492.
47. Houghson RL, Smyth GA. Slower adaptation of VO_2 to steady state of submaximal exercise with beta adrenergic blockade. Eur J Appl Physiol 1983;52:107–110.
48. McConnell TR, Clark BA. Prediction of maximal oxygen consuption during handrail-supported treadmill exercise. J Cardiopulm Rehabil 1987;7:324–331.
49. Zeimetz G, McNeill J, Hall J, Moss R. Quantifiable changes in oxygen uptake, heart rate, and time to target heart rate when handrail support is allowed during treadmill exercise. J Cardiopulm Rehabil 1985; 5:525–539.
50. Wilkoff B, Corey J, Blackburn G. A mathematical model of the cardiac chronotropic response to exercise. J Electrophysiol 1989;3:176–180.

51. Borg GA. Physiological bases of perceived exertion. Med Sci Sports Exer 1982;14:377–381.
52. Borg G, Linderholm H. Perceived exertion and pulse rate during graded exercise in various age groups. Acta Med Scand 1967;472:194–206.
53. Brubaker PH, Rejeski WJ, Law HC, et al. Cardiac patients' preception of work intensity during graded exercise testing: do they generalize to field settings? J Cardiopulm Rehabil 1994;14:127–133.
54. Robertson RJ, Goss FL, Auble TE, et al. Cross-modal exercise prescription at absolute and relative oxygen uptake using perceived exertion. Med Sci Sports Exer 1990;22:653–659.
55. Oldbridge NB, Pashkow FJ. Adherence and motivation in cardiac rehabilitation. In: Pashkow FJ, Dafoe WA, eds. Clinical Cardiac Rehabilitation: a Cardiologist's Guide. Williams and Wilkins, Baltimore, MD, 1999, pp. 467–503.

9

Obesity and Coronary Artery Disease

Implications and Interventions

Kristine Napier, MPH, RD

CONTENTS

INTRODUCTION

Obesity increases the risk of disease and death. With now one-third of Americans classified as obese *(1,2)*, and the prevalence increasing, it is evident that obesity and its consequences have become one of the country's most urgent health care concerns. As we move into the 21st century, obesity-induced diseases will claim an increasing percentage of health care resources, as well as medical efforts.

It has been clearly demonstrated that obesity greatly increases the risk of diabetes mellitus, hypertension, dyslipidemia, coronary artery disease (CAD) *(3)*, and some cancers. Women who are more than 40% overweight have higher rates of fatal endometrial, ovarian, cervical, breast, and gallbladder cancers *(4)*. According to the American Cancer Society, increasing weight is directly related to risk of cancer in men who have never smoked.

This chapter discusses the relationship of obesity to coronary artery disease (CAD), reviewing the epidemiological evidence that obesity increases the potency of risk factors for CAD. Although there has been general agreement that extreme obesity increases the risk of CAD as well as all-cause mortality *(5)*, it is only in more recent years that there is a consensus that even modest degrees of weight gain and obesity significantly increase the risk of CAD. The chapter also reviews the proposed mechanisms by which obesity inflates these risks, and the association of body fat distribution vs. total body fat content to CAD risk. The chapter concludes with practical and candid strategies for weight reduction.

From: *Contemporary Cardiology: Preventive Cardiology:*
Strategies for the Prevention and Treatment of Coronary Artery Disease
Edited by: J. Foody © Humana Press Inc., Totowa, NJ

DEFINITION AND PREVALENCE OF OBESITY

Officially in the United States a person is said to be obese when body mass index (BMI) exceeds 27.8 kg/m^2 in men and 27.3 kg/m^2 in women (1), which corresponds to 120% of desirable body weight (6). According to these standards, the National Health and Nutritional Examination Survey found 24% of adult men and 28% of adult women to be obese in the survey period from 1978–1980 (7). Just a decade later, in the survey period from 1988–1991, the percentages rose alarmingly to 31% and 34%, respectively (1,8). Prevalence varies by race, with rates considerably higher among black women and Hispanics of both genders (1,9).

It is important to differentiate between the official definition of obesity and the metabolic point in time at which being overweight contributes to CAD risk. The latter occurs at lower body weights than are defined by the official definitions of obesity, especially with central or truncal adiposity. Taking into account such metabolic consequences, it seems more appropriate to define three stages of obesity and institute more aggressive weight loss strategies accordingly. According to these more aggressive standards, a person is said to be moderately obese when BMI is in the range of 25–26.9; obese when BMI is 27–30.9; and markedly obese when BMI equals or exceeds 31 (10).

Refer to Tables 1–3 for ideal body weights, and Table 4 for BMIs; BMI is a far more powerful tool in describing how body weight impacts disease risk.

Weight patterning, or fat distribution, can lower the threshold at which the cardiovascular consequences of adiposity begin. Persons with truncal or central adiposity are at significantly greater risk, as will be discussed shortly. In addition, in persons genetically predisposed to cardiovascular disease, gaining weight accentuates their genetically programmed risk factors, rendering weight gain for them of far greater consequence (11). For example, a certain subset of genetically susceptible people will become hypertensive upon gaining weight; another dyslipidemic; and another will acquire type 2 diabetes, each a potent risk factor for CAD.

METABOLIC COMPLICATIONS OF OBESITY

Many of the metabolic abnormalities engendered by obesity occur in the cardiovascular system, increasing the risk for developing CAD. The major metabolic changes, and therefore risk factors, for CAD resulting from obesity include:

1. Atherogenic dyslipidemia, which includes
    a. Elevated total cholesterol
    b. Increased serum triglyceride
    c. Decreased low-density lipoprotein (LDL) particle size
    d. Reduced serum high-density lipoprotein (HDL)
2. Hypertension
3. Insulin resistance and glucose intolerance
4. Abnormalities in the coagulation system (procoagulant state) (12)

Some investigators believe that insulin resistance is the root cause of this group of risk factors; hence, they favor the term *insulin resistance syndrome (13–15)*. A reduction in insulin sensitivity, however, may be but one of several abnormalities resulting from a generalized metabolic derangement induced by obesity. Thus, a more generic term for the syndrome of multiple metabolic risk factors, *metabolic syndrome (12)* seems more

Table 1
Desirable Weights for Men

Height Without Shoes	Frame Size*	Desirable Weight (pounds)	Overweight (≥20% over desirable weight)	Obese (≥30% over desirable weight)
5'5"	Small	124-133	≥155	≥168
5'5"	Medium	130-143	≥164	≥178
5'5"	Large	138-156	≥176	≥191
5'6"	Small	128-137	≥160	≥173
5'6"	Medium	134-147	≥169	≥183
5'6"	Large	142-161	≥182	≥198
5'7"	Small	132-141	≥164	≥178
5'7"	Medium	138-152	≥174	≥189
5'7"	Large	147-156	≥188	≥204
5'8"	Small	136-145	≥169	≥183
5'8"	Medium	142-156	≥179	≥194
5'8"	Large	151-170	≥193	≥209
5'9"	Small	140-150	≥174	≥189
5'9"	Medium	146-160	≥184	≥200
5'9"	Large	155-174	≥198	≥214
5'10"	Small	144-154	≥179	≥194
5'10"	Medium	150-165	≥190	≥205
5'10"	Large	159-179	≥203	≥220
5'11"	Small	148-158	≥184	≥199
5'11"	Medium	154-170	≥194	≥211
5'11"	Large	164-184	≥209	≥226
6'0"	Small	152-162	≥188	≥204
6'0"	Medium	158-175	≥200	≥217
6'0"	Large	168-189	≥215	≥233
6'1"	Small	156-167	≥194	≥211
6'1"	Medium	162-180	≥205	≥222
6'1"	Large	173-194	≥221	≥239
6'2"	Small	160-171	≥199	≥216
6'2"	Medium	167-185	≥211	≥229
6'2"	Large	178-199	≥227	≥246
6'3"	Small	164-175	≥204	≥221
6'3"	Medium	172-190	≥217	≥235
6'3"	Large	182-204	≥232	≥302

*Use Table 3 to calculate frame size. Adapted from ref. *(16)*.

appropriate and is used in this chapter to denote the constellation of risk factors commonly associated with obesity.

The genesis of metabolic syndrome begins with energy imbalance leading to energy overload, which results in excess fat being stored inertly in adipose tissue *(17–19)*. But an energy overload state also results in high fasting concentrations of nonesterified fatty

Table 2
Desirable Weights for Women

Height Without Shoes	Frame Size*	Desirable Weight (pounds)	Overweight (≥20% over desirable weight)	Obese (≥30% over desirable weight)
5'0"	Small	102-110	≥127	≥138
5'0"	Medium	107-119	≥136	≥147
5'0"	Large	115-131	≥148	≥160
5'1"	Small	105-113	≥131	≥142
5'1"	Medium	110-122	≥139	≥151
5'1"	Large	118-134	≥151	≥164
5'2"	Small	108-116	≥134	≥146
5'2"	Medium	113-126	≥143	≥155
5'2"	Large	121-138	≥155	≥168
5'3"	Small	111-119	≥138	≥150
5'3"	Medium	116-130	≥148	≥160
5'3"	Large	125-142	≥160	≥173
5'4"	Small	114-123	≥142	≥153
5'4"	Medium	120-135	≥152	≥165
5'4"	Large	129-146	≥164	≥178
5'5"	Small	118-127	≥146	≥159
5'5"	Medium	124-139	≥157	≥170
5'5"	Large	133-150	≥169	≥183
5'6"	Small	122-131	≥151	≥164
5'6"	Medium	128-143	≥162	≥176
5'6"	Large	137-154	≥174	≥188
5'7"	Small	126-135	≥156	≥169
5'7"	Medium	132-147	≥167	≥181
5'7"	Large	141-158	≥179	≥194
5'8"	Small	130-140	≥162	≥176
5'8"	Medium	136-151	≥172	≥186
5'8"	Large	145-163	≥185	≥200
5'9"	Small	134-144	≥167	≥181
5'9"	Medium	140-155	≥176	≥191
5'9"	Large	149-168	≥190	≥205
5'10"	Small	138-148	≥172	≥186
5'10"	Medium	144-159	≥181	≥196
5'10"	Large	153-173	≥196	≥212

*Use Table 3 to calculate frame size. Adapted from ref. *(16)*.

acids. Several tissues bear the brunt of the effects of excess nonesterified fatty acids, including skeletal muscle; it is the major site of nonesterified fatty acid utilization *(18)*. According to Randle and colleagues *(20)*, increased muscle uptake of nonesterified fatty acids in obese persons shifts energy utilization from carbohydrates to fatty acids. This shift leads to resistance to the action of insulin in muscle *(21,22)*, which creates a tendency for hyperglycemia.

Table 3
Frame Size According to Wrist Measurement

Height in inches	Wrist size in inches that indicates small frame	Wrist size in inches that indicates medium frame	Wrist size in inches that indicates large frame
Under 5'3"	Less than 5 1/2"	5 1/2"–5 3/4"	Greater than 5 3/4"
5'3" to 5'4"	Less than 6"	6"–6 3/4"	Greater than 6 1/4"
Over 5'4"	Less than 6 1/4"	6 1/4"–6 1/2"	Greater than 6 1/2"

Adapted from ref. *(16)*.

In turn, peripheral insulin resistance secondary to obesity is accompanied by hyper-insulinemia *(23,24)*. High nonesterified fatty acid concentrations may act directly on the pancreatic β-cells to prime them for enhanced insulin secretion in response to any given increasing serum glucose concentration *(25)*. Prolonged overstimulation of insulin secretion by β-cells may eventually impair β-cell function, thereby reducing insulin secretion and leading to type 2 diabetes *(26,27)*.

A third major target of energy overload is the liver *(28–31)*. The increased concentration of very-low-density lipoprotein (VLDL) particles entering the bloodstream raise both plasma triglycerol and cholesterol concentrations *(12,29)*. The higher triglycerol concentrations in turn cause the creation of smaller LDL particles *(32,33)* and decrease concentrations of HDL cholesterol *(34)*. In addition, obesity apparently increases the activity of hepatic triglycerol lipase *(35,36)*. This change may also reduce LDL particle size *(37)* and lower HDL cholesterol concentrations further *(38,39)*.

THE GENESIS OF OBESITY

The cause of obesity is multifaceted and complex, but shares a common global link: industrialization and the adoption of a Western lifestyle. This industrialization of Asia and even Africa and the Middle East show a trend toward obesity *(40–43)*. Asians, for example, have traditionally lived in rural environments with a lifestyle that supported a lean habitus: they commonly performed heavy physical labor and had a limited food supply. Their lifestyle is changing, however, as their societies grow more urbanized and industrialized. Today, with an increasingly generous food supply and decreasingly physical labor-intensive employment, their incidence of weight gain increases steadily *(44)*. In tandem is a steady and proportionate rise in several CAD risk factors, including LDL cholesterol, insulin resistance, and glucose intolerance, as well as a definite increased frequency of CAD *(45)*.

Although industrialization is a significant factor for weight gain around the world, increasing age is another. Certainly, the two causes are interrelated, with industrialization the root of some of the factors leading to the weight gain of aging. In the United States, the average American gains approximately 10 kg (22 lb) between age 20 and age 50 *(46)*. Several factors are thought to contribute to what has been termed the weight gain of aging, including a decline in metabolic rate, decreased physical activity, and genetics. Although at one time high-fat diets were thought to contribute to weight gain, this is now a point of considerable controversy.

The major reason for the well-documented age-associated decrease in resting metabolic rate (RMR) *(47–51)* is most likely the decline in muscle mass that also occurs with

Table 4
Body Mass Index and How to Calculate

Height (inches)	Body Mass Index*																
	19	20	21	22	23	24	25	26	27	28	29	30	31	32	33	34	35
	Normal Weight						Moderately Obese		Obese				Markedly Obese				
	Body Weight (pounds)																
58	91	96	100	105	110	115	119	124	129	134	138	143	148	153	158	162	167
59	94	99	104	109	114	119	124	128	133	138	143	148	153	158	163	168	173
60	97	102	107	112	118	123	128	133	138	143	148	153	158	163	168	174	179
61	100	106	111	116	122	127	132	137	143	148	153	158	164	169	174	180	185
62	104	109	115	120	126	131	136	142	147	153	158	164	169	175	180	186	191
63	107	113	118	124	130	135	141	146	152	158	163	169	175	180	186	191	197
64	110	116	122	128	134	140	145	151	157	163	169	174	180	186	192	197	204
65	114	120	126	132	138	144	150	156	162	168	174	180	186	192	198	204	210
66	118	124	130	136	142	148	155	161	167	173	179	186	192	198	204	210	216
67	121	127	134	140	146	153	159	166	172	178	185	191	198	204	211	217	223
68	125	131	138	144	151	158	164	171	177	184	190	197	203	210	216	223	230
69	128	135	142	149	155	162	169	176	182	189	196	203	209	216	223	230	236
70	132	139	146	153	160	167	174	181	188	195	202	209	216	222	229	236	243
71	136	143	150	157	165	172	179	186	193	200	208	215	222	229	236	243	250
72	140	147	154	162	169	177	184	191	199	206	213	221	228	235	242	250	258
73	144	151	159	166	174	182	189	197	204	212	219	227	235	242	250	257	265
74	148	155	163	171	179	186	194	202	210	218	225	233	241	249	256	264	272
75	152	160	168	176	184	192	200	208	216	224	232	240	248	256	264	272	279
76	156	164	172	180	189	197	205	213	220	230	238	246	254	263	271	279	287

*Body Mass Index (BMI) is usually measured with the Quetelet index as follows: weight divided by height squared (W/H^2 [kg/m^2]). To use the table, find your height in the left-hand column. Move across the row to your weight; the number at the top of the column is the BMI for your height and weight. Adapted from ref. (16).

164

aging. Muscle mass has a much higher RMR than fat mass, and when muscle mass falls, so, too does RMR. Other factors may also contribute to age-associated declines in RMR, including the possibility that as we age, we waste less metabolic energy *(52,53)*. Fortunately, increases in physical activity, especially in weight training, can counter the decline in RMR, as is discussed later in the section on weight control strategy.

According to the National Institutes of Health Consensus Development Panel on Physical Activity and Cardiovascular Health, physical activity is at an all-time low in the United States *(54)*. The latest Surgeon General's report, Physical Activity and Health, found that more than 60% of American adults are not regularly active; in fact, 25% of adults report absolutely no physical activity. Of even greater concern is the trend toward decreased physical activity at younger ages. The Surgeon General's report found that nearly half of American youths 12–21 yr of age are not vigorously active on a regular basis, and that physical activity declines dramatically during adolescence. Now that high school students have a choice regarding physical education classes, daily enrollment in physical education classes has declined from 42% in 1991 to 25% in 1995. In terms of decreased calorie expenditure, this is disastrous in combination with an increasingly enhanced industrialized society relying more on mechanization rather than physical labor.

Body weight is not influenced solely by behavior and culture. Two lines of research support the theory that body weight is under genetic control: studies in identical twins *(55)* and genetic epidemiology *(56)*. The latter suggests that as much as one-fourth to one-half of the variability on body weight in the general population is explained by genetics. Currently, it is unknown if genetic factors influence appetite and the amount of food ingested, the rate of energy expenditure, or both *(57)*. It should be emphasized that although simply having the genetic profile that predisposes to obesity does not imply that such people will automatically become obese. In this population, environment and behavior also play significant roles in the determination of body weight.

WEIGHT PATTERNS VS. OVERALL ADIPOSITY IN CAD

Body fat distribution appears to play an important and independent role in enhancing cardiovascular disease risk factors. People with more central fat accumulation having a heightened risk of CAD risk factors than those with fat in the peripheral regions, such as the gluteal-femoral area. Central adiposity is strongly related to insulin resistance and the associated metabolic abnormalities, including insulin resistance, hyperinsulinemia and elevated triglycerides. As a result, the risks of type 2 diabetes, dyslipidemia and hypertension are increased *(52)*. Cancer mortality also seems to be related to central adiposity *(58)*.

Two measures are used to describe the risk associated with central adiposity: the waist-to-hip ratio and waist circumference. Traditionally, the waist-to-hip ratio (WHR) was the more commonly used method, and, in fact, most studies published to date have used that measure. According to the 1998 Evidence Report on obesity from the National Institutes of Health, however, the waist circumference has recently been found to be the better marker of abdominal fat content and carries greater prognostic significance. Ideal waist circumference varies by gender. Men should strive for a waist circumference of less than 40 in. (102 cm) and women 35 in. (88 cm). Waist circumference may not applicable in people under 5 ft tall *(52)*.

Whether central adiposity remains a risk factor after taking total adiposity into account has been a subject of controversy. The Nurses' Health study evaluated this issue, studying the relationship in 44, 702 women aged 40–65 yr of age. Researchers adjusted for BMI and other cardiac risk factors, and confirmed an independent association between the risk of CAD in women and central adiposity as measured by WHR and waist circumference. Women with a WHR of 0.88 or higher had a relative risk of 3.25 for CAD compared with women with a WHR of less than 0.72. A waist circumference of 96.5 cm (38 in.) or more was associated with a relative risk (RR) of 3.06. After adjustment for reported hypertension, diabetes and high cholesterol level, a WHR of 0.76 or higher or waist circumference of 76.2 cm (30 in.) or more was associated with more than a twofold higher risk of CHD *(59)*.

THE EPIDEMIOLOGICAL EVIDENCE FOR OBESITY IN CAD

A number of studies have confirmed the association of obesity with increased CAD risk in several populations. In the late 1960s and early 1970s, epidemiologists noted that CAD was higher in heavier persons, but there was little evidence that any obesity index made an additional contribution to risk once coexisting risk factors were taken into account *(60–62)*. Until the early 1980s, the consensus was that the increased CAD risk among the obese was due primarily to the influence of the associated risk factor profile and not to obesity itself.

In 1983, investigators from the Framingham Heart Study and the National Heart, Lung and Blood Institute reexamined data from a subset of patients in the Framingham Heart Study specifically to study the obesity–CAD risk question. The initial analysis had suggested that the degree of obesity is not a potent independent risk factor for CAD, particularly in women *(63,64)*. The researchers were spurred to reanalyze the data for two reasons: there were upward revisions to the Metropolitan Life Insurance Company desirable weight tables, essentially because of new data suggesting that it was healthier to be heavier than once thought. In addition, the researchers realized that the original analysis of the Framingham Heart Study data was based on analyses of the influence of relative weight over shorter periods of follow-up and may not have conveyed the true impact of disease risk *(65)*.

The reanalysis examined data from 5209 men and women from the original Framingham study, a population followed biennially for 26 yr for the development of CAD. The reanalysis showed that obesity was a significant independent predictor of CAD, particularly among women. Percentage of desirable weight predicted the 26-yr incidence of CAD, coronary death and congestive heart failure (CHF), after controlling for age, cholesterol, systolic blood pressure, cigarette smoking, left ventricular hypertrophy, and glucose intolerance. Relative weight in women was also positively and independently associated with coronary disease, stroke, congestive failure, and coronary and CAD death. In addition, the reanalysis showed that weight gain after the early adult years conveyed an increased risk of CAD in both men and women, a risk that could not be attributed to initial weight or the levels of the risk factors that may have resulted from weight gain. So, nearly two decades ago, researchers first confirmed that obesity is an independent risk factor for CAD *(65)*.

Five years later, investigators from the Framingham Heart Study reported on the relationship of obesity and CAD risk in a subset of older, nonsmoking persons. At that time, there were 3630 people from the original Framingham study who survived to age 65 yr by the 16th biennial examination. Current and ex-smokers were excluded from the study, resulting in a final study population of 1723 people who had been followed from 1–23 yr. The major independent variable was BMI, based on weight measurements taken at the examination at which an individual attained age 65 yr and on height measurements taken closest to that examination. Among men, four classes of BMI were created: (1) BMI less than 23.0 kg/m^2; (2) BMI between 23.0 and 25.2 kg/m^2; (3) BMI between 25.3 and 28.3 kg/m^2; and (4) BMI 28.4 kg/m^2 and greater. For women, the four groups were: (1) BMI less than 24.2 kg/m^2; (2) BMI between 24.2 and 26.1 kg/m^2; (3) BMI between 26.2 and 28.6 kg/m^2; and (4) BMI of 28.7 kg/m^2 or greater *(66)*.

The researchers found that men with a BMI 28.4 kg/m^2 and greater had a relative risk for all-cause mortality of 1.7, and those with a BMI between 25.3 and 28.3 kg/m^2 a relative risk of 1.3. Among women, the relative risk for all-cause mortality was 2.0 for those with a BMI 28.7 kg/m^2 or greater and 1.4 for women with a BMI between 26.2 and 28.6 kg/m^2. The authors concluded that, after controlling for cardiovascular risk factors, being overweight is a serious health problem for older people. This relationship was even stronger for those with long-standing weight problems.

As noted earlier, there are significant differences in the prevalence of both CAD and obesity by race. As such, it is important to determine if there are differences in the impact of risk factors, such as obesity, on CAD. Investigators from the University of Minnesota examined the relationship between obesity and CAD in blacks and whites in two populations, young and middle-aged adults *(67)*.

One sample was the Coronary Artery Risk Development in Young Adults (CARDIA) study, which consisted of 5115 adults aged 18–30 yr of age living in three cities (Birmingham, AL; Chicago; and Minneapolis); there were approximately equal numbers of whites and blacks in this study. The second sample, the Atherosclerosis Risk in Communities (ARIC) investigation studied 12,681 people aged 45–64 from Forsyth County, NC; Jackson, MS; suburban Minneapolis and Washington County, MD. In both populations, obesity was defined as the sum of subscapular and triceps skinfold measurements. Prevalence of CAD in blacks aged 45–65 was associated with obesity; after adjusting for age and cigarette smoking, the odds ratio was 1.3 for both black men and women. Further analysis showed that central adiposity conferred increased risk.

The authors also examined the relationship between the sum of subscapular and triceps skinfold measurements and levels of atherogenic plasma lipids, systolic blood pressure, serum glucose, serum insulin, and the prevalence of diabetes mellitus, finding a positive association. Interestingly, although they found that the strength of these relationships was similar in blacks and whites, the also found that with each unit increase in sum of skinfold thicknesses, plasma triglyceride concentrations in blacks appeared to increase only one-third to one-half as much as in whites.

In contrast, the Charleston Heart Study did not find that BMI nor fat patterning predicted mortality in black women, although it did in the cohort of white women in the study *(68)*. BMI and body girths were examined as predictors of all-cause and CHD mortality during 25–28 yr of follow-up in a subset of 312 white and 243 black women. Body girth was measured at the chest, abdomen, and midarm. The black women had a significantly greater mean BMI than the white women (27.7 kg/m^2 vs. 24.7 kg/m^2), which meant that 25% of the white and 46% of the black women were obese. All of the girths in the black women were greater than in the white women, although white women had more central adiposity than did the black women.

BMI was associated with both all-cause and coronary heart disease mortality in white, but not black women. After controlling for differences in BMI, the risk of all-cause mortality was greater in white women with larger chest and abdominal girths. In black women, the girths were not predictive of either all-cause or CHD mortality.

The relationship of adiposity to CAD and stroke risk was studied in Japanese men in the Honolulu Heart Program, a study that followed 8006 Japanese men for 18–20 yr; all men were of Japanese ancestry and born between 1900 and 1919 and living on the island of Oahu in 1965. BMI, subscapular skinfold thickness, and centrality index (subscapular skinfold thickness/triceps skinfold thickness) were measured at baseline and at follow-up. After controlling for other cardiovascular risk factors, the authors found that all three indicators of obesity were predictive of CAD risk, indicating an independent contribution of body fat to CAD risk *(69)*.

Of particular interest is the study by Fraser and colleagues *(70)*, examining the association of traditional risk factors on Seventh Day Adventists, a population at low-risk of CAD because of their characteristically low-risk lifestyle, which also found a clear association of obesity on CAD risk. This was the first study to examine the association between traditional risk factors and CAD events in Adventists. Over 10,000 men and 17,000 women, ranging in age from 25 to 99, with approximately one-quarter over age 65, were followed for 6 yr for the occurrence of myocardial infarction and CAD-related deaths. Overall, the authors found that even in this low-risk lifestyle population, traditional coronary risk factors (hypertension, diabetes mellitus, body height, body weight, smoking, and exercise habits) exhibit their usual associations with the risk of CAD-associated events. Obesity, examined by weight tertiles, was more clearly associated with myocardial infarction than with fatal events. The relative risks were 1.0, 1.18, and 1.83 for increasing tertiles of obesity.

The impact of modest degrees of overweight was examined in a cohort of 115,818 women from the Nurses' Health Study *(71)*. The women were between the ages of 30 and 55 yr at enrollment in 1976 and then followed for 14 yr for changes in weight and the incidence of CAD, which the investigators defined as nonfatal MI or fatal CAD. After controlling for age, smoking, menopausal status, postmenopausal hormone use, and parental history of CAD, the authors found that even modest increases in weight increase the risk of CAD. Among women within the BMI range of 18–25 kg/m^2, weight gain after age 18 yr of age remained a strong predictor of CAD risk. Comparing women with stable weight after age 18 (defined as ±5 kg of weight at age 18), women who gained 5–7.9 kg had a relative risk of CAD of 1.25; those who gained 8–10.9 kg, RR = 1.64; 11–19 kg weight gain, RR = 1.92; and weight gain greater than 20 kg, RR = 2.65. The authors emphasize that even modest weight gains during adult life and levels of body weight not generally considered to be overweight are associated with important increases in the risk of CAD.

This study by researchers from the Harvard School of Public Health and the Brigham and Women's Hospital was one of the first to call to attention the dangerously false reassurance that small amounts of weight gain are "normal" and expected, a reassurance fueled by the 1990 upward changes in US weight guidelines that allowed for weight gain with age. The revisions were increased to correspond to so-called normal body mass indexes of 21–27 kg/m^2, in contrast to the 1985 guidelines, which corresponded to a BMI between 19 and 24 kg/m^2. The 1990 changes in weight tables implied that weight gains of 4.5–6.8 kg were consistent with good health. Also of concern was the other implication of the revised weight tables: that a BMI less than 21 kg/m^2 is unhealthy. Finally, these 1990 changes brought false reassurance about overweight in one additional way: they indicated that the seriousness of a person's degree of overweight should be evaluated by the presence of comorbid conditions such as hypertension, diabetes—rather than respond to the degree of overweight to prevent such complications *(72,73)*.

The Harvard researchers also examined the effect of obesity and body fat distribution in a cohort of 29,122 U.S. middle-aged and older men from the Health Professionals Follow-up Study, a prospective study of 51,529 US male health professionals who were 40–75 yr old in 1986 *(74)*. They confirmed that weight is an independent risk factor for CAD, but also found that although BMI predicted CAD risk in men younger than age 65, body fat distribution (as measured by WHR) was more predictive of risk in men aged 65 and older.

The investigators measured BMI, WHR, and height at entrance into this study in 1987, and also inquired about weight gain since age 21. They then followed the men for 3 yr for the occurrence of CAD events, defined as fatal CAD, nonfatal MI, coronary artery bypass grafting, or percutaneous transluminal coronary angioplasty. Men were excluded if they had a history of myocardial infarction, angina, stroke, coronary artery bypass graft, or coronary angioplasty; the authors controlled for alcohol use, vitamin E supplementation, smoking, total energy intake, family history of myocardial infarction, profession, and three dietary factors (intake of total and type of fat, cholesterol, and fiber).

The authors found that BMI, WHR, short stature, and weight gain since age 21 were associated with an increased risk of CHD. They reported their results by age of study participants at time of enrollment: men less than age 65 and those age 65 and older, comparing both with lean men with a BMI less than 23.0 kg/m^2. The association of increased weight (as described by increasing BMI) was strongest for the younger men. Among men younger than 65, after adjusting for the other coronary risk factors noted, the relative risk for CAD events was 1.72 for men with BMI 25–28.9 kg/m^2; 2.61 for BMI 29–32.9 kg/m^2, and 3.44 for BMI greater than or equal to 33 kg/m^2. Although the relative risks were much lower in the group of men aged 65 and older in each BMI category, the WHR was a much stronger predictor of risk. Those with WHRs in the highest quintiles had a relative risk 2.76 compared to men with WHRs in the lowest quintile.

WEIGHT CONTROL STRATEGIES: A POSITIVE RATHER THAN A NEGATIVE SPIN

Helping patients lose weight is difficult. Assisting them in maintaining lost weight is certainly the more difficult task, with recidivism rates exceptionally high, often over 95%, depending on the series one examines. Still, given the cardiovascular and other disease burdens imposed by obesity, it is essential to try new strategies to help patients achieve and maintain weight loss. Health care professionals, especially nutrition professionals, are challenged to redefine efforts that historically have not worked to help patients achieve and maintain weights compatible with better health. The following is a candid, practical discussion of strategies that should improve your patients' odds of success.

Imposing a positive spin on dietary changes necessary in controlling weight is the basis of all efforts. Historically, nutrition counseling has been negatively focused, with advice centered on what patients should avoid. For the patient, this translates into deprivation. This author maintains that nutrition counseling must have a positive focus. As such, our program of nutrition intervention in the Preventive Cardiology and Rehabilitation Program is named "The Nutrition Enhancement Project," after the concept that nutritional intervention should enhance rather than deprive patients' lifestyles. Certainly, CAD patients must be instructed on how to limit dietary fats, especially saturated fats, but this, too, can be accomplished under the guise of enhancing one's lifestyle rather than avoiding the forbidden fruit.

This author divides weight loss strategies into three categories: behavioral, food, and exercise. The first two are certainly intimately related to each other, but for purposes of discussion, they are discussed separately here.

Behavioral Strategies

APPROPRIATE WEIGHT GOAL SETTING

Weight loss goal setting is dual pronged: health care professionals must help patients set both reasonable weight loss goals and an appropriate and flexible calorie level. Although the ultimate goal is to help patients achieve a BMI below that which defines obesity (27.8 kg/m² for men and 27.3 kg/m² for women), this may not be a reasonable initial goal. This is especially true when it translates into weight loss needs in excess of 20% of a person's current weight. Some clients may consider such weight loss demands daunting and unachievable, feelings that prevent some people from making any changes at all. Instead, set smaller weight loss increments for patients, encouraging them to approach weight loss in smaller goals. According to the NIH Evidence Report on Obesity, a weight loss goal of 10% is realistic and achievable. It is better, says the NIH Evidence Report, to maintain a moderate weight loss over a prolonged period than to regain after a marked weight loss. After maintaining a moderate weight loss for 6 mo, patients with more weight to lose should be encouraged to lose an additional 10%; if necessary, they can take another break and continue as needed to achieve the healthiest weight for them.

In addition to changing a seemingly impossible task to an achievable one, the benefits of losing 10% of body weight have been well documented in their ability to reduce obesity-associated risk factors *(52)*.

APPROPRIATE CALORIE GOAL SETTING

As health care professionals, we have failed to communicate one of the most critical pieces of the weight loss algorithm: only modest reductions in calorie intake are necessary to achieve weight loss. We are guilty of handing out 1200 or 1300 calorie diet sheets, calorie levels too low to maintain over any extended period. Not only are such calories levels exceedingly difficult to maintain, but they are unnecessary to achieve weight loss goals.

Grundy *(75)* has noted that the degree of energy imbalance leading to obesity is relatively small, He calculates, from standard estimates of energy requirements per kilogram of body weight, that an excess of only 300 cal/d (1255 kJ/d) of excess energy maintains approximately 10 lb kg (22 lb) of excess weight. In other words, the middle-aged person who has gained 10 kg of excess weight since age 25 has only 300 calories of energy imbalance. Grundy similarly calculates that 600 cal/d (2510 kJ) sustains approximately 20 kg (44 lb) of excess weight.

Calorie levels in the range of 1400–1700 are far more reasonable to sustain, and will result in the desired weight loss over the long haul. This may be difficult to convey to patients once they become motivated and want to realize immediate results. It may be useful to have them work with a registered dietitian, who can calculate with them the caloric content of the diet they had been following, and the relatively insignificant daily changes necessary to achieve a 300-calorie deficit. Empowering patients with this type of knowledge is quintessential in helping them achieve both their short-term goal of losing weight steadily and their long-term goal of maintaining lost weight.

THREE IMPORTANT MOTIVATION STRATEGIES

Persevering with weight loss requires an inordinate amount of self-motivation. This author finds three strategies particularly important to convey and continuously review with patients in need of losing weight.

1. Help patients realize that tomorrow is today, or, simply put, helping them not wait for the proverbial tomorrow to begin the lifestyle modifications necessary to lose weight. Be aware that some clients may not want to begin weight loss efforts for fear of failing.

2. Give patients permission to forgive their transgressions. Help clients realize ahead of time that their weight loss program will not be perfect and strategize with them on how they will deal with such transgressions. Research confirms that people who recover quickly from their transgressions realize more weight loss success. This author suggests a simple scheme to use with patients in teaching them how to handle transgressions: help patients that they can fall forward (i.e., learn from their mistake and move forward), or fall backward (i.e., fall down and never recover) after eating something they had not planned to.

3. The final behavioral strategy bridges to the food strategies: encourage patients to eat only food they enjoy, and to enjoy every bite they eat. The last strategy is so important that it warrants additional discussion.

Nutrition professionals know from experience that one of the most expedient ways for clients to surrender dieting motivation is to eat food they do not like. A recent survey, the 1999 Health Focus Trend Report *(76)*, found that fewer shoppers than ever before are willing to compromise taste for health benefits. Also, the survey reported that fewer shoppers are willing to avoid favorite foods in order to eat healthier.

Practically speaking, health care professionals wishing to help clients achieve success must find ways to make this a reality, including becoming students themselves of gourmet healthy cooking and eating. This facilitates assisting patients in seeking gourmet healthy food and cooking classes.

Food Strategies

This author encourages the use of food strategies for losing weight that shift the focus from the negative to the positive. The Health Focus Trend Report, confirms the consumer demand for this paradigm shift to positive-based nutrition information, with consumers reporting they want "Positive nutrition, with little or no downside." The Trend Report also noted that consumers want to understand the science behind the advice, and in a format they can assimilate: understandable bites. In fact, the survey found that the market for health and nutrition information is less satisfied and more demanding than ever before. This provides support for empowering patients with another critical piece of the weight loss algorithm: how food affects their disease. It follows, then, that consumers, with their focus on longevity with good health and good quality of life, believe that prevention benefits are about health management through disease and symptom prevention.

Given this important background information, let's take a brief look at the main food strategies that should be addressed with CAD patients embarking on weight loss programs:

1. Include protein at each meal and snack: Research confirms that of the three macronutrients, protein is the most satiating *(77)*, which may help avoid excessive eating. Clients should be instructed in how to choose protein foods, which tend to be sources of fat, especially saturated fat. Vegetable and marine sources of protein should be encouraged.

Clients should be advised to include at least two fish meals and two vegetable protein meals weekly; all lunch protein should be vegetable based.

2. Increase fiber intake: Including high-fiber foods is advantageous to clients with CAD for several reasons. From a weight loss point of view there is now evidence that increasing fiber intake may decrease the metabolizable energy content of the diet, especially of fat *(78)*. In addition, high-fiber foods lead to earlier satiety and also to decreased unplanned snacking *(79)*. High-fiber foods tend to be replete with the nutrients and phytochemicals that may help decrease CAD risk factors, including folate, B_6, vitamin C, vitamin E, carotenoids, flavonoids, potassium, and other minerals.

3. Front load calories: Dieters tend to start the day with their greatest willpower, which often works against them. Practically speaking, this means they often eat a very-low-calorie breakfast and lunch. Often, this brings them to midday or early evening with excessive hunger; in turn, this leads to overeating at day's end. By front loading calories, or eating the calorically heavier meals at the beginning of the day, patients are more satisfied at the end of the day. Taking in enough calories at the beginning of the day may reduce the feeling of fatigue that often troubles dieters.

4. Divide calories into six meals rather than three.

Preliminary evidence indicates that consuming calories in six smaller meals rather than three larger ones may assist with weight loss. Researchers from Tufts University studied the fat-burning ability of two groups of women: one in their twenties and another that was postmenopausal. Each age group of women was fed three test-size meals of varying calories—250 calories, 500 calories, and 1000 calories. After each test meal, the researchers measured the amount of energy each age group burned. The metabolic response to the 250- and 500-calorie meals was similar between the two groups, but quite disparate after the 1000-calorie meal. The postmenopausal women burned about 30% less fat than the younger women. In addition to giving clients the metabolic edge in losing weight, eating six smaller meals may also help reduce total and LDL cholesterol levels.

EXERCISE STRATEGIES

Clients need to engage regularly in two forms of exercise to improve the chances of weight loss success and maintain lost weight: aerobic and weight training. According to the latest Surgeon General's report on Physical Activity and Health, all Americans should exercise 30 min most, and preferably all, days of the week to improve cardiovascular fitness *(80)*. In addition, concludes the report, there may become additional benefit gained through engaging in even greater amounts of exercise. This is also the minimum amount of exercise needed to maintain muscle mass. Cross training, or performing more than one type of aerobic exercise helps build muscles throughout the body, and therefore keeps total muscle mass greater—and metabolism higher.

Although the Surgeon General's report concluded that consumers can derive much the same benefit from dividing 30 min of exercise into two or three shorter sessions, it also states that people who can maintain a regular regiment of activity that is of longer duration or of more vigorous intensity are likely to derive greater benefits.

It is worthwhile to review with clients the multiple benefits of exercise. In addition to boosting metabolism and assisting with weight loss, physical activity greatly reduces the risk of premature mortality in general and of CAD, hypertension, colon cancer, and diabetes mellitus in particular. Physical activity also improves mental health and is important for the health of muscles, bones, and joints.

The second form of physical activity—weight training, or resistance training—is also key to maintaining muscle mass, especially with increasing age. According to the American College of Sports Medicine (ACSM), resistance training should be progressive in nature, and provide a stimulus to all major muscle groups; it should also be individualized. The ACSM recommends performing one set of 8–10 exercises 2–3 d/wk; if time allows, clients are advised to perform a second set of the same exercise, which may provide greater benefits. Older and more frail persons (those over age 50–60) may benefit from 10–15 repetitions using less weight *(81)*.

CONCLUSION

In most people, weight gain is insidious. Health care professionals should take this as a positive factor and also a call to action. Rather than waiting for patients to reach obesity, health care professionals should follow their weight over time and encourage patients to act early when weight loss is not so daunting. Because the health consequences of being overweight begin prior to being defined as obesity, it is critically important for the health care professional to follow patients' weight over time and assist them in preventing the excessive weight gain that defines obesity.

REFERENCES

1. Kuczmarski RG, Flegal KM, Campbell SM, Johnson CL. Increasing prevalence of overweight among US adults. The National Health and Nutrition Examination Surveys, 1960–1991. JAMA 1994;273: 205–211.
2. Federation of American Societies for Experimental Biology Life Sciences Research Office. Third report on nutrition monitoring in the United States. US Government Printing Office, Washington, DC, 1995.
3. Solomon CF, Manson JE. Obesity and mortality: a review of the epidemiologic data. Am J Clin Nutr 1997;66(Suppl):1044S–1050S.
4. Lew EA, Garfinkel L. Variations in mortality by weight among 750,000 men and women. J Chronic Dis 1979;32:564–576.
5. Manson JE, Stampfer MH, Hennekens CH, et al. Body weight and longevity, a reassessment. JAMA 1987:257:353–358.
6. Metropolitan Life Insurance Company. 1983 height and weight tables. Stat Bull Metropol Insur Co 1984:64:2–9.
7. Najjar MF, Rowland M. Anthropometric reference data and prevalence of overweight, United States, 1976–1980. Vital Health Stat 1987;11:238.
8. Federation of American Societies for Experimental Biology Life Sciences Research Office, 1995.
9. Federation of American Societies for Experimental Biology Life Sciences Research Office. 1995.
10. Metropolitan Life Insurance Company. Metropolitan height and weight tables. Stat Bull Metropol Life Insur Co 1983:64:1–9.
11. Garrison RJ, Kannel WB. A new approach for estimating healthy body weights. Int J Obes 1993:17: 417–423.
12. Grundy SM. Atherogenic dyslipidemia and the metabolic syndrome: pathogenesis and the challenge of therapy. In: Gotto AM Jr, ed. Drugs Affecting Lipid Metabolism. Kluwer Academic Publishers, Dordrecht, Netherlands, 1996, pp. 237–247.
13. Reaven GM. Insulin resistance and its consequences: non-insulin-dependent diabetes mellltus and coronary heart disease. In: LeRoith D, Taylor SI, Olefsky JM, eds. Diabetes Mellitus. Lippincott-Raven, Philadelphia, PA, 1966, pp. 509–519.
14. DeFronzo RA. The triumvirate: β-cell, muscle, liver. A collusion responsible for NIDDM. Diabetes 1998;37:667–687.
15. Howard G, O'Leary DH, Zaccaro D, et al. Insulin sensitivity and atherosclerosis. Circulation 1996:93: 1809–1817.
16. NIH. Clinical Guidelines on the identification, evaluation, and treatment of overweight and obesity in adults: the evidence report. June 1998. US Department of Health and Human Services.

17. Bjorntorp P. Bergman H, Varnauskas E. Plasma free fatty acid turnover rate in obesity. Acta Med Scand 1969;185:351–356.
18. Jenson MD, Haymond MW, Rizza RA, et al. Influence of body fat distribution on free fatty acid metabolism in obesity. J Clin Invest 1989:83:1168–1173.
19. Campbell PJ, Carlson MG, Nurjhan N. Fat metabolism in human obesity. Am J Physiol 1994:266: E600–E605.
20. Randle PI, Priestman DA, Mistry S, Halsall A. Mechanisms modifying glucose oxidation in diabetes mellitus. Diabetologia 1994:37:S155–161.
21. Abate N, Garg A, Peshock RM, et al. Relationship of generalized and regional adiposy to insulin sensitivity in men. J Clin Invest 1995:96:88–98.
22. Abate N, Garg A, Peshock RM, et al. Relationship of generalized and regional adiposy to insulin sensitivity in men with NIDDM. Diabetes 1996:45:1684–1693.
23. Elahi D, Nagulesparan N, Herscopf, RJ. Feedback inhibition of insulin secretion by insulin: the hyperinsulinemia of obesity. N Engl J Med 1989;306:1196–1202.
24. Saad MF, Knowler WC, Pettitt DJ, et al. The natural history of impaired glucose tolerance in the Pima Indians. NJEM 1998;319:1500–1506.
25. Stein DT, Esser V, Stevenson BE, et al. Essentiality (sic) of circulating fatty acids for glucose-stimulated insulin secretion in the fasted rat. J Clin Invest 1996;97:2728–2735.
26. Zimmet P, Dowse G, Bennett PH. Hyperinsulinemia is a predictor of non-insulin-dependent diabetes mellitus. Diabetes Metab Rev 1991:17:101–118.
27. Garg A, Chandalia M, Vuituh F. Severe islet amyloidosis in congenital generalized lipodystrophy. Diabetes Care 1996;19:28–31.
28. Grundy SM, Mok HY, Zech L, et al. Transport of very low density lipoprotein triglycerides in varying degrees of obesity and hypertriglyceridemia. J Clin invest 1979:63:1274–1283.
29. Kesaniemi YA, Bells WF, Grundy SM. Comparison of metabolism of alipoprotein B in normal subjects, obese patients, and patients with coronary heart disease. J Clin Invest 1985;76:586–595.
30. Egusa G, Beltz WP, Grundy SM, Howard BV. Influence of obesity on the metabolism of alipoprotein B in man. J Clin Invest 1985;76:596–603.
31. Miettinen TA. Cholesterol production in obesity. Circulation 1971;44:842–250.
32. Austin MA, Kokanson JE, Brunzell JD. Characterization of low-density lipoprotein subclasses: methodologic approaches and clinical relevance. Curr Opin Lipidol 1994;5:395–403.
33. Richards EG, Grundy SM, Cooper K. Influence of plasma triglycerides on lipoprotein patterns in normal subjects and in patients with coronary artery disease. Am J Cardiol 1989:63:1214–1220.
34. Schaefer EJ, Levy RI, Anderson DW, et al. Plasma triglycerides in regulation of HDL-cholesterol. Lancet 1978:2:391–393.
35. Katzel LI, Coon PJ, Busby MJ, et al. Reduced HDL_2 cholesterol subspecies and elevated postherapin hepatic lipase activity in older men with abdominal obesity and asymptomatic myocardial ischemia. Arterioscler Thromb 1992:12:814–823.
36. Depres JP, Ferland M, Joorjani S, et al. Role of hepatic-triglyceride lipase activity in the association between intra-abdominal fat and plasma HDL cholesterol in obese women. Arteriosclerosis 1989:9:485–492.
37. Zambon A, Austin MA, Brown BG, et al. Effect of hepatic lipase on LDL in normal men and those with coronary artery disease. Arterioscler Thromb 1993;13:147–153.
38. Kuusi T. Saarinen P, Nikkila EA. Evidence for the roll of hepatic endothelial lipase in the metabolism of plasma high density lipoprotein$_2$ in man. Atherosclerosis 1980;36:589–593.
39. Blades B, Vega GL, Grundy SM. Activities of lipoprotein lipase and hepatic triglyceride lipase in postheparin plasma of patients with low concentrations of HDL cholesterol. Arterioscler Thromb 1993;13: 1227–1235.
40. Gopinath N, Chadu SL, Jain P, et al. An epidemiological study of obesity in adults in the urban population of Delhi. J Assoc Physicians India 1994:42:212–215.
41. Popkin BM, Paeratakul S, Zhai F, Ge K. A review of dietary and environmental correlates of obesity with emphasis on developing countries. Obes Res 1995:3(Suppl 2):89S–93S.
42. el Mugamer IT, Alizayat AS, Hossain MM, Pugh RN. Diabetes, obesity, and hypertension in urban and rural people of Bedouin origin in the United Arab Emirates. J Trop Med Hyg 1995:98:407–415.
43. Amine EK, Samy M. Obesity among female university students in the United Arab Emirates. J Royal Soc Health 1996;116:91–96.
44. Singh RB, Niza MA, Agarwal P, et al. Epidemiologic study of central obesity, insulin resistance and associated disturbances in the urbal (sic) population of North India. Acta Cardiol 1995:50:215–225.

45. Bhatnager D, Anand IS, Durrington PN, et al. Coronary risk factors in people from the Indian sub-continent living in West London and their siblings in India. Lancet 1997;331:397–398.
46. National Institute of Health. The Lipid Research Clinics population studies data book: the prevalence study. NIH, Bethesda, MD, 1979 (Publication no 79-1527).
47. Visser M, Deurenberg P, van Staveren WA, Hautvast JGAJ. Resting metabolic rate and diet-induced thermogenesis in young and elderly subjects: relationship with body composition, fat distribution, and physical activity level. Am J Clin Nutr 1995:61:772–778.
48. Tzankoff SP, Norris AH. Longitudinal changes in basal metabolism in man. J Appl Physiol 1978;45: 536–539.
49. Poehlman ET, Toth MJ. Mathematical ratios lead to spurious conclusions regarding age and sex-related differences in resting metabolic rate. Am J Clin Nutr 1995:61:482–485.
50. Poehlman ET, Berke EM, Joseph JR, et al. Influence of aerobic capacity, body composition, and thyroid hormones on the age-related decline of resting metabolic rate. Metabolism 1992:41:915–921.
51. Poehlman ET. Regulation of energy expenditure in aging humans. J Am Geriatric Soc 1993:41:552–559.
52. NIH Clinical Guidelines on the identification, evaluation, and treatment of overweight and obesity in adults: the evidence report. June 1998. US Department of Health and Human Services.
53. Garrow JS. Modern methods of measuring body composition. In: Whitehead RG, Prentice A. New Techniques in Nutritional Research. Academic, San Diego, 1991, pp. 233–239.
54. NIH Consensus Development Panel on Physical Activity and Cardiovascular Health. Physical activity and cardiovascular health. JAMA 1996;276:241–246.
55. Bouchard C, Tremblay Y, Despres J. The response to long-term overfeeding on identical twins. N Engl J Med 1990:322:1477–1482.
56. Bluchard (sic) C, Perusse L. Genetics of obesity. Annu Rev Nutr 1993:13:337–354.
57. Grundy SM. Multifactorial causation of obesity: implications for prevention. Am J Clin Nutr 1998; 67(Suppl):563S–572S.
58. Folsom AR, Kay SA, Sellers TA, et al. Body fat distribution and 5-year risk of death in older women. JAMA 1993;269:483–487.
59. Rexrode KM, Carey VJ, Hennekens CH, et al. Admoninal adiposity and coronary heart disease in women. JAMA 1998;280:1843–1848.
60. Rabkin SW, Mathewson FA, Hsu PH. Relation of body weight to development of ischemic heart disease in a cohort of young North American men after a 26 year observation period. The Manitoba Study. Am J Cardiol 1977:39:452.
61. Robertson TL, Kato H, Gordon TM, et al. Epidemiologic studies of coronary heart disease and stroke on japanese men living in Japan, Hawaii, and California. Am J Cardiol 1977;39:244.
62. Chapman JM, Coulson AH, Clark VA. Borun ER. The differential effect of serum cholesterol, blood pressure and weight on the incidence of miocardial infarction and angine pectoris. J Chronic Dis 1971; 23:631.
63. Truett J, Cornfield J, Kannel W. A muitivariate analysis of the risk of coronary heart disease in Framingham. J Chronic Dis 1967;20:511.
64. Kannel WB, Gordon T. Obesity and cardiovascular disease. The Framingham Study. In; Burland WL, Samuel PD, Yudkin J, eds. Obsesity Symposium. Proceedings of a Survier Research Institute Symposium, Churchill-Livingstone, Edinburgh, 1974, p. 24.
65. Hubert HB, Feinleib M, McNamara PM, Castelli WP. Obesity as an independent risk factor for cardio-vascular disease: a 26-year follow-up of participants in the Framingham Heart Study. Circulation 1983; 67:968–977.
66. Harris T, Cook F, Garrison R, et al. Body mass index and mortality among nonsmoking older persons. The Framingham Heart Study. JAMA 1988;259:1520–1524.
67. Folsom AR, Burke GL, Byers CL, et al. Implications of obesity for cardiovascular disease in blacks: the CARDIA and ARIC studies. Am J Clin Nutr 1991;53:1604S–1611S.
68. Steven J, Keil JE, Rust PF, et al. Body mass index and body girths as predictors of mortality in black and white women. Arch Intern Med 1992;152:1257–1262.
69. Curb JD, Marcus EB. Body fat, coronary heart disease, and stroke in Japanese men. Am J Clin Nutr 1991; 53:1612S–1615S.
70. Fraser GE, Strahan M, Sabate J, et al. Effects of traditional coronary risk factors on rates of incident coronary events in a low-risk population. Circulation 1992;86:406–413.
71. Willett WC, Manson JE, Stampfer MJ, et al. Weight, weight change and coronary heart disease in women. JAMA 1995;273:461–465.

72. US Department of Agriculture, US Dept. of Health and Human Services. Nutrition and Your Health: Dietary Guidelines for Americans, 3rd ed. Washington DC: US Government Printing Office, 1990.
73. US Department of Agriculture, US Dept. of Health and Human Services. Nutrition and Your Health: Dietary Guidelines for Americans, 2nd ed. Washington DC: US Government Printing Office, 1985.
74. Rimm EB, Stampfer MJ, Giovannucci E, et al. Body size and fat distribution as predictors of coronary heart disease among middle-aged and older US men. Am J Epidemiol 1995;141:1117–1127.
75. Grundy SM. Multifactorial causation of obesity: implication for prevention. Am J Clin Nutr 1998; 67(Suppl):563S–572S.
76. HealthFocus, Inc. 1999 HealthFocus Trend Report. Published by HealthFocus, Inc. P.O. Box 7174, Des Moines, IA 50309-7174.
77. Poppitt SD, McCormack D, Buffenstein R. Short-term effects of macronutrient preloads on appetite and energy intake in lean women. Physiol Behav 1998;64:279–284.
78. Baer DJ, Rumpler WV, Miles CW, Fahey GC. Dietary fiber decreases the metabolizable energy content and nutrient digestibility of mixed diets fed to humans. J Nutr 1997;127:579–586.
79. Delargy HJ, O'Sullivan KR, Fletcher RJ, Blundell JE. Effects of amount and type of dietary fibre (soluble and insoluble) on short-term control of appetite. Int J Food Sci Nutr 1997;48:67–77.
80. US Department of Health and Human Services, Centers for Disease Control and Prevention. Physical Activity and Health: A Report of the Surgeon General Executive Summary.
81. Pollock ML, Gaesser GA, Butcher JD, et al. The recommended quantity and quality of exercise for developing and maintaining cardiorespiratory and muscular fitness and flexibility in health adults. Med Sci Sports Exer 1998, pp. 975–991.

10

Tobacco as a Cardiovascular Risk Factor

Robyn Bergman Buchsbaum, MHS, CHES
and Jeffrey Craig Buchsbaum, MD, PHD

CONTENTS

INTRODUCTION

Tobacco use in the form of cigarettes has long been established as a major risk factor for coronary heart disease (CHD). It is the most preventable cause of mortality. Each year, cigarette smoking causes more than 400,000 deaths in the United States alone, more than the number of American lives lost during World War I, Korea, and Vietnam combined *(1)*. Not only does this modifiable behavior cause pain and suffering, but it poses a significant economic burden. Total US Medicaid expenses due to tobacco are over $6 billion a year *(2)*. Total direct health care costs are in excess of $50 billion a year. Indirect losses, usually due to lost productivity, increase that figure by another $50 billion a year *(2)*. Since the mid-1990s, state attorneys general have participated in legal action with tobacco companies in hopes of winning back money spent on Medicaid expenses. In 1998, an out-of-court settlement was reached giving states billions of dollars. In addition to state-sponsored legal action, civil lawsuits in which individual smokers sue tobacco companies have become more and more commonplace.

Despite the legal battles taking place on state and federal levels, personal battles with tobacco are still being waged. Although smoking prevalence is the lowest it has been in decades, approximately 26% of Americans still smoke. This percentage is still higher than the 15% national goal outlined in Healthy People 2000 *(3)*. Additionally, the decrease in smoking prevalence is not being seen across all groups. Specifically, cigarette smoking

From: *Contemporary Cardiology: Preventive Cardiology:*
Strategies for the Prevention and Treatment of Coronary Artery Disease
Edited by: J. Foody © Humana Press Inc., Totowa, NJ

continues to be a problem with young, African-American men and women, whose rates are increasing or maintaining, respectively, at their current levels. An inverse relationship between education level and smoking status has also been seen. Prevalence among college graduates is far less than those with less than a high school education *(4)*. Although more than 40 million Americans have quit smoking, each day approximately 3000 people, usually teenagers, start *(4)*. Worldwide, cigarette smoking is linked to the deaths of some 3 million a year. Due to tobacco's allure, it is fast becoming one of the leading killers in developing countries *(5)*.

HISTORY

Cigarette smoking reached its fashionable peak in the 1950s when smoking was advertised as a health benefit. In fact, physicians were the primary endorsers. Ads portrayed cigarettes as "physician tested" or the "brand of physicians" *(6)*. These ads had some truth to them. Physicians and other allied health workers continued to smoke tobacco in spite of early evidence that cigarettes were linked to increased incidence of carcinoma *(7)*. Even in the early 1950s, cigarette ads were still prominent in leading medical journals such as *the Journal of the American Medical Association*, *The Lancet*, and the *British Medical Journal (7)*.

Cigarettes were fashionable and trendy. Soon smoking became what some call "the most overpracticed addiction in the world" *(8)*. It was around that time in 1964 that the Surgeon General and his advisory committee released their report, entitled Smoking and Health, a strong condemnation of tobacco use. The committee had reviewed 7000 scientific articles in the process of developing the report. Since then, there have been over 30,000 articles published connecting tobacco use with a vast array of medical problems *(9)*.

Despite the overwhelming evidence that tobacco use in any form is connected with morbidity and mortality, the tobacco industry continues to deny any real harm from their product. Only recently has there been some weakening of this position and only after secret memoranda and documents were released to the press. For the first time ever, the tobacco companies are under careful scrutiny with the threat of Food and Drug Administration (FDA) regulation looming closer.

BIOCHEMISTRY AND PATHOPHYSIOLOGY

Since the Surgeon General's first report in 1964, subsequent reports have found tobacco use to be associated with a long list of medical issues, not the least of which is coronary heart disease (CHD). The various mechanisms related to smoking and cardiac disease cross broad categories including decreased oxygen-carrying capacity secondary to carbon monoxide's direct effects on hemoglobin *(10)*, vasoconstriction, platelet adhesion and hypercoagulability, catecholamine release, and endothelial dysfunction secondary to complex molecular mechanisms *(11)*. Of the thousands of ingredients *(12)* contained within a cigarette, nicotine and carbon monoxide appear to be the most lethal culprits. By smoking a single cigarette, the body reacts by increasing myocardial oxygen demand secondary to increased heart rate, blood pressure, peripheral resistance, and cardiac output *(13,14)*. Yet, the very same cigarette decreases the amount of coronary blood flow and myocardial oxygen supply. The elevated carboxyhemoglobin levels due to smoking decrease the oxygen-carrying capacity of the blood resulting in myocardial ischemia *(13,15)*. Studies have shown that smoking increases the blood's ability to coagulate while

---

Key Points

- Cigarette smoking has been proven to be a powerful predictor of cardiovascular mortality.
  Each year, cigarette smoking causes more than 400,000 deaths in the US alone
- Total direct health care costs related to tobacco are in excess of $50 billion a year
- Smoking causes decreased oxygen-carrying capacity, vasoconstriction, platelet adhesion and hypercoagulability, catecholamine release, and endothelial dysfunction
- Passive smoke increases a person's risk of coronary heart disease, most likely in a dose-dependent manner
- There are substantial benefits to smoking cessation:
  - Smoking cessation results in immediate, substantial health benefits with people of all age groups and differing disease states
  - Individuals who quit smoking live longer
  - Smoking cessation decreases the risk of lung cancer, other cancers, heart attack, stroke, and chronic lung disease
  - The health benefits resulting from smoking cessation far outweigh the risks of gaining a small to moderate amount of weight following quitting

---

also enhancing platelet aggregation and adhesiveness *(16–19)*, even in the presence of aspirin *(20)*. In addition, smoking causes endothelial cell dysfunction, thus potentiating possible injury to the blood vessel wall *(13,21)*. The smoking of one cigarette appears to cause acute endothelial dysfunction for at least 60 min without the development of tolerance *(13)*. Additionally, chronic exposure to cigarette smoke has been shown to cause localized hypoxia, allowing for subendothelial edema and lipid accumulation in the vessel walls. Chronic smoking also lowers fibrinolytic function, allowing further plaque formation *(22)*. Because chronic smoking is also associated with increased serum cholesterol and reduced high-density lipoproteins, the damage to the blood vessel walls provides ample opportunity for exposure to lipids and thrombosis. Recently, smoking has been shown to lower the amount of endothelial derived nitric oxide (NO) produced *(23–25)*. Many current areas of pathophysiological investigation relating heart disease and smoking go beyond the scope of this chapter, including both traditional approaches in areas like the role of homocysteine *(26,27)* and an increasing role for molecular biology and genetics.

EPIDEMIOLOGY

Cigarette smoking has been proven to be a powerful predictor of cardiovascular mortality. The Framingham Study showed a 10-fold increase in relative risk of sudden cardiac death in men who smoked than in nonsmoking men. This also held true for women with a relative risk 4.5 times higher in women smokers *(28)*. Risk from cigarette smoking is dose dependent. Quantity and duration of a smoking habit are the factors most contributory to the development of disease. An individual's risk for cardiac events depends on the age at which the person started smoking, the number of cigarettes smoked per day, and the depth of inhalation *(15)*. Studies have shown that low-yield cigarettes make little difference in regard to risk *(29)*. Although even younger smokers have more raised plaque lesions than do nonsmokers *(30)*, middle age is when both men and women's risk for CHD doubles that of their nonsmoking counterparts *(15)*. Because overall smoking history in pack-years is important in determining risk, smoking as little as 1–4 cigarettes a day over a long duration can double the risk of CHD *(31)*.

Patients who have established heart disease and yet continue to smoke suffer severe consequences. The Coronary Artery Surgery Study (CASS) provided evidence showing that 5- yr mortality is significantly higher for smokers than quitters, 22% vs. 15% *(32)*. Patients who had quit smoking had a survival rate around 80% compared with a 69% survival rate for those who continued to smoke *(33)*. In addition, after a 10-yr follow-up, smokers had a lower quality of life compared to former or nonsmokers. Smokers were more likely to have angina, be limited in their activity level, be unemployed, and, overall, have more hospital admissions *(33)*.

In a study by Daly and associates *(33)*, smokers were observed for over 7 yr after their hospital admission, either for myocardial infarction or unstable angina. Mortality in individuals who continued smoking was 82%, whereas those who stopped smoking had mortality rates around 37%. The continuation of smoking was most pronounced in patients with unstable angina where higher rates of sudden death were seen *(34)*.

Although the evidence for increased morbidity and mortality resulting from cigarette smoking is overwhelming, there are some areas in which smoking use is not associated with increased risk, emphasizing the need for more understanding of the pathophysiology of smoking. There is mixed evidence regarding smoking and postangioplasty restenosis. Several studies have shown no relationship between smoking status and restenosis, whereas two other studies have shown that smoking was an independent predictor of restenosis *(35–39)*. Additionally, smoking has a questionable relationship with the incidence of angina *(40)*. In both the Framingham Study and the Goteborg Primary Prevention Study, the risk of angina was not significantly higher for smokers than nonsmokers *(28,40)*. Additionally, although there is a strong belief that there is a synergistic interaction between smoking and other major risk factors, the exact relationship is not clearly understood *(1,40)*.

PASSIVE SMOKING

Recently, the issue of environmental exposure to cigarette smoke has gotten a great deal of attention. For years, observational data suggested that environmental tobacco smoke was related to a host of medical problems including CHD. Up until recently, however, no definitive studies were published linking environmental tobacco smoke to morbidity and mortality. The problem was due to the difficulty in proving causality in exposed people. In 1986, after the US Surgeon General and the National Academy of Sciences determined that this was clearly an issue that needed to be resolved, epidemiologic studies began showing a definite negative relationship between environmental tobacco smoke and CHD *(41)*. In almost all of these studies, the relative risks and/or odds ratios for nonsmoker spouses of smokers were greater than 1 *(41)*.

One of the strongest studies to date, published by Kawachi and colleagues *(41)*, followed over 32,000 nonsmoking women between the ages of 36 and 71 for 10 yr. The results were clear. For nonsmoking women exposed to cigarette smoke in either the workplace or at home, relative risk (RR) of developing coronary heart disease increased. Specifically, for women who reported only occasional exposure to cigarette smoke, the relative risk rose to 1.58. For those with regular exposure to cigarette smoke, the relative risk increased to 1.91 *(42)*. Not only was this study important due to its prospective nature, it was also due to the fact that a causal relationship was taking shape *(43)*.

Although the major epidemiologic studies have differed with regard to endpoints and/ or methodology, the results have been consistent. Passive smoke increases a person's risk of CHD and most likely in a dose-dependent manner. All of the major studies controlled for one or more confounding factors such as age, high blood pressure, high cholesterol, body mass, socioeconomic status, and education. Despite this attempt to disprove the relationship, the consistent outcome is that environmental tobacco smoke increases RR for CHD with nonsmokers.

Translated into real numbers, approximately 37,000 deaths a year from CHD are attributable to passive smoking in the US *(41)*. Beyond our borders, it is estimated that 18% of people living in developed nations will die from the effects of environmental smoke exposure *(5)*.

The mechanisms by which environmental tobacco smoke cause morbidity and mortality are similar to those of current smokers. Nonsmokers exposed to tobacco smoke on a regular basis are found to have an increased myocardial oxygen demand, oftentimes resulting in ischemia and increased platelet aggregation *(41)*. Although this increase in oxygen demand is considerably smaller than that of primary smokers, the effects can clearly be seen during exercise, a time in which the body uses large amounts of its oxygen from the blood *(41)*. In a study by Leone and colleagues *(43)*, healthy young adults were more easily exhausted during exercise after being experimentally exposed to tobacco smoke *(44)*. For adults with established heart disease, exposure to passive smoke results in decreased ability to exercise and a greater likelihood of developing arrhythmias during exercise *(41)*. During the same time that there is an increase in oxygen demand, the carbon monoxide in tobacco smoke reduces the oxygen-carrying ability of the blood by forming carboxyhemoglobin. In addition, the oxygen that is received is not as efficiently used by the myocardium after repeated exposure to passive smoke *(41)*. Other deleterious effects from environmental tobacco smoke include increased resting heart rate and blood pressure (both systolic and diastolic) *(41)*.

Blood platelets are negatively impacted by environmental tobacco smoke increasing the risk of thrombus, damaging the lining of the coronary arteries, and contributing to plaque lesion formation *(45)*. In a study done by Burghuber and associates *(45)*, smokers and nonsmokers were exposed to cigarette smoke for 20 min in a waiting room. The results found that nonsmokers had significant changes in their platelet activity, almost equal to that of a smoker. The smoker, on the other hand, had very few changes in their platelet activity after additional exposure to smoke *(46)*. This study, in addition to other similar studies *(47–50)*, have found that nonsmokers' platelet activity is much more sensitive to even low levels of passive smoke than platelet activity of smokers *(45)*.

There has also been evidence that passive smoking causes damage to the endothelial cells, leaving them open to increased platelet adherence and eventually increased atherosclerosis. Additionally, it has been shown that passive smoking negatively affects high-density lipoprotein cholesterol (HDL-C), leaving exposed nonsmokers at higher risk of developing CHD than nonexposed, nonsmokers *(45)*.

In a recent study by Howard and co-workers *(50)*, 10,814 carotid ultrasounds were compared by smoking classification and passive smoking classification. In addition to finding higher rates of atherosclerosis progression among current smokers as expected, the results also showed a 20% increase in atherosclerosis progression in individuals exposed to passive smoke. The effects of passive smoke in this study appeared to be cumulative and irreversible, prompting more debate over banning smoking in all public places *(51)*.

SMOKING CESSATION

It has long been understood that nicotine is one of the all-time most addictive substances. No doubt that is the reason so many people continue to smoke. Since 1964, when the landmark Surgeon General's report on smoking and health was released, the number of ex-smokers has increased tremendously, allowing for thorough study of smoking cessation to occur. In 1990 the Surgeon General released another report entitled, "The Health Benefits of Smoking Cessation." There were four major conclusions regarding heart disease in the report:

1. Smoking cessation results in immediate, substantial health benefits with people of all age groups and differing disease states.
2. Those who quit smoking live longer.
3. Smoking cessation decreases the risk of lung cancer, other cancers, heart attack, stroke, and chronic lung disease.
4. The health benefits resulting from smoking cessation far outweigh the risks of gaining a small- to-moderate amount of weight following quitting (52).

The benefits from quitting smoking are staggering. In a study looking at women, smoking and incidence of myocardial infarction (MI), those who had not smoked for 3–4 yr had an RR virtually identical to nonsmokers' relative risk. This remained true regardless of the amount smoked, the duration of smoking, the age of the woman, or the presence of other cardiac risk factors (53). Many studies have come to the same conclusions (54,55). There have been other studies suggesting upwards of 10 yr smoke free to see a significant decrease in risk (42).

Clearly, smoking cessation is essential in maintaining health. In spite of all the information regarding benefits to quitting, millions continue to smoke. According to a recent study by Ayanian and Cleary (55), smokers do not see themselves at increased risk of heart disease or cancer despite the general knowledge that smoking "isn't good" (56). Yet, it is estimated that approximately 70% of current smokers desire to quit, but only 8% a year have some success. Of those 8%, only 10% will maintain their new nonsmoking status (57). Physician involvement in the cessation process is a key factor. Several studies have shown that encouragement from the physician regarding smoking cessation is effective (58,59). Yet according to a study in the early 1980s, less than half of all smokers had received advice from their physician to quit, a figure that still holds true today (60). More disturbingly is the fact that there are clear demographic differences between smokers who are counseled and those who are not. Specifically, men with heart disease were counseled more often than women with heart disease. Non-Hispanic whites also had higher rates of smoking cessation counseling than their Hispanic counterparts. Adolescents were very rarely counseled even though they had more potential opportunities compared to adult smokers. Income level was a significant predictor of counseling with white collar workers receiving advice more often than blue collar workers. On a positive note, two thirds of heavier smokers were counseled despite the fact that they had fewer physician visits per year than lighter smokers (60). In a meta-analysis study looking at 39 smoking cessation, controlled trials, the results showed that there is nothing novel about successful intervention programs. Personalized advice and assistance from the physician and other members of the staff over a long period of time was the key to increasing cessation rates (61). It also appears that withdrawing this assistance after cessation results in higher rates of relapse than if the message continues to be given at each physician visit (61).

Stages of Change and the Physician

The stages-of-change model, well accepted within the field of public health, has long been the basis for smoking cessation intervention. Understanding and working within the model's framework allows both the patient and the physician a guide through the "jungle" of cessation. Many physicians believe success on their parts is cessation on the patient's. This kind of thinking only leads to frustration for both the patient and the physician. Within the stages-of-change framework, there is a middle ground. The stages-of-change model includes five stages; precontemplation, contemplation, preparation, action, and maintenance *(62)*. As opposed to other models that are linear in thinking, the stages of change model is circular. All smokers fit into one of the following categories.

Precontemplation—The patient has no intention of trying to quit in the next 6 mo. He or she avoids communication regarding the topic and is usually uninformed or under-informed regarding personal risk.

Contemplation—The patient is fairly aware of the risks and is seriously thinking of quitting within the next 6 mo. However, the patient is still not convinced of the long-term benefits and thinks more about the short-term costs. Many patients get stuck in the "thinking" phase without impetus to move forward.

Preparation—The patient is getting ready to quit within the next month. He or she is already making small changes in preparation for his or her quit date.

Action—The patient has made major and substantial change to his or her risky behavior and is most at risk of relapse during this time period, lasting about 6 mo.

Maintenance—The patient is actively working on maintaining a smoke-free environment *(62)*.

It is important to assess a patient's stage at each visit so that the physician can tailor the smoking cessation message. Instead of defining success as cessation, success becomes moving the patient forward on the road to cessation *(62)*. Patients who are precontemplative are not interested in setting quit dates or hearing about nicotine replacement. A more effective use of the physician's time is to discuss the patient's personal risk from smoking. Oftentimes patients get stuck in the contemplative stage. They know the risks of smoking in abstract, but the discomfort and irritation that comes with cessation is too high a price to pay *(62)*. These patients need firm warnings from the physician as well as information on programs and nicotine replacement.

The reality of smoking cessation is that for every 100 patients counseled to cessation, 75 will relapse *(62)*. The circular nature of the stages-of-change model is important because patients who relapse will return usually to the precontemplative or contemplative stage. On average, it takes a smoker three to four cycles through the stages before true cessation occurs *(62)*. With this understanding, physicians can reduce the frustration associated with cessation advice and continue to help the patient move along toward the ultimate goal of cessation. Prochaska and Goldstein *(61)* suggest the following simple three-question assessment of a patient's stage regarding smoking cessation.

Assessment of Patient's Stage Regarding Smoking Cessation

Are you intending to quit smoking in the next 6 months? If the answer is no, the patient is precontemplative.

Are you intending to quit smoking in the next month? If the answer is no but the patient answered yes to question one, the patient is contemplative.

Did you try to quit smoking in the past year? If yes, and the patient is planning to quit within the next month, the patient is in the preparation stage (61).

Cessation and Relapse Prevention and Techniques

Techniques to decrease physiologic addiction
- Nicotine fading: Reduce nicotine consumption by changing to a lower tar and nicotine brands; cutting down in other ways
- Nicotine gum/patch: Substitute nicotine gum for nicotine from cigarettes while adjusting to nonsmoking status
- Bupropion: Treatment of dependence with non-addicting agent
- Stop smoking

Techniques to decrease physiologic dependency
- Create a dislike for smoking:
- Rapid smoking: Smoke rapidly until ill effects occur
- Smoke holding: Hold smoke in mouth while concentrating on unpleasant sensations
- Covert sensitization: Concentrate on unpleasant aspects of smoking, e.g., keep a butt jar visible
- Hypnosis
- Accupuncture

Relapse prevention methods
- Coping skills: Patient learns to cope with environmental, psychologic, and physiologic cues that stimulate desire to smoke
- Stress cues: Learn relaxation, stress management
- Friends offering cigarettes: Practicing saying no
- Urges: Learn to let them peak and pass
- Cognitive restructuring: Patient learns to view him or herself as a nonsmoker, change attitudes
- Social support: Patient enlists the help of family and friends to provide encouragement
- Alcohol codependence and treatment
- Time

For persons who have already quit, it is important not to stop asking about their smoking status. Patients need to be asked how long ago they quit and if this is less than 6 mo, they are in the action stage and are at high risk for relapse. If they are more than 6 mo smoke free, they are in maintenance and support needs to continue *(62)*.

INTERVENTIONS

The American Heart Association, the American Cancer Society, and the American Lung Association, along with thousands of local programs, offer behavior modification programs trying to help the millions of people looking to quit smoking every year. These techniques are useful and can be initiated in the physician's office. Techniques such as logging each cigarette smoked in a diary while noting the "triggering" event or the feelings associated with the cigarette (i.e., stress, coffee consumption, and so on) are useful in helping patients understand when they smoke most. Helping the patient set a quit date is often effective in moving them into a state of action. Preparing patients for what they and their families can expect during nicotine withdrawal is also important. Insufficient social support is one of the leading predictors of relapse *(63)*. In addition to behavior modification, physicians now have at their disposal a variety of pharmacologic smoking cessation aids.

Nicotine Gum

Nicotine gum (nicotine polacrilex) was the first pharmacologic aid for those attempting to quit smoking and was approved by the FDA in 1985. The gum comes in two different doses, 2 mg, the more common dose, and 4 mg and is now sold over the counter. The goal of nicotine gum is to deliver a short burst of nicotine to overcome nicotine cravings while helping the patient to discontinue the habit of smoking. In early studies looking at 2 mg gum vs. 4 mg gum, the results showed the two doses to be comparable in efficacy *(64,65)*. In later studies, however, when more nicotine-dependent smokers were analyzed separately, it was found that the 4-mg dose of the gum was much more effective *(65)*. It is believed that the 2-mg dose of gum actually translates into 0.8–1.0 mg of nicotine, which is bioavailable to the smoker. For smokers with increased levels of nicotine dependence, this is inadequate to control nicotine cravings *(66)*. In a study by Herrera and associates *(66)*, the 6-wk, 1-yr, and 2-yr chemically verified quit rates for high nicotine dependent smokers on the 4-mg gum were 60, 39, and 34%, respectively *(67)*. Side effects noted with all doses of nicotine gum use include gastric upset, hiccups, and/or jaw ache *(68)*. In addition, it has also been noted that coffee and carbonated beverages can block absorption of nicotine from the gum, a concern for some patients *(69)*. Table 1 gives additional information and usage guidelines.

Nicotine Patch

The transdermal nicotine patch was first available for prescription in late 1991, approved for over-the-counter use in 1996, and has since become one of the most widely used pharmacologic aids in smoking cessation. The patch delivers a steady dose of nicotine to the bloodstream eliminating the nicotine cravings that accompany smoking cessation. In 1994, Fiore and colleagues *(69)* conducted a meta-analysis of 23 clinical trials involving the nicotine patch. Overall, the study saw a 22% abstinence rate 6 mo poststudy vs. a 9% abstinence rate of subjects on placebo. Additionally, the researchers found that the nicotine patch was fairly effective without intense adjuvant therapy, although subjects involved in behavioral counseling were more likely to be abstinent at 6 mo poststudy *(70)*. The study also found that both the 16-h and the 24-h patches were effective. Various versions of the patch are now sold over the counter after multiple studies proved its efficacy, safety, and cost effectiveness *(71)*.

The biggest benefit of patch use as opposed to gum use is the steady stream of nicotine into the blood system. Contrary to preliminary data, smoking cigarettes while wearing the patch is not cardiotoxic. Instead, the risk associated with simultaneous use of patch and cigarettes is no more than risk from cigarette smoking alone. Although cigarette smoking increases blood coagulability, transdermal nicotine does not appear to have the same effect *(11)*. The nicotine gum and patch are commonly used together and have shown greater success in achieving smoking cessation than either alone. However very few studies have looked at the combination use *(72)*.

The patch comes over the counter as Nicotrol® and Nicoderm CQ®. Nicotrol is a one-dose patch, whereas Nicoderm CQ is a stepped approach with three varied-dose patches. There has not been any evidence that one brand is more effective than the other, as there are pros and cons to each *(72)* *(see* Table 1 for additional information and usage guidelines).

Nicotine Nasal Spray

The nicotine nasal spray was first approved by the FDA for prescription use in 1996. The goal of its introduction was to deliver nicotine more rapidly so as to better handle smokers' cravings. Studies have consistently found that the nasal spray doubles the quit rates of smokers when compared to the use of placebo *(72)*. The spray is successful at increasing peak levels of nicotine faster than either the nicotine gum or the patch, yet not as rapidly as a cigarette *(73)*. The dose is one spray into each nostril or 1 mg of nicotine. It is recommended that patients start with 1–2 doses per hour with a minimum of 8 doses per day and a maximum of 40 doses per day. This should be reduced after 6–8 wk of continuous treatment *(74)*. The side effects from the nasal spray are significant. The most common are runny nose, nasal irritation, throat irritation, watery eyes, sneezing, and coughing *(75)*. However, most side effects disappear within 1 wk. There has been some evidence that weight gain normally seen after cessation is delayed in patients using the nasal spray consistently *(75)*. More studies are needed to clarify the issue of weight gain and nasal spray. There has been some concern regarding treatment dependence with the nicotine nasal spray due to its rapid nature. Recent studies have not shown abuse liability *(76,77)* (*see* Table 1 for additional information and usage guidelines).

Nicotine Inhaler

In 1998, the inhaler became the fourth addition to the nicotine replacement family. As with other nicotine replacement products, the inhaler doubles quit rates when compared to placebo *(78,79)*. It is currently available only by prescription. The inhaler is a small plastic rod containing a nicotine plug that delivers a nicotine vapor each time a patient takes a "puff." Although resembling a cigarette, the inhaler contains considerably less nicotine than a true cigarette. It takes approximately 80 puffs from the inhaler to equal the amount of nicotine in one cigarette. Patients are instructed to take frequent continuous "puffs" each time they have a nicotine craving, using the inhaler for about 20 min per craving *(80)*. The vapors are then absorbed through the lining of the mouth. The major benefit associated with the inhaler is the similar hand–mouth ritual to which smokers are accustomed *(72)*. For a pack-a-day smoker, this hand–mouth action is repeated almost 200 times a day *(81)*, sometimes making the habit more difficult to break than the nicotine addiction. The side effects are relatively mild with mouth and throat irritation being the most common *(72)* (*see* Table 1 for additional information and usage guidelines).

Bupropion

Bupropion, or Zyban®, is a slow-release formulation of the antidepressant more commonly known as Welbutrin® *(82)*. For many years researchers believed there to be a relationship between dopamine, norepinephrine, other neurotransmitters and nicotine *(83)*. Early studies with doxepin, clonidine, and nortriptyline showed promise as adjuncts to smoking cessation therapy *(84–86)*. In the early 1990s, two small double-blind studies using the immediate release version of bupropion at 300 mg found efficacy *(83)*. Bupropion, an inhibitor of neuronal uptake of norepinephrine and dopamine, is believed to help smokers quit in two ways *(83)*. The first is by affecting dopaminergic activity in the brain where reinforcement of addictive drugs occurs. The second is by working on noradrenergic activity affecting nicotine withdrawal *(83)*.

Table 1

Pharmacotherapy Summary

Product	Dosage	Guidelines	Duration of use	Advantages	Disadvantages
Nicotine gum	2 mg or 4 mg Persons who smoke less than 25 cigarettes a day should use the 2-mg gum, otherwise use the 4-mg. No more than 24 pieces per day.	Bite the gum slowly until it tingles, then park it in between the cheek and gum for a minute. Continue this chewing and parking for 30 min.	Weeks 1–6, 1 piece every 1–2 h Weeks 7–9, 1 piece every 2–4 h Weeks 10–12 1 piece every 4–8 h	The gum is convenient, sold over the counter, and flexible to the patient.	Nicotine is slow to absorb in the system. Must be chewed correctly to avoid gastric distress and to achieve nicotine levels. It is contraindicated for those with jaw or dental problems.
Nicotine patch	Stepped-dose approach = 21 mg, 14 mg, and 7 mg. One-dose approach = 15 mg.	The patch must be rotated to different locations on the body that have minimal hair	6–10 wk depending on the brand. No study has found one brand to be more effective than the other.	There are few side effects to the patch. It is easy to use and only needs to be applied once a day.	Nicotine is delivered slowly to the brain with no flexibility in dose. In addition, skin rashes can occur.
Nicotine nasal spray	1–2 sprays per hour.	The nasal spray works best with a minimum of 8 doses/d and a maximum of 40 doses/d.	6–8 wk is appropriate use. Abuse liability does not seem to be a problem. Risks of long-term use are less than risks from continued cigarette use for highly dependent smokers.	The nasal spray delivers nicotine quickly for rapid relief of cravings. It is easy to use and it may decrease weight gain during use.	The side effects (nose and throat irritation, sneezing, coughing, watery eyes) can be hard to tolerate, although they typically disappear within about 1 wk.
Nicotine Inhaler	One cartridge equals 80 deep draws or 300 shallow puffs per craving. No more than 16 cartridges should be used per day.	Twenty minutes of continuous, active puffing was found to be most effective in achieving appropriate nicotine levels.	Up to 3 mo with gradual reduction over 6–12 wk if needed.	The inhaler substitutes the hand–mouth behavior to which smokers have been habituated.	It must be used frequently throughout the day. Mild side effects (mouth and throat irritation) may occur.
Bupropion	150 mg, 300 mg	Patients should start with 150 mg daily 3 d prior to quitting. Patients should then increase the dose to 150 mg twice a day.	7–12 wk is the recommended treatment period.	Bupropion is nonnicotinic and can be used with the patch. It is a pill and is taken once a day. Weight gain may be less with bupropion.	There is a slight risk of seizure and should not be taken if there is a history of seizure, anorexia, heavy alcohol use, or head trauma. Dry mouth and insomnia are the most common side effects.

As with other nicotine replacement treatments, clinical studies found bupropion consistently doubling quit rates when compared to placebo *(83,87)*. Interestingly enough, extended-release bupropion worked equally well for smokers with and without a history of depression, bolstering the notion that buproprion works differently for each condition *(72)*. In a recent study by Jorenby and associates *(87)*, higher quit rates were seen with a combination of bupropion and nicotine patch *(88)*. The recommended dosage for smoking cessation is 300 mg/d for 7–12 wk, beginning 1 wk prior to smoking cessation. The most common side effects include dry mouth, insomnia, and headache. Hurt and colleagues *(82)* also found reduced weight gain for patients on a higher dose of bupropion (300 mg). This appeared only to last for the duration of the drug treatment *(83)*. Earlier trials with bupropion found evidence of increased seizures *(89)*. However, more recent studies have found that risk to be no more than with other antidepressants. It is recommended, however, to screen patients for seizure possibility prior to bupropion treatment. It is advised that patients with seizure disorders, anorexia, heavy alcohol use, or head trauma should use other pharmacologic agents for smoking cessation *(72)* (*see* Table 1 for additional information and usage guidelines).

REFERENCES

1. Fielding J. Smoking: health effects and control. N Engl J Med 1985;313:491–497.
2. Centers for Disease Control and Prevention. Medical care expenditures attributable to cigarette smoking —United States, 1993. MMWR 1994;43:469–472.
3. Office of Disease Prevention and Health Promotion. Healthy people 2000: midcourse review and 1995 revisions. US Department of Health and Human Services, 1995, Washington, DC.
4. Pierce J, Fiore MC, Novotny TE, et al. Trends in cigarette smoking in the United States—projections to the year 2000. JAMA 1989;261:61–65.
5. Peto R, Lopez AD, Boreham J, et al. Mortality from smoking worldwide. Br Med Bull 1996;52:12–21.
6. Mahaney F. Oldtime ads tout health benefits of smoking: tobacco industry had doctors' help. J Natl Cancer Inst 1994;86:1048–1049.
7. Bartrip P. Pushing the weed: the editorializing and advertising of tobacco in the Lancet and the British Medical Journal, 1880–1958. Clio Med 1998;46:100–126.
8. DeNelsky G. Smoking: what it's all about, what to do about it. Presentation February 2, 1998; Preventive Cardiology and Rehabilitation Group, Cleveland Clinic Foundation, Cleveland, OH.
9. Terry L. The Surgeon General's first report on smoking and health—a challenge to the medical profession. NY St J Med 1983;83:1254–1255.
10. Adams KF, Koch G, Chatterjee B, et al. Acute elevation of blood carboxyhemoglobin to 6% impairs exercise performance and aggravates symptoms in patients with ischemic heart disease. J Am Coll Cardiol 1988;12:900–909.
11. Benowitz N, Gourlay SG. Cardiovascular toxicity of nicotine: implications for nicotine replacement therapy. J Am Coll Cardiol 1997;29:1422–1431.
12. Johnstone RA, Plimmer JR. The chemical constituents of tobacco and tobacco smoke. Chem Rev 1959; 59:885–936.
13. Lekakis J, Papamichael C, Vemmos C, et al. Effects of acute cigarette smoking on endothelium-dependent arterial dilatation in normal subjects. Am J Cardiol 1998;81:1225–1228.
14. Thomas CB, Murphy E. Circulatory responses to smoking in healthy young men. Ann NY Acad Sci 1960;90:266–276.
15. Tresch D, Aronow WS. Smoking and coronary artery disease. Clin Geriatr Med 1996;12:23–32.
16. Nowak J, Andersson K, Benthin G, et al. Effect of nicotine infusion in humans on platelet. Acta Physiol Scand 1996;157:101–107.
17. Gleerup G, Winther K. Smoking further increases platelet. Eur J Clin Invest 1996;26:49–52.
18. Nowak J, Andersson K, Benthin G, et al. Effect of nicotine infusion in humans on platelet aggregation and urinary excretion of a major thromboxane metabolite. Acta Physiol Scand 1996;157:101–107.
19. de Padua Mansur A, Caramelli B, Vianna CB, et al. Smoking and lipoprotein abnormalities on. Int J Cardiol 1997;62:151–154.

20. Hung J, Lam JY, Lacoste L, Letchacovski G. Cigarette smoking acutely increases. Circulation 1995;92: 2432–2436.

21. Reinders JH, Brinkman HM, van Mourik JA, de Groot PG. Cigarette smoke impairs endothelial cell prostacyclin production. Arteriosclerosis 1985;6:15–23.

22. Allen RA, Kluft C, Brommer JP. Effect of chronic smoking on fibrinolysis. Atherosclerosis 1985;5: 443–450.

23. Rangemark C, Wennmalm A. Smoke-derived nitric oxide and vascular prostacyclin are unable to counteract the platelet effect of increased thromboxane formation in healthy female smokers. Clin Physiol 1996;16:301–315.

24. Ichiki K, Ikeda H, Haramaki N, et al. Long-term smoking impairs platelet-derived. Circulation 1996;94: 3109–3114.

25. Randi ML, Fabris F, Cella G, Rossi C, Girolami A. Cerebral vascular accidents in young patients with essential. Angiology 1998;49:477–481.

26. Jensen OK, Ingerslev J. Increased p-homocysteine—a risk factor for thrombosis. Ugeskr Laeger 1998; 160:4405–4410.

27. Miller GJ, Bauer KA, Cooper JA, Roseberg RD. Activation of the coagulant pathway in cigarette smokers. Thromb Haemost 1998;79:549–553.

28. Kannel W, McGee D, Castelli WP. Latest perspective on cigarette smoking and cardiovascular disease: the Framingham Study. J Cardiac Rehabil 1984;4:267–277.

29. Strong J, Malcom GT, McMahan CA, et al., for the Pathobiological Determinants of Atherosclerosis in Youth Research Group. Prevalence and extent of atherosclerosis in adolescents and young adults: implications for prevention from the pathobiological determinants of atherosclerosis in youth study. JAMA 1999;281:727–735.

30. Willett W, Green A, Stampfer MJ, et al. Relative and absolute risks of coronary heart disease among women who smoke cigarettes. N Engl J Med 1987;317:1303–1309.

31. Vlieststra R, Kronmal RA, Oberman A, et al. Effect of cigarette smoking on survival of patients with angiographically documented coronary artery disease—report from the CASS registry. JAMA 1986; 255:1023–1027.

32. Cavender J, Rogers WJ, Fisher LD, et al., for the CASS Investigators. Effects of smoking on survival and morbidity in patients randomized to medical or surgical therapy in the Coronary Artery Surgery Study (CASS): 10-year follow-up. J Am Coll Cardiol 1992;20:287–294.

33. Daly L, Mulcahy R, Graham IM, Hickey N. Long term effect on mortality of stopping smoking after unstable angina and myocardial infarction. Br Med J 1983;287:324–326.

34. Macdonald R, Henderson MA, Hirshfeld JW Jr, et al. Patient-related variables and restenosis after percutaneous transluminal coronary angioplasty—a report from the M-HEART group. Am J Cardiol 1990; 66:926–931.

35. Arora R, Konrad K, Badhwar K, Hollman J. Restenosis after transluminal coronary angioplasty: a risk factor analysis. Cathet Cardiovasc Diagn 1990;19:17–22.

36. Benchimol D, Benchimol H, Bonnet J, et al. Risk factors for progression of atherosclerosis six months after balloon angioplasty of coronary stenosis. Am J Cardiol 1990;65:980–985.

37. Galan K, Deligonul U, Kern MJ, et al. Increased frequency of restenosis in patients continuing to smoke cigarettes after percutaneous transluminal coronary angioplasty. Am J Cardiol 1988;61:260–263.

38. Myler R, Topol EJ, Shaw RE, et al. Multiple vessel coronary angioplasty: classification, results and patterns of restenosis in 494 consecutive patients. Cathet Cardiovasc Diagn 1987;13:1–15.

39. Wilhelmsen L. Coronary heart disease: epidemiology of smoking and intervention studies of smoking. Am Heart J 1988;115:242–249.

40. Glantz S, Parmley WW. Passive smoking and heart disease—epidemiology, physiology and biochemistry. Circulation 1995;83:1–11.

41. Kawachi I, Colditz GA, Speizer FE, et al. A prospective study of passive smoking and coronary heart disease. Circulation 1997;95:2374–2379.

42. Dwyer J. Exposure to environmental tobacco smoke and coronary risk. Circulation 1997;96:1367–1369.

43. Leone A, Mori L, Bertanelli F, et al. Indoor passive smoking: its effect on cardiac performance. Int J Cardiol 1991;33:247–252.

44. Glantz S, Parmley WW. Passive smoking and heart disease—mechanisms and risk. JAMA 1995;273: 1047–1053.

45. Burghuber O, Punzengruber C, Sinzinger H, et al. Platelet sensitivity to prostacyclin in smokers and non-smokers. Chest 1986;90:34–38.

46. Davis J, Hartman CR, Lewis HD, et al. Cigarette smoking-induced enhancement of platelet function: lack of prevention by aspirin in men with coronary artery disease. J Lab Clin Med 1985;105:479–483.

47. Davis J, Shelton L, Eigenberg DA, et al. Effects of tobacco and non-tobacco cigarette smoke on endothelium and platelets. Clin Pharmacol Therap 1985;37:529–533.

48. Davis J, Shelton L, Eigenberg DA, Ruttinger HA. Smoking-induced changes in endothelium and platelets are not affected by hydroxyethlrutosides. Br J Exp Pathol 1986;67:765–771.

49. Davis J, Shelton L, Eigenberg DA, Hignite CE. Lack of effect of aspirin on cigarette smoke-induced increase in circulating endothelial cells. Haemostasis 1987;17:66–69.

50. Howard G, Wagenknecht LE, Burke GL, et al. Cigarette smoking and progression of atherosclerosis: the atherosclerosis risk in communities (ARIC) study. JAMA 1998;279:119–124.

51. United States Department of Health, Education and Welfare, Public Health Service. The health benefits of smoking cessation. Report of the Surgeon General, Washington, DC, 1990.

52. Rosenberg L, Palmer JR, Shapiro S. Decline in the risk of myocardial infarction among women who stop smoking. N Engl J Med 1990;322:214–217.

53. Rosenberg L, Kaufman DW, Helmrich SP, Shapiro S. The risk of myocardial infarction after quitting smoking in men under 55 years of age. N Engl J Med 1990;313:1512–1514.

54. Dobson A, Alexander HM, Heller RF, Lloyd DM. How soon after quitting smoking does risk of heart attack decline? J Clin Epidemiol 1991;44:1247–1253.

55. Ayanian J, Cleary PD. Perceived risks of heart disease and cancer among cigarette smokers. JAMA 1999;281:1019–1021.

56. Health and Human Services Agency for Health Care Policy and Research (AHCPR). Smoking cessation: clinical practice guideline. Deparatment of Health and Human Services, Washington, DC, 1996.

57. Ockene J, Kristeller J, Goldberg R, et al. Increasing the efficacy of physician-delivered smoking intervention: a randomized clinical trial. J Gen Intern Med 1991;6:1–8.

58. Glynn T, Manley MW, Pechacek TF. Physician-initiated smoking cessation program: the National Cancer Institute trials. In: Engrstrom P, Rimer, B, Mortenson, LE, eds. Advances in Cancer Control. Wiley, New York, 1990, pp. 11–26.

59. Frank E, Winkleby MA, Altman DG, et al. Predictors of physicians' smoking cessation advice. JAMA 1991;266:3139–3144.

60. Kottke T, Battista RN, DeFriese GH, Brekke ML. Attributes of successful smoking cessation interventions in medical practice—a meta-analysis of 39 controlled trials. JAMA 1988;259:2883–2889.

61. Prochaska J, Goldstein MG. Process of smoking cessation—implications for clinicians. Clin Chest Med 1991;12:727–735.

62. Hughes J, Hatsukami DK. Signs and symptoms of tobacco withdrawal. Arch Gen Psychiatry 1986;43:289–294.

63. Kornitzer M, Kittel F, Dramaix M, Bourdoux P. A double-blind study of 2 mg vs 4 mg nicotine gum in an industrial setting. J Psychosom Res 1988;31:171–176.

64. Tonnesen P, Fryd V, Hansen M, et al. Two and 4-mg nicotine chewing gum and group counselling in smoking cessation: an open randomized controlled trial with a 22 month follow-up. Addict Behav 1988;13:17–27.

65. Benowitz N, Jacob P, Savanapridi C. Determinants of nicotine intake while chewing nicotine polacrilex gum. Clin Pharmacol Ther 1987;41:457–473.

66. Herrera N, Franco R, Herrera L, et al. Nicotine gum, 2 and 4 mg for nicotine dependence: a double-blind placebo-controlled trial within a behavior modification support program. Chest 1995;108:447–451.

67. Lee E, D'Alonzo, GE. Cigarette smoking, nicotine addiction and its pharmacologic treatment. Arch Intern Med 993;153:34–48.

68. Henningfield J, Radzius A, Cooper TM, Clayton RR. Drinking coffee and carbonated beverages blocks absorption of nicotine from nicotine polacrilex gum. JAMA 1990;264:1560–1564.

69. Fiore M, Smith SS, Jorenby DE, Baker TB. The effectiveness of the nicotine patch for smoking cessation—a meta-analysis. JAMA 1994;271:1940–1947.

70. Wasley M, McNagny SE, Phillips VL, et al. The cost-effectiveness of the nicotine transdermal patch for smoking cessation. Prev Med 1997;26:264–270.

71. Hughes J, Goldstein MG, Hurt RD, Shiffman S. Recent advances in the pharmacotherapy of smoking. JAMA 1999;281:72–76.

72. Schneider N, Lunell, E, Olmstead, RE, Fagerstrom KO. Clinical pharmacokinetics of nasal nicotine delivery—a review and comparison to other nicotine systems. Clin Pharmacokinet 1996;31:65–80.

73. McNeil Consumer Products. Nicotrol nasal spray prescribing information. McNeil Consumer Products, Fort Washington, PA, 1996.

74. Sutherland G, Stapleton JA, Russell MA, et al. Randomized controlled trial of nasal nicotine spray in smoking cessation. Lancet 1992;340:324–329.
75. Hughes J. Dependence on and abuse of nicotine replacement: an update. In: Benowitz N, ed. Nicotine Safety and Toxicity. Oxford University Press, New York, 1998, pp. 147–160.
76. Schuh K, Schuh LM, Henningfield JE, Stitzer ML. Nicotine nasal spray and vapor inhaler: abuse liability assessment. Psychopharmacology 1997;130:352–361.
77. Leischow S, Nilsson F, Franzon M, et al. Efficacy of the nicotine inhaler as an adjunct to smoking cessation. Am J Health Behav 1996;20:364–371.
78. Tonnesen P, Norregaard J, Mikkelsen K, et al. A double-blind trial of a nicotine inhaler for smoking cessation. JAMA 1993;269:1268–1271.
79. McNeil Consumer Products. Nicotrol inhaler prescribing information. McNeil Consumer Products, Fort Washington, PA, 1999.
80. McNeil Consumer Products. Nicotrol inhaler patient information. McNeil Consumer Products, Fort Washington, PA, 1999.
81. Glaxo Wellcome Inc. Zyban prescribing information. Glaxo Wellcome, Research Triangle Park, NC, 1998.
82. Hurt R, Sachs DP, Glover ED, et al. A comparison of sustained-release bupropion and placebo for smoking cessation. N Engl J Med 1997;337:1195–1202.
83. Prochazka A, Petty TL, Nett L, et al. Transdermal clonidine reduced some withdrawal symptoms but did not increase smoking cessation. Arch Intern Med 1992;152:2065–2069.
84. Prochazka A, Weaver MJ, Keller RT, et al. A randomized trial of nortriptyline for smoking cessation. Arch Intern Med 1998;158:2035–2039.
85. Edwards N, Murphy JK, Downs AD, et al. Doxepin as an adjunct to smoking cessation: a double-blind pilot study. Am J Psychiatry 1989;146:373–376.
86. Ferry L, Burchette RJ. Efficacy of bupropion for smoking cessation in non-depressed smokers. J Addict Disord 1994;13:249.
87. Jorenby D, Leischow SJ, Nides MA, et al. A controlled trial of sustained-release bupropion, a nicotine patch, or both for smoking cessation. N Engl J Med 1999;340:685–691.
88. Ascher J, Cole JO, Colin JN, et al. Bupropion: a review of its mechanism of antidepressant activity. J Clin Psychiatry 1995;56:395–401.

11 Women and Coronary Artery Disease

JoAnne Micale Foody, MD
and Cynthia Pordon, DO

CONTENTS

INTRODUCTION

Cardiovascular disease (CVD) is the leading cause of mortality among women in the United States—500,000 women each year die of coronary heart disease (CHD). CHD is more age dependent in women than in men: women are usually 10 yr older than men when coronary manifestations first appear and MI may occur as much as 20 yr later. One in eight women aged 45–64 yr has clinical evidence of CHD and this increase to nearly 1 in 3 in women older than 65. With the aging of the American population, more women than men now die each year of CHD *(1)*.

Deaths in women from cardiovascular disease are almost twice that of deaths due to cancer. Approximately one out of every two women in the United States will die from some cardiovascular event—most likely, myocardial infarction (MI), hypertensive heart disease, or stroke (Fig. 1).

The impact of CVD is even greater for black women in whom the overall annual mortality rate due to cardiovascular disease is approximately 67% higher than in white women (2.25/1000 vs. 1.35/1000, respectively).

Coronary risk factors are highly prevalent in women in the United States *(2–7)*. In women aged 20–74, 33% have hypertension, more than one quarter have hypercholesterolemia, more than one quarter are cigarette smokers, more than a quarter are overweight, and more than a quarter report sedentary lifestyles. Although these risk factors are more prevalent

From: *Contemporary Cardiology: Preventive Cardiology:*
Strategies for the Prevention and Treatment of Coronary Artery Disease
Edited by: J. Foody © Humana Press Inc., Totowa, NJ

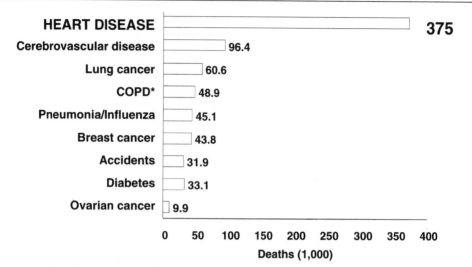

Fig. 1. CAD: leading cause of death in US women in 1995. *COPD = chronic obstructive pulmonary disease. Adapted from ref. *1*.

in men than in women, as women age their risk factor profile approaches and, in some instances, surpasses that of their male counterparts.

Although risk factors for CAD are similar in men and women (Table 1), the impact of individual coronary risk factors and the results of their interventions differ dramatically by gender *(2–7)*. Special emphasis must also be placed on those uniquely female attributes that modify coronary risk: specifically oral contraceptives, pregnancy, menopausal status, and the use of postmenopausal hormone therapy.

CLINICAL PRESENTATION OF CAD IN WOMEN

Angina pectoris (AP) is the main initial and subsequent presenting symptom of coronary heart disease (CHD) in women, while myocardial infarction (MI) and sudden caridac death (SCD) are the more common presentations in men. Women with AP are likely to be older than men and to have hypertension, diabetes mellitus (DM), and congestive heart failure (CHF) more commonly. They are also less likely than men to have a prior history of either MI or a percutaneous coronary intervention.

Myocardial infaction is more ominous in women than in men. Hospital mortality is higher for MI in women than in men. Although the presentations are identical, women are less likely to be treated aggressively; they are half as likely to have acute catheterization, angioplasty, thrombolysis, or coronary artery bypass grafting (CABG). Women who survive have earlier and more frequent recurrence of MI and their 1-yr mortality is greater. Although sex differences lessen when older age and comorbidity in women are considered, these differences do not completely disappear. Women who present with MI have higher Killip classes, more tachyarrythmias, more atrial ventricular (AV) block, CHF, shock, recurrent angina, and rupture.

Survival benefit from thrombolysis for acute myocardial infarction (AMI) was similar in women and men even though women tended to have more bleeding complications. Nonetheless, the mortality difference between sexes persist. Primary percutaneous transluminal coronary angioplasty (PTCA) provides an alternative to thrombolysis in women as women, appear to have equally good outcomes when compared to men.

Table 1
Risk Factors for Cardiovascular Disease in Women

Modifiable risk factors	Unmodifiable risk factors
Dyslipidemias	Increasing Age
Hypertension	Gender
Diabetes mellitus	Genetics
Cigarette smoking	Race
Obesity	Menopause (?)
Physical inactivity	
Genetics (?)	

CARDIOVASCULAR RISK FACTORS IN WOMEN

Cholesterol and Dyslipidemia

It is well established that the higher the level of serum cholesterol, the higher the risk of CHD *(8)*. Multiple studies have borne out these results. Lipid and lipoprotein concentrations vary according to a woman's ovarian function. Women who have undergone natural menopause or oophorectomy have significantly higher concentrations of total cholesterol (TC) when compared to menstruating women or those who have undergone hysterectomy with preservation of ovarian function. Similar findings have been observed for changes in low-density lipoprotein cholesterol (LDL-C) levels.

Lipids are uniquely affected by gender. Lipid subfractions change predictably with aging in both men and women, but not at all in the same way. The effects of endogenous gonadal hormones in life-cycle changes in women is evident. Furthermore, compositional differences in lipid particles between men and women have been observed.

Total Cholesterol

Plasma TC level is similar up to 20 yr of age in both sexes. Then, TC level increases progressively but at a slower rate for women until the sixth decade. Thus, men's level generally remains slightly higher. After the sixth decade, women's TC levels generally increase faster, exceeding those of men of similar age *(9)*. This is attributable to the rise in LDL-C in women postmenopause and the persistent discrepancy in high-density lipoprotein cholesterol (HDL-C). Although the relatively larger contribution of HDL-C to TC in premenopausal women is commonly appreciated by medical professionals, the general public does not, and the discovery of an elevated TC in a premenopausal woman usually by public screening can lead to confusion and unwarranted concern.

Although TC, HDL-C, and LDL-C levels have been demonstrated to be independent predictors of CAD in men *(10–13)*, less is known about the effect of lipid concentrations on CAD in women. When comparing data by gender, serum cholesterol is associated with CAD in women similarly to men. At each level of cholesterol, however, men have higher rates of disease than do women, thus, women may be at high risk for CAD at different levels of cholesterol than men *(14)*. For example, the Framingham Study investigators found that women with total cholesterol levels above 295 mg/dL had only 60% the rate of myocardial infarction compared with men with TC < 204 mg/dL *(7)*.

But the data convincingly show that women who have a total serum cholesterol above 260 mg/dL are two or three times at risk of developing CAD than are women whose TC level is below 200 mg/dL. Only The Lipid Research Clinics (LRC) found increased mortality at lower cholesterol levels (>235 mg/dL).

In the Evans County Study, TC is predictive of cardiovascular disease mortality in white women younger than 65 *(15)*. Among black women, cholesterol was negatively associated with all-cause mortality. In a study published the same year, the Charleston Heart Study, a lack of consistency of results by different statistical analyses in black women make conclusions concerning the nature of the relationship between cholesterol and CHD mortality less strong in black women than in white women. White women having a cholesterol value one standard deviation above the mean (sd = 52.5 mg/dL) had a 60% higher CHD mortality rate (hazard ratio = 1.6, 95% CI: 1.2–2.1). In black women, the estimated hazard ratio for a one standard deviation (sd = 47.8 mg/dL) increase in cholesterol is 1.4 (95% CI: 1.03-1.8). The results suggest that the relationship of cholesterol to CHD mortality is different in white and black women *(16)*.

Some studies demonstrate gender differences in the elderly for TC as a risk factor for death from CAD. Serum TC level predicted fatal CAD outcomes in middle-aged (<65 yr) and older (65 yr) men and women; however, the strength and consistency of these relationships in older women were diminished *(17)*. Analysis of the Rancho Bernardo Study data suggests that in the elderly, TC level predicts fatal coronary events in men but not in women *(6)*. These results are not unexpected given the TC value is calculated from HDL-C, LDL-C, and TG (TC = HDL-C + LDL-C + TG/5) and that LDL level was found to be no better a predictor of fatal CHD than total cholesterol in either gender, and that women had higher levels of HDL than men, explaining the usually higher TC levels.

The Donolo-Tel Aviv study also noted that the adverse effects of a high TC level may be balanced by a high HDL-C level: women with high HDL-C had similar low rates of CHD regardless of their level of TC. No such relationship was observed in the male participants. In the same way, the investigators demonstrated a two- to-fivefold higher risk of CHD in women whose HDL-C level was less than 23% of their TC, even in those individuals whose TC was less than 200 mg/dL *(18)*.

Thus there appears to be virtually no risk of CHD in women with a "desirable " level of total cholesterol (<205), whereas even a slight elevation in cholesterol (up to a "borderline" high level of 220–250 mg/dL) results in an approximate doubling of risk. The incidence of CHD continues to rise steeply as cholesterol concentrations reach the "high" level (>280 mg/dL). The annual rate of CHD in women also rises sharply in relation to age, plateauing at the age of 65–74 and then begins to decline. Fewer than 10/1000 women under the age of 55 (presumed to be pre- or perimenopausal) develop CHD, whereas the rate of CHD jumps to almost 25/1000 in women between the ages of 55 and 64 (presumed to be postmenopausal) and to more than 30/1000 in women between the ages of 65 and 74. Thus the risk of CHD is strongly correlated to both increasing age and serum TC level in women.

HDL-C

The HDL-C levels of male children are slightly higher than those of female children until puberty, but as girls pass through puberty, HDL-C levels do not fall as they do in boys of the same age. After puberty, HDL-C levels in women increase slowly until before menopause while they remain constant in men. Thus, the average HDL-C values in adult women are approximately 20% higher than those of men *(19)*. Women prospectively followed through menopause demonstrate a decline in the mean HDL-C levels of approx-

Table 2
Changes in HDL Cholesterol in Premenopausal vs. Postmenopausal Women

Elevated levels of HDL are cardioprotective in men and women
HDL-C is a key predictor of CHD mortality in women
Menopausal women have significantly lower HDL-C levels than premenopausal
    women, independent of other biologic characteristics
This may place postmenopausal women at greater risk for CHD

imately 3.5 mg/dL. However, HDL-C levels generally remain higher in women than men throughout life (20).

Compositional differences in HDL-C between men and women also have been observed. HDL-C, which seems to exert a protective effect on the development of atherosclerosis (21), has two subfractions: HDL-C-2 and HDL-C-3. Most studies show that high HDL-C-2 levels are associated with reduced risk of CHD (22,23), whereas high levels of another component, HDL-C-3 (HDL-C-3B), might be associated with increased CAD risk. Women have higher HDL-C-2 and lower HDL-C-3 than men (24). In 1988, Otha and colleagues showed that in women, HDL-C has a higher content of apolipoprotein A_1 (apo A_1), cholesterol and phospholipid, particularly in the so-called apolipoprotein A_1-containing fraction (25). This fraction is very roughly equivalent to HDL-C-2, which is thought to be the protective fraction of HDL-C.

The effects of endogenous gonadal hormones during normal life-cycle changes for HDL-C has been elucidated. In pregnancy, HDL-C rises (as well as LDL-C and TG) until the 24th week and then it begins to fall. Interestingly, this fall in HDL-C is not accompanied by a fall in apo A_1 levels, implying a change in HDL-C composition during the last period of pregnancy. After menopause, HDL-C declines again, but the decline occurs gradually over the 2 yr preceding cessation of menses (26). This decline is accompanied by a rise in apo A_1 levels, implying again a change in HDL-C composition (27).

Elevated HDL-C levels play a key role in protecting both men and women against the development of CHD (Table 2). Stensvold and co-workers, in a screening for CVD performed in three Norwegian counties on a population of 23,680 men and 23,425 women (6.8 yr mean follow-up), showed that CVD mortality decreased with increasing HDL-C (28). The inverse association between mortality and HDL-C in women was stronger than in men. HDL-C appears to have greater relative predictive value as well. Not only are total HDL-C levels higher, but there is a greater difference in CAD risk per milligram difference in HDL-C in women (29). Data from the Framingham Study also demonstrate that HDL-C level is a more powerful predictor in women: for every 10 mg/dL change in HDL-C, a 40–50% change in coronary risk was noted and the Framingham investigators suggest that the protective effect of HDL-C in women is approximately twice the atherogenic effect of LDL-C (30). In a more recent review of data from the Framingham population, Kannel and Wilson confirmed that among men and women, the risk of CHD-related events increases steeply with each increment in the ratio TC/HDL-C and in women, a ratio higher than 7.5 appears to attenuate greatly the risk advantage over men and resulting in almost the same incidence rate observed in men (31). Bass and co-workers recently reported on a population of 1405 women aged 50–69 yr selected from the Lipid Research Clinic's follow-up data (32). Higher CVD death was seen at elevated levels of TC in women with low HDL-C levels but not among women with high HDL-C levels. Women with high HDL-C levels had similar CVD mortality rates at all levels of TC. Women with

Table 3
Ratio of TC: HDL Cholesterol in Women by Age:
The Framingham Study

Age (yr)	Mean	Standard deviation
15–24	3.4	0.9
25–34	3.4	1.1
35–44	3.6	1.2
45–54	4.0	1.5
55–64	4.5	1.5
65–74	4.6	1.5
75–79	4.7	1.4

low HDL-C levels had a three-fold increased risk of CVD death when compared with women with high HDL-C levels. Hong and colleagues studied the usefulness of the ratio TC/HDL-C in predicting angiographic artery disease in women *(33)*. TC levels did not correlate with the presence of CAD. However, TC/HDL-C was higher among women with CAD and this ratio was the most predictive factor of the presence, extensiveness, and severity of CAD.

It is important to consider the absolute value of the HDL. Most women have mean HDL-C levels of 50 mg/dL or higher. Both the Framingham Study and the Donolo-Tel Aviv Study have documented increased CVD incidence and mortality in women whose HDL-C levels are greater than 35 mg/dL, but less than 50 mg/dL. Considering these data, Bass *(32)* defined a low HDL-C level for values less than 50 mg/dL, and a high HDL-C level for values >50 mg/dL, resulting in an increased mortality relative risk of 1.7 with an HDL-C level less than 50 mg/dL in women (compared to an HDL-C over 50 mg/dL). Thus, the cutoff of 35 mg/dL for HDL-C levels as recommended in the NCEP Adult Treatment Panel II (ATPII) Report to identify individuals at high risk of CVD appears to be appropriate for men but not for women *(34)*.

The LRC follow-up study showed that HDL-C was the major lipid predictor of CHD mortality in women. Some recent data suggest that HDL-C levels decline in association with natural menopause, thus placing postmenopausal women at greater risk for CHD than their male counterparts. The ratio of TC: HDL-C should be 4.0 or less. The Framingham Study illustrated that the ratio rises steadily with age in women (Table 3).

LDL-C

LDL-C levels are lower in women than in men throughout the first two thirds of the life span. After the middle of the fifth decade, as a result of menopause, LDL-C levels in women rise abruptly, whereas LDL-C levels in men remain stable. In the last third of life, women generally have higher LDL-C levels *(35)*. Again, compositional differences in LDL-C exist between pre- and postmenopausal women: postmenopausal women tend to have increasing levels of a smaller, denser type of LDL-C *(36)*, which is thought to be particularly atherogenic because it may be more susceptible to oxidation *(37)*. It is interesting to note that high HDL-C-3 is often associated with higher concentrations of small dense LDL-C particles and a low LDL-C peak particle diameter *(38)*. This association characterizes the recently described LDL-C subclass as phenotype B, which is a coronary risk factor *(39)*.

The NCEP ATPII Report indicates an LDL-C level of 130 mg/dL or higher as a risk factor for CHD in both men and women. In fact, the role of LDL-C as a risk factor in women is somewhat controversial. Few prospective studies have examined LDL-C and CHD risk in women. Very-high LDL-C (VHLDL-C) concentrations carry the same poor prognosis in both sexes. However, women who are heterozygous have a lower risk attributable to LDL-C compared with heterozygous men *(40)*. This finding may be merely due to the higher HDL-C levels found in women. Another, possibility is supported by at least one animal study *(41)*. In this investigation, the arterial wall LDL-C content of estrogen-treated monkeys was considerably lower than that of non-estrogen-treated control animals, implying that estrogen may, in some way inhibit the arterial wall uptake of LDL-C cholesterol. This possibility is especially relevant to premenopausal women, and could explain why LDL-C level is a less stronger predictor of CHD for them.

Postmenopausal women with high levels of LDL-C are not protected by estrogen, nor by the generally higher level of HDL-C. The higher levels of LDL-C are most likely associated with a greater percentage of small dense LDL-C particles. Premenopausal women are relatively protected by estrogen and high level of HDL-C, but for postmenopausal women, LDL-C level might be a stronger and perhaps more independent risk factor.

Lipoprotein(a)

Lp(a) consists of two components: an LDL-C-like particle with apo-protein B-100 and a hydrophobic protein moiety known as apolipoprotein (a) [apo(a)] linked by a disulfide bond *(28)*. Apo(a) is synthesized in the liver and is about 80% analogous to plasminogen. Thus, Lp(a) is a molecule with both lipoprotein and clotting potential. Lp(a) can be bound by LDL-C receptors and apparently also by plasminogen receptors. Lp(a) is now felt to be an atherogenic lipoprotein *(43,44)*. A prospective investigation of elevated Lp(a) detected by electrophoresis in the Framingham Heart Study revealed that elevated plasma Lp(a) was a strong, independent predictor of myocardial infarction in women *(45)*.

Regarding potential gender differences in Lp(a) levels and coronary risk, the published studies are inconsistent. Age and sex were not found to influence the plasma levels of Lp(a) according to Maeda and co-workers *(46)*. In general, Lp(a) levels are higher in women than in men throughout most of the life span, particularly during the postmenopausal period. Steinmetz and colleagues noted that menopause as a risk factor correlated with increased Lp(a), but this increase was not significant *(47)*. Solymoss and associates docu-mented that Lp(a) was a significant risk in older women particularly when it was associated with a high TC to HDL-C-ratio *(48)*.

VLDL-Cholesterol and Triglycerides

Triglycerides (TG) are secreted together with cholesterol and phospholipid in the form of very-low-density lipoprotein-cholesterol (VLDL-C) such that 60 to 70% of VLDL-C is TG and 20% cholesterol. Little difference in TG concentrations is noted between genders until puberty. Then, TG increases in both sexes with increasing age, although at a much slower rate in women. TG levels in men actually decrease in middle age, whereas they continue to increase gradually in women. Thus, mean levels in women equal those of men by the age of 70 yr. There are age and, again, gender-related compositional differences in VLDL-C as well. In middle-aged women, the VLDL-C is larger, lighter, and lower in free cholesterol content than the VLDL-C in men of comparable age *(49)*. The

Table 4
CHD Risk Factors in Diabetic vs. Nondiabetic Women:
The Framingham Study

Risk factor	Diabetic	Nondiabetic
Serum cholesterol (mg/dL)	259	250
HDL-C (mg/dL)	54*	58
LDL-C (mg/dL)	157	155
TGs (mg/dL)	141**	133
Systolic blood prssure (mmHg)	150**	139
Relative weight (% ideal)	129**	121
Cigarettes/d	6	5

*$p < 0.05$.
**$p < 0.01$.

VLDL-C precursors in post-menopausal women are relatively protein and cholesterol-poor and richer in TG and thus, potentially more atherogenic.

The role of TG in the development of CHD is still the subject of some debate. For the most part, TGs have not been shown to be a statistically independent predictor of CAD risk when HDL-C and LDL-C are considered in a multivariate analysis. But studies have demonstrated TG as a strong and independent risk factor for women and some experts feel they should be conscientiously addressed.

Elevated TGs are a significant risk factor for CVD even after adjustment for multiple risk factors, including TC levels. Elevated TG levels are likely to be prevalent in post-menopausal women where they may be markers for the presence of other atherogenic lipoproteins. We see that as women age and as they progress through menopause, the percentage of smaller, denser LDL-C rises; and the occurrence of small dense LDL-C has been associated with hypertriglyceridemia. We know that small dense LDL-C may be more susceptible to oxidation and thus more atherogenic, and thus, its association with TG may explain the predictive power of TG in older postmenopausal women.

DIABETES MELLITUS

DM is the single, most powerful risk factor for CAD in women. Its impact is greater in women than in men (Chapter 7, Figure 1). Women with diabetes have a fivefold increase in cardiovascular disease than in women without diabetes. Follow-up data from the Framingham Study have shown that the prevalence of diabetes among women rises sharply with age (Table 4).

High blood glucose levels are a strong predictor of CHD risk, independent of whether or not the individual has clinical diabetes. The annual incidence of CHD increases with blood glucose levels and increasing age. There is, for example, little risk of CHD in women with blood glucose levels <60 mg/dL ("low"). Above about 130 mg/dL, however, the CHD risk escalates sharply—doubling and even tripling over that associated with lower glucose levels.

Women with diabetes have been found to have twice the risk of MI as nondiabetic women of the same age; the risk of MI in diabetic women equals that of nondiabetic men of the same age. In diabetic women, the incidence of CAD is almost three times that of nondiabetic women as compared with a twofold increase in incidence in men. Diabetes cancels the female hormonal advantage over males. There is also some indication that

DM predisposes women to more lethal coronary events, almost doubling the case fatality rates. The presence of diabetes tends to attenuate any gender-related differences in cardiovascular morbidity and mortality. In fact, the risk of CHD in diabetic women is higher than that of both diabetic men and nondiabetic women, even after adjustment has been made for age and other CHD risk factors.

The higher risk among diabetic women may be partially explained by the "clustering" of multiple risk factors in diabetic individuals, such as hypertension, smoking, and obesity. Diabetic women have significantly higher levels of four CHD risk factors (other than diabetes or high blood glucose levels): (1) HDL-C, (2) TGs, (3) systolic blood pressure, and (4) relative body weight (Table 4). Compared with nondiabetic individuals, diabetics have an adverse lipid profile. TC, LDL-C, and TG levels are higher. HDL-C levels are lower. Interestingly, these differences in lipoprotein levels between diabetics and controls are much more dramatic in women than in men *(50)* (Chapter 7, Figure 2). Numerous other studies *(51–54)* confirm Walden's observations. Moreover, compared with gender-matched nondiabetics, diabetic women have a greater risk of CAD than do diabetic men *(55)*. Thus, diabetes seems to neutralize much of the protection against CAD conferred in women by their initially favorable lipoprotein profile, which is largely explained by insulin activity. In men and women, insulin promotes lipoprotein lipase-mediated TG removal. Thus, a deficiency of insulin results in hypertriglyceridemia. Diabetes increases endogenous hepatic VLDL-C secretion. Activity of the LDL-C-receptors is also insulin dependent and is downregulated in the absence of insulin. Concentrations of HDL-C are increased by insulin administration in men and women with insulin-dependent diabetes *(56,57)*.

HYPERTENSION

The two other leading causes of cardiovascular mortality and morbidity in women are stroke and hypertension. Stroke is the second leading cause of cardiovascular mortality in women, accounting for nearly 100,000 deaths among women in the US *(1)*. This was substantially higher than the number of men who died from stroke in that year. The incidence of both fatal and nonfatal stroke rises steadily with age in both genders. Among women aged 30–44 the estimated incidence of stroke is only 8000 annually. This figure rises sharply to 50,000 in women between the ages of 45 and 65 and more than triples to 179,000 in women over the age of 65. Thus, postmenopausal women are at significantly higher risk of stroke than are premenopausal women. Although the incidence of stroke is higher for men of all ages compared to women of all ages, the mortality rate is higher in women. This is due in large part to almost an 80% higher death rate from stoke in black women than in white women.

The epidemiology, natural history and therapy of hypertension are impacted by gender. Although premenopausal women are less likely than men to have hypertension, one in four Caucasian women aged 20 or greater have hypertension. The tendency of women to have lower blood pressure than men early in life is counterbalanced by the fact that a women's blood pressure increases more steeply with aging than it does in men. Prior to menopause, women are at risk for hypertension due predominantly to two gender specific exposures: contraceptive use and pregnancy. With menopause, women, in particular, African-American women, develop hypertension. By age 65 more than half of all women are hypertensive and nearly three-quarters of women over the age of 75 are hypertensive.

OBESITY

The Nurses' Health Study (5) showed that women with a body mass index (BMI) 25–29 kg/m^2 compared with the leanest women, had an age-adjusted relative risk for CHD of 1.8, whereas morbidly obese women (BMI >29 kg/m^2) had a relative risk for CHD of 3.3. In 115,886 American women 30–55 yr of age who were followed in the Nurses' Health Study, 40% of coronary events were attributable to excess body weight. Twenty-five percent of American women 35–64 yr of age have BMIs of 29 or higher—the category of women having relative risks of nonfatal MI and fatal CHD of 3.2 and 3.5, respectively.

Obesity has been shown to be an independent risk factor for the development of CAD in women. In a 26-yr follow-up of participants in the Framingham Heart Study, relative weight in women was positively and independently associated with coronary disease, and coronary and CVD death. The study further showed that weight gain after the young adult years conveyed an increased risk of CVD in both genders that could not be attributed either to the initial weight or the levels of the risk factors that may have resulted from weight gain. Based on other epidemiological studies, 30% of the CAD occurring in obese women can be attributed to the excess weight alone, and even mild-to-moderate overweight increases the risk of coronary disease in middle-aged women.

Truncal, android, or male pattern obesity, manifested as a rise in the waist-to-hip ratio, correlates with higher LDL-C and lower HDL-C levels. Truncal obesity is associated with both higher blood pressure and hyperinsulinemia, which leads to increases in atherogenic lipoproteins and decreases in HDL-C. The mechanism for this is unclear, although it has been hypothesized that it may somehow be related to an increase in peripheral insulin resistance: the portal venous drainage of abdominal fat may induce hepatic insulin resistance, elevated circulating insulin, higher TG levels, and lower HDL-C levels.

Obesity has been strongly associated in women with three major risk factors for CAD: non-insulin-dependent DM, hypercholesterolemia, and hypertension (58). In multiple studies, obesity was found to be associated with significant modifications of the lipid profile, especially higher TG and LDL-C levels (59–61). These modifications appear to be relatively more important in women (60–62). Moreover, HDL-C has also been shown to be negatively associated with obesity (63). Some cross-sectional studies, however, suggest that a higher relative weight, or percentage body fat (64) must be present in women, relative to men, in order to observe these abnormalities in the serum lipids.

In fact, more than generalized obesity, an increase in truncal fat (also called "android" or male pattern obesity) is manifested as a rise in the waist-to-hip ratio, and correlates with higher LDL-C and lower HDL-C levels (65). Central or truncal obesity is associated with both higher blood pressure and hyperinsulinemia, which is thought to result in increases in atherogenic lipoproteins and decreases in HDL-C (66). The mechanism for this is unclear, although it has been hypothesized that it may somehow be related to an increase in peripheral insulin resistance: the portal venous drainage of abdominal fat may induce hepatic insulin resistance, elevated circulating insulin, higher TG levels , and lower HDL-C levels (67).

Here, again, sexual hormones may play an important role. Although obese premenopausal women tend to have "gynecoid" or gluteal-femoral fat distribution, menopause has been found to promote the development of android or truncal obesity (68,69). This may be another mechanism by which menopause further influences the atherogenic potential of the lipid profile. In young men, but not in younger women, waist-to-hip ratio correlated with an increase in insulin and was inversely related to HDL-C (70). This relationship appeared to be largely independent of body mass index and triglycerides. The more efficient insulin-mediated glucose homeostasis in women imparts a distinct advantage to child-bearing women that is lost in the diabetic state and at least partly explains the gender differential in the atherosclerotic process (70).

Evidence suggests that the distribution of body fat may be a more determining factor of cardiovascular risk than absolute weight (69,71). The distribution of adiposity as assessed by waist-to-hip ratio is significantly related to coronary atherosclerosis in both females and males and waist-to-hip ratio was significantly greater in females with CAD (71). Other investigators have similarly observed that individuals with a truncal (android) distribution are at higher risk than those with a gynecoid or peripheral distribution of body fat (72,73). Lapidus and associates showed that an increased waist-to-hip ratio correlates with increased risk of both MI and CVD death in women (74).

However, the modification of blood lipid levels is not the only factor involved for CAD risk in truncal obesity, because the waist-to-hip ratio remains positively correlated with CAD even after controlling for smoking, hypertension, glucose intolerance, BMI, and especially, blood lipids (72). Perhaps it simply reflects the relative accessibility of omental and peritoneal abdominal fat to the circulation in truncal obesity. For males, the close proximity of the intestinal fat to the circulation can give rapid access to TG-rich lipoproteins such as the chylomicrons, which can be efficiently metabolized for muscle energy providing an important survival advantage for the otherwise less metabolically efficient male.

SMOKING

Although diabetes is the most biologically gender-differentiated risk factor for coronary disease in women, cigarette smoking may be the most psychologically and sociologically distinguishing risk behavior for men and women. Cigarette smoking in women is an especially serious risk. Cigarette smoking carries an especially increased hazard for young women because it is often accompanied by oral contraceptive use, a combination that promotes thrombogenesis.

Smoking is deadly, claiming nearly 200,000 lives in the United States in 1994, or nearly one-fifth of all heart disease deaths. Among adult Americans, the prevalence of cigarette smoking declined markedly since its peak in 1965, when 40% smoked. Smoking prevalence has declined more rapidly among men than women, so that the gender gap in smoking prevalence has narrowed considerably. This difference is likely to continue to narrow, because adolescent females are starting to smoke at the same rate as males. This is likely to contribute to a substantially greater female burden of cardiovascular disease.

A dose-response relationship exists between the number of cigarettes smoked per day and increasing levels of plasma cholesterol for both men and women under the age of 60 yr (75). The increase is significantly greater in women: on average, TC increases by 0.33 mg/dL for each cigarette smoked in men, but by 0.48 mg/dL in women. Possible mechanisms include enhanced lipolysis, increased levels of plasma-free fatty acids, and an antiestrogenic effect of cigarette smoking (75).

That cigarette smoking increases hepatic reesterification of free fatty acids has been confirmed (76). This explains the observed smoking-induced increases in serum-free fatty concentrations and helps clarify the atherogenic effects of smoking on serum lipids. Insulin resistance syndrome is likely to be an important reason for the increased atherogenicity observed in smokers (77). Chronic cigarette smokers are insulin resistant, hyperinsulinemic, and dyslipidemic compared with nonsmokers. Furthermore, normo-triglyceridemic smokers exhibit an abnormal postprandial lipid metabolism consistent with lipid intolerance. The postprandial hyperlipidemia is characteristic of the insulin resistance syndrome and Axelsen suggests that the defect in lipid removal could be related to the low HDL-C in this syndrome *(78)*.

Finally, it appears that smoking enhances lipid peroxidation. Lipid peroxidation by-products were increased in smokers and fell in those withdrawn from cigarettes *(79)*. It is quite possible that smoking can cause the oxidative modification of important biologic molecules in vivo. Thus, through multiple mechanisms it appears that smoking impacts the lipid profile and the pathophysiologic alteration of lipid. From the gender perspective, smoking neutralizes the advantage of increased HDL-C in both premenopausal and postmenopausal women. Furthermore, the insulin resistance attributable to smoking has profound implications for the woman who has the combination of truncal obesity, glucose intolerance, hypertriglyceridemia, and hypertension.

New evidence points to the significant role of passive smoking in the development of CAD. Women are seriously threatened by this new, emerging risk factor for CAD. Passive smoke reduces the ability of the blood to deliver oxygen to the myocardium and impairs the heart's ability to utilize oxygen. After inhaling only two cigarettes, nonsmokers' platelet activity matches that of a habitual smoker. Second-hand smoke causes increased intimal wall damage, accelerates atherosclerotic lesions, and increases intimal wall damage folowing ischemia or myocardial infarction.

For several decades it has been clear that smoking is associated with an elevated risk of CHD among men. For some time, it was believed that cigarette smoking was not associated with CHD among women. However, positive correlations have been observed in both case-control and prospective-cohort studies of nonfatal MI, and of fatal coronary disease.

The Nurses Health Study *(5)*, a large prospective cohort study of women examined the incidence of CHD in relation to cigarette smoking in a cohort of 119,404 female nurses from the age of 30–55. The number of cigarettes smoked per day was positively correlated with the risk of CHD (relative risk [RR] = 5.5 for >25 cigarettes per day), nonfatal myocardial infarction (RR = 5.8), and angina pectoris (relative risk = 2.6) Overall, cigarette smoking accounted for approximately half these events. This attributable risk was highest among women who were already at increased risk because of older age, family history of MI, obesity, hypertension, hypercholesterolemia or diabetes. These data emphasize the importance of cigarette smoking as a determinant of CHD in women, as well as the markedly increased hazards associated with this habit in combination with other risk factors for this disease.

HOMOCYSTEINE

Hyperhomocysteinemia is caused by genetic and lifestyle influences. This may include the low intake of folate and vitamin B_6. The importance of hyperhomocysteinemia in the pathogenesis of atherosclerosis was first demonstrated in studying vascular disease in children with two different enzyme abnormalities of homocysteine metabolism. It was felt that perhaps homocysteine caused atherosclerosis by a direct effect on the arterial cells *(80,81)*. No prospective data are available regarding the intake of these vitamins and the prevention of CAD.

The Nurses Health Study evaluated 80,082 women with no previous history of CAD, cancer, hypercholesterolemia, or diabetes who completed a detailed food frequency questionnaire. They were followed for 14 yr, during which there 658 cases of nonfatal MI and 281 cases of fatal CHD. From the food questionnaire, the intake of folate and vitamin B_6 were estimated. After controlling for cardiovascular risk factors, including smoking, HTN, intake of alcohol, vitamin E, fiber, and saturated and polysaturated fats, the relative risks of CHD for these two vitamins were assessed. The relative risks for CHD were less for those women with higher intakes of folate and vitamin B_6, suggesting they may play an important role in the preventation of CHD (82).

Physical Activity

Sedentary lifestyle is now recognized as a major risk for CAD. However, studies that specifically address the effects of increased physical activity on coronary disease risk factors beyond lipids, are uncommon and up to recently the findings have been equivocal. Even moderately fit women demonstrate significantly better blood sugar, blood pressure, and anthropometric indices in addition to improvement in the lipid profile when compared to women in the lowest-fitness category.

Increasing evidence shows that inactivity and a sedentary lifestyle may be independent risk factors for the development of CAD in both men and women. Few studies have addressed the relationship between physical fitness or habitual activity level to cardiovascular disease in women.

Cross-sectional studies comparing active and sedentary women report a positive association between exercise and HDL-C in both pre- and postmenopausal women. Significant differences between groups remained for HDL-C values when results were adapted for differences in percent of body fat. Two studies compared plasma lipids with menopausal status in females runners. They showed no differences in HDL-C between pre- and postmenopausal women who exercised, but when inactive and exercising women were compared, it appeared that younger premenopausal women responded with lipoprotein changes less strongly than older postmenopausal women. Hence, exercise appeared to attenuate the age-related increase in LDL-C and decrease in HDL-C. Otherwise, in these cross-sectional studies, women on hormone replacement therapy who reported exercising had higher HDL-C than sedentary women not on HRT.

Psychosocial Aspects of Heart Disease in Women

Over the past decade, a large body of evidence has accumulated regarding the relationship of socioeconomic status, employment, type A behavior, hostility, depression, and social support to cardiovascular disease.

Socioeconomic factors, including educational attainment are an important contributing factor to coronary disease risk. Women with a low educational level had a significantly increased age-specific incidence of angina pectoris. There was no significant correlation between marital status or number of children and incidence of ischemic heart disease or overall mortality. Multivariate analyses showed that the association between low educational level and incidence of angina pectoris was independent of socioeconomic group itself, cigarette smoking, systolic blood pressure, indices of obesity, serum TGs, and serum cholesterol.

As women have assumed different roles in the workplace, the impact of these roles on cardiovascular and women's health in general has come in question. Working women appear to be healthier than nonworking/nonemployed women according to several health indicators. Several additional studies have confirmed these results. Employed women, in general, have less risk factors: they smoke fewer cigarettes, have lower fasting glucose levels, drink less alcohol, and exercise more than their unemployed counterparts. Mean high-density lipoprotein cholesterol level was significantly higher in employed women compared with homemakers.

Menopause as a Risk Factor

No risk factor is as specific for women as hormonal status. Menopause, or the permanent cessation of menses resulting from the loss of ovarian function, coincides with an increase in several comorbidities including cardiovascular disease. As defined by WHO, menopause is clinically defined as the absence of menses for at least 1 yr. The perimenopause is the period immediately before menopause that is characterized by progressive alterations in endocrine and reproductive functions.

Menopause evokes several endocrine changes that have a dramatic impact on postmenopausal health. Ovarian secretion of estrogen, progesterone, and inhibin progressively decline as ovarian function ceases. As a result, the secretion of both FSH and LH is altered. In contrast to estrogen, androgen production from the ovary is less affected by menopause. The adrenal gland continues to secrete large amounts of the precursor steroids such as dehydroepiandosterone-sulfate (DHEA-S) and androstenedione, which can be converted into androgens and/or estrogens in the peripheral tissues. The conversion of these precursor steroids to estrone by adipose tissue is the major source of estrogen in postmenopausal women. As a result of these modifications the ratios of estrone and estradiol and of androgens to estrogens is increased in the postmenopausal woman.

The increase in the prevalence of cardiovascular disease in the postmenopausal years has been partially attributed to the adverse effects of estrogen deficiency on plasma lipid and lipoprotein levels, to direct effects of estrogen deficiency on the cardiovascular system, and finally due to an increase in central obesity. Multiple studies show that a direct relationship does exist between menopause and risk of CAD in women (83–86).

More recently, investigators have focused on the role of menopause in the development of the constellation of metabolic abnormalities including central obesity and insulin resistance. Review of cross-sectional and longitudinal studies suggest that the menopause transition is associated with an increase in abdominal and visceral adipose tissue accumulation. These results appear to be independent of the aging process and total body fat distribution. The majority of interventional studies involving the use of HRT show that hormone replacement therapy attenuates the accumulation of central fat in postmenopausal women compared to controls. Retrospective comparisons of users and nonusers of HRT also demonstrate a protective effect of HRT on fat distribution. In general, little data exist regarding the role of menopause in the development of insulin resistance. However, there appears to be a moderate effect of menopause on its development. Moderate effects of estrogen therapy on were found on insulin resistance in postmenopausal women, although long-term clinical trials are lacking. Treatment with progestins appears to have a deleterious effect on insulin sensitivity. It has been hypothesized that a portion of the adverse cardiovascular risk associated with menopause may be associated with metabolic derangements resulting in an increase in central obesity and insulin resistance.

RISK FACTOR MODIFICATION IN WOMEN

Modification of Blood Lipids

PRIMARY PREVENTION

The majority of primary prevention trials have focussed on middle-aged men. Limited data are available in women and this provides a barrier to the implementation of strategies to reduce risk in women. The Air Force/Texas Coronary Atherosclerosis Prevention Study (AFCAPS/TexCAPS) *(81)* is the first primary prevention statin study to include a large number of women (997/6605). Therapy with the cholesterol-lowering drug lovastatin (Mevacor) reduced the risk of first acute major coronary events in healthy adults with average to mildly elevated cholesterol levels and low HDL by 36%. The trial included 6,605 healthy adults aged 45 to 73 (997 women, 487 Hispanic Americans, and 206 African-Americans). Inclusion criteria for the study included no evidence of CAD, an LDL cholesterol between 130 and 190 mg/dL, HDL less than 45 mg/dL (less than 47 mg/dL for women), and TG levels less than 400 mg/dL. None of the participants had evidence of heart disease; 22% had hypertension, 2% had diabetes, and 12% were smokers. Preliminary results indicate that patients taking lovastatin had reduced risk for coronary events. Their risk of first acute coronary event (sudden death, MI, unstable angina) was reduced by 36 percent, risk of first coronary events was reduced by 54 percent in women, 34% in men, 43% in hypertensive patients and diabetic patients, and 29% in the elderly. Patients in the lovastatin group also had a 33% reduction in procedures such as angioplasty and bypass, and a 34% reduction in hospitalization due to unstable angina.

These results are significant for several reasons. It included a large number of minorities, and in general, included patients that would not ordinarily have been considered candidates for cholesterol-lowering therapy based on precious NCEP guidelines. This group however represent the majority of persons who eventually develop heart disease. This study represents a significant advance in our understanding of the role of reducing cholesterol in preventing new onset of heart disease in apparently healthy persons. The WOSCOPS study *(88)* demonstrated that treatment of relatively high risk men with clearly elevated cholesterol levels significantly reduced their risk of heart attack and death from heart disease, The AFCAPS/TexCAPS dramatically expands the number of persons who are possibly candidates for drug therapy for their cholesterol levels to include women, diabetics, and minorities.

SECONDARY PREVENTION

Recent trials have demonstrated that the most significant benefit for lipid lowering in women is those with existing CAD. Although few studies include women, and very few analyze women in a separate group, recent data suggest a significant decrease in coronary morbidity and mortality with the aggressive lowering of cholesterol levels in women. The impact of drug therapy appears comparable or even more effective in altering lipid levels in women, compared with men in both primary and secondary prevention. A consistent, albeit limited, set of data exists in women. Recent data from the 4S *(89)*, CARE *(90)*, and LIPID *(91)* studies have expanded our knowledge regarding the importance of lipid lowering with statins in women.

In the 4S trial *(89)* of 4444 patients, 18% of whom were women, simvastatin produced mean changes in TC, LDL-C, and HDL-C of −25%, −35%, and +8%, respectively. The probability that a woman avoided a major coronary event was 77.5% in the placebo group and 85.1% in the treatment group. Total mortality and risk for a major coronary event were similar for both genders. Other benefits of treatment included a 37% reduction ($p < 0.00001$) in the risk of undergoing myocardial revascularization procedures.

In the Cholesterol and Recurrent Events (CARE) Study *(90)*, designed to address the question of whether LDL-C lowering with pravastatin in patients with CHD and normal or only mildly elevated LDL-C concentrations provided clinical benefit, a greater reduction in CHD death and nonfatal MI was observed in the subset of women in this study as compared with men. These data corroborate the findings from other trials that the benefits of lipid lowering therapy start to appear relatively soon after the initiation of therapy. Women may have a greater benefit from cholesterol reduction interventions.

The LIPID study *(91)*, performed in New Zealand and Australia, was a double-blind, random, placebo-control study on 9014 subjects (1511 of whom were women, one-third over age 65 yr, 777 diabetics) using pravastatin 40 mg/d. Subjects age 31–75 yr, who experienced an acute MI or unstable angina within the previous 3 mo–3 yr, and had TC values from 155–270 mg/dL, triglycerides less than 445 mg/dL, were eligible for participation. The primary endpoint, coronary mortality, was reduced by 24% ($p < 0.0005$). Secondary objectives, total mortality (reduced by 23%, $p < 0.0001$), and overall cardiac events (23% reduction, $p < 0.0001$) were also met with demonstrated positive results. The risk reduction in MI incidence was 29%, $p < 0.00001$. Procedure rates of CABG and PTCA were also reduced by 24% and 18%, respectively. Stroke incidence was reduced by 20% ($p = 0.022$).

Although the Scandinavian Simvastatin Survival Study (4S) *(89)* trial was the first secondary prevention trial to clearly demonstrated a reduction in total mortality, the Long-Term Intervention with Pravastatian in Ischaemic Disease (LIPID) *(91)* trial has significant differences in design and hypotheses. Important differences, exist between the LIPID study and 4S cohort. Fully 80% of the LIPID enrollees were not candidates for 4S based on their cholesterol level, age, or history of CAD. LIPID is the first study to examine the use of an HMG CoA reductase inhibitor in patients with a history of unstable angina. The LIPID study provides important data on noncoronary mortality and on other groups such as women and diabetic patients who, to date, were underrepresented in clinical trials.

Postmenopausal women with a history of CHD may need more aggressive treatment for elevated cholesterol, according to a recent study. The Heart and Estrogen/Progestin Replacement Study (HERS) *(92)*, involving 2763 women with a known history of CAD, found that although 47% of the HERS participants were currently receiving some form of cholesterol-lowering medication, 63% had LDL-C levels, which exceeded the National Cholesterol Education Program (NCEP) *(34)* guidelines. Therefore, many of the women who were eligible to receive cholesterol lowering drug therapy based on their elevated cholesterol levels either were not receiving drug treatment, or were not treated aggressively enough. Fully 91% of the study's participants had LDL-C levels which exceeded the 1993 ATP goal of less than 100 mg/dL.

Most of the women were white (88.7% white, 7.9% African-American, 2% Hispanic) and generally, most were inactive and overweight. Many were ex-smokers (49%) and over 13% still smoked. More than half (59.5%) had high blood pressure and 23% had diabetes. The researchers found that women with one or more of the following conditions were less likely to be on a cholesterol-lowering agent: African-American, Hispanic, or other ethnic identity, higher BMI, were sedentary, consumer of alcohol or tobacco, and persons with a diagnosis of CAD that preceded 1985. Women with lower LDL-C levels tended to have postgraduate education, participated in an exercise program, and were never married.

Cholesterol should be treated in women as in men and women may benefit more. The fact that premenopausal women are at lower risk of heart disease than men of the same age has been misinterpreted by many to mean that risk factors are not as important to treat in women as in men.

Despite ample data on the benefits of lipid-lowering data from the HERS study in women with heart disease indicate less than half (47%) of women were being treated with lipid-lowering therapy and of these, less than one tenth (8%) reached the goal LDL-C of 100 mg/dL.

Dietary Modification and Weight Loss in Women

Efforts to prevent or treat obesity have had only limited success. Striking excesses in morbidity and mortality from CHD attributable to obesity in middle-aged women have stimulated greater efforts to understand and treat the problem of obesity in women. The presence of excess truncal fat in both men and women correlates with increases in LDL-C and decreases in HDL-C, accounting for the increase risk of CHD observed in central obesity. Adipose tissue in postmenopausal women can serve as a source of estrogen synthesis. Thus, the benefits of weight reduction in older women may be offset by the loss of estrogen-producing adipose tissue. As an additional consequence, the expected increases in HDL-C and decline in LDL-C with weight loss may be less evident than in men.

The NCEP *(34)* dietary intervention recommends that dietary changes should be made in two steps. Step I involves an intake of saturated fat of 8–10% of total calories, 30% or less of the total calories should be derived from fat, and less than 300 mg of cholesterol per day. If this diet proves inadequate to achieve the goals, the patient should proceed to the Step II diet. Step II calls for further reductions in saturated fat intake to less than 7% of calories and in cholesterol to less than 200 mg per day. The polyunsaturated/saturated fat ratio (P/S) should thus be increased.

All reduced fat diets have a beneficial effect on LDL-C, but they consistently also reduce HDL-C, which is disadvantageous for women. Furthermore, the literature observes specific gender differences for diet responsiveness. Furthermore, menopausal status may affect dietary responsiveness. Men have a greater decline in LDL-C and TG levels than in postmenopausal women, whereas postmenopausal women have a greater decline in HDL-C levels than in men when following a low-fat diet.

From the woman's perspective, the most important problem with diet therapy appears to be the accompanying decrease of HDL-C. The decrease is more severe in women, and even more extreme in postmenopausal women. Given that the inverse relationship of HDL-C to cardiac events may be more emphatic in women than the adverse risk imparted by LDL-C, the conclusion is that diet may have opposite the desired effect. As suggested, for women with a very high LDL-C and who are at risk for CHD all available techniques must be used to lower LDL-C. For low-risk women, unless they have a weight problem, the benefits of a low-fat diet are far from clear.

In addition to caloric restriction and behavior modification, exercise is one of the most methods of weight loss for the obese patient. The greatest weight losses have been reported in a combined regime of diet and exercise rather than diet or exercise alone. Two issues important to weight loss effectiveness are degree of loss and duration of loss. Even if weight is lost, studies indicate that in the vast majority of cases, weight loss maintenance frequently fails due to the many physiologic factors that contribute to obesity. Approximately two thirds of persons who lose weight will regain it within 1 yr, and almost all persons who lose weight will regain it within 5 yr. As evidenced by a substantial research, this short-term weight loss is ineffective in modifying coronary risk factors. Additional health risks that accompany weight cycling are increased cardiovascular morbidity and mortality, as well as increased abdominal fat, blood pressure, and insulin resistance.

EXERCISE

Exercise is generally accepted as a mechanism to increase HDL-C and to lower LDL-C levels in men. Although a number of studies have been carried out in women, they unfortunately fail to consider potential confounders such as hormonal status and body composition. Cross-sectional studies comparing active and sedentary women report a positive association between exercise and HDL-C in both pre- and postmenopausal women. Results from longitudinal training studies are more difficult to interpret because of experimental design, inadequate type, duration, and intensity of the exercise interventions or lipid measurements made without regard to the phase of the menstrual cycle or when studies were carried out in women with high baseline HDL-C. Because lipids vary approximately 10–25% through the course of the menstrual cycle, menstrual phase should be controlled in premenopausal women when determining lipid changes after an exercise intervention.

Generally, intervention studies suggest that exercise training programs in the absence of other interventions attenuate the age-related increase in TC level but do not cause HDL-C levels to rise appreciably in older women. In younger women, high volumes of exercise (accompanied by decreased body fat) may increase HDL-C.

In conclusion, exercise improves the lipid profile but probably less strongly for women than for men. Again, hormonal status may influence the response. Post-menopausal women seem to exhibit a greater response to exercise, even if some training studies are controversial. Exercise at least seems to attenuate the age-related modifications in the lipid profile.

ANTIOXIDANT THERAPY

Antioxidants may suppress the formation of oxidized LDL and thereby influence the formation of atherosclerotic plaque. Both epidemiological and laboratory studies suggest that antioxidants can provide a protective effect on coronary arteries.

The Nurses' Health Study assessed the relative risk of a major CAD event in 87,245 female nurses followed for up to 8 yr. Relative risk of major coronary disease of nurses in the lowest quintile of vitamin E intake was compared with risk in the highest quintile (relative risk, 0.66 after adjustment for age and smoking). Adjustment for a variety of other coronary risk factors and nutrients, including other antioxidants, had little effect on the results. As the authors point out: "Although these prospective data do not prove a cause-and-effect relation, they suggest that among middle-aged women the use of vitamin E supplements is associated with a reduced risk of coronary heart disease." No large randomized clinical trials of antioxidants have yet been reported, albeit two such trials, the Women's Health Initiative and an ancillary Trial of Antioxidant Therapy, are in progress.

SMOKING CESSATION

Significant gender differences exist in smoking-cessation behavior. Some are ascribed to chemistry, others to a lack of confidence in the ability to quit, and still others are concerns regarding postcessation weight gain. In addition, nicotine may have different effects on women and men.

Cigarette smoking carries an especially increased hazard for young women because it is often accompanied by oral contraceptive use, a combination that promotes thrombogenesis. In general, women are less likely to contemplate smoking cessation than men, are likely to smoke to reduce tension and control weight. Although women quit smoking at the same rate as men, they are less able to maintain cessation over the long term. Women's anxiety about postcessation weight gain is a major impediment to their even attempting to quit smoking. Smoking cessation has also been suggested as a possible contributing factor to the increase in prevalence of overweight in the US. Postcessation weight gain, an average of 10 lb more over a 10-yr period, appears to be due to both increased eating and the metabolic changes produced by nicotine withdrawal. Nicotine gum has been shown to partially reduce or delay gain.

The clinical implications are that smoking-cessation programs for women may have to emphasize strategies to help them develop confidence to stop smoking, to make a commitment to quitting, and to develop strategies for maintaining cessation for extended periods of time. Smoking-cessation programs for women should emphasize techniques for reducing tension and for weight control.

Former smokers live longer than continuing smokers and that a person 50 yr or younger who quits smoking has a 50% reduction in mortality over the next 15 yr vs. a smoker. In the Nurse's Health Study, the CHD risk is decreased by 30% within only 2 yr after cessation. These benefits extend to the population with diagnosed CAD. Overall, the bulk of studies in indicate a 30–50% reduction in CHD mortality in the first 2 yr and a more gradual decline in the next 10–20 yr before the smoker mirrors the CHD mortality risk of a never smoker.

Twelve-year follow-up data from the Nurse' Health Study examined the relationship of time since smoking with reduction in CHD incidence and mortality in middle-aged women. On stopping smoking, one third of the excess risk of CHD was eliminated within 2 yr of cessation. Thereafter, the excess risk returned to the level of those who had never smoked during the interval 10–14 yr following cessation.

HORMONE REPLACEMENT THERAPY AND CAD

Nearly all of the evidence that hormonal replacement therapy (HRT) might be cardioprotective in the postmenopausal woman comes from observational studies. Long-term clinical studies to evaluate the potential benefit of HRT in primary prevention are currently underway. The studies suggest that the risk of CHD is reduced by about 35–50% among healthy, postmenopausal women who take estrogen. In the Nurses' Health Study, the largest prospective study published to date involving more than 48,000 postmenopausal women, a highly significant reduction in myocardial infarction or death was noted (relative risk 0.56) among postmenopausal estrogen users. Significant reductions were noted even after adjustment for other risk factors and regardless of cause of menopause (natural or surgical), duration of estrogen use, or age. Indeed, several studies suggest that postmenopausal estrogen use may be associated with lower risk of CHD in women well into the eighth decade of life.

Hormonal status must be carefully considered because of the important effects of estrogen not only on lipids, but also on endothelial function and other risk factors. After menopause, women often have an increase in weight, higher levels of LDL-C, and lower

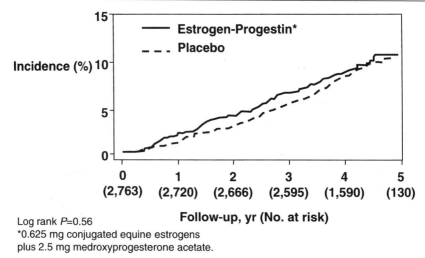

Log rank *P*=0.56
*0.625 mg conjugated equine estrogens
plus 2.5 mg medroxyprogesterone acetate.

Fig. 2. HERS: combined HRT does not increase all-cause mortality. Log rank *p* = 0.56. *0.625 mg conjugated equine estrogens plus 2.5 mg medroxyprogesterone acetate. Adapted from ref. 92.

levels of HDL-C. Oral estrogen replacement is useful in improving the lipid profiles in women, with falls in LDL-C and rises in HDL-C.

Progestins have opposite effects from estrogens and thus may limit the desirable effects of estrogens. The addition of a progestin to estrogen replacement regimens to prevent uterine hyperplasia is now widely accepted as necessary in women with an intact uterus. Furthermore, the effects of added progestins is a function of the dose and androgenicity of the particular preparation. The C-21 progestins, including medroxyprogesterone, which is the most commonly used noncontraceptive progestin in the US, are less androgenic than the 19-NOR agents. The stronger the progestin, the less the LDL-C decrease and HDL-C increase induced by the estrogen.

HERS *(92)* is the first randomized, double-blind, placebo controlled trial was performed to assess the role of estrogen plus progestin in secondary prevention. This trial of 2763 women younger than 80 yr with known CAD found no significant difference between groups in the primary outcome of MI or CAD death or in any of the secondary outcomes. HERS failed to show that HRT could prevent coronary disease events in women with CHD over a mean follow-up of 4 yr (Figs. 2 and 3). Although there was a strong trend for benefit in years 4 and 5 of the study with a 33% decrease in CHD events, there was, however, a disturbing 4.1% incidence of CHD events in the HRT group in year 1 compared with a 2.7% incidence in the placebo group. The study was somewhat underpowered because there was a greater than expected dropout rate in year 1 of the study and a greater than expected crossover rate from the placebo to HRT arm. Moreover, the average follow-up of the patients was 6 mo shorter than expected. Based on the findings of no overall cardiovascular benefit and a pattern of early increase in risk of CAD events, the study raised further questions about the role of HRT in the acute setting and demonstrated an early adverse event profile in women with CAD receiving HRT.

In order to examine the representativeness of the HERS cohort to the general population of postmenopausal women with CHD, the baseline cardiovascular risk factor data from HERS was compared to similar data from women presumed to have CHD from the NHANES III *(16)*. In general, the HERS cohort had fewer CHD risk factors than women with myocardial or angina in NHANES III, although comparison is hindered by differ-

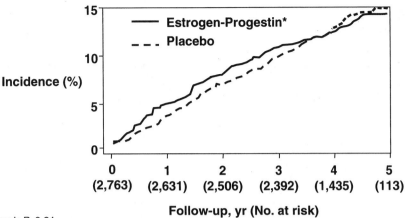

Log rank *P*=0.91.
* Combined incidence of nonfatal MI and CHD death.
† 0.625 mg conjugated equine estrogens plus
2.5 mg medroxyprogesterone acetate.

Fig. 3. HERS: combined HRT does not reduce primary CHD endpoints. *Combined incidence of nonfatal MI and CHD death. 0.625 mg conjugated equine estrogens plus 2.5 mg medroxyprogesterone acetate. Adapted from ref. *92*.

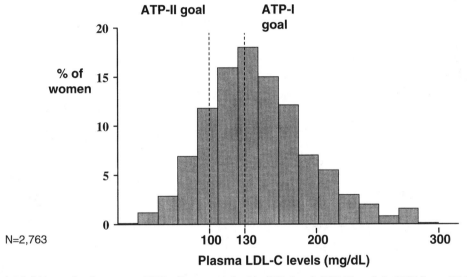

Fig. 4. Lipid lowering in women: LDL-C compared with ATP-I and ATP-II goals in HERS. *n* = 2763. Adapted from National Lipid Education Council, www.lipidhealth.org.

ences in selection criteria. there were substantially fewer women with diabetes and hypertriglyceridemia in HERS.

Furthermore, women enrolled in the HERS trial were not optimally treated with regard to NCEP Adult Treatment Panel (ATP) goals for lipid lowering *(17)*. In a cross-sectional analysis of women enrolled in HERS, only 47% of participants were taking a lipid-lowering medication, 63% did not meet the 1988 treatment goal of LDL-C level less than 130 mg/dL and 91% did not meet the 1993 goal of LDL-C less than 100 mg/dL (Fig. 4). Better implementation of these guidelines among women with coronary disease would by highly desirable and may impact on their ultimate cardiovascular event rate.

ERA is a three-armed trial comparing estrogen, estrogen plus progestin, and placebo in 309 postmenopausal women with CHD. Initial results of this study showed no benefit of estrogen, estrogen plus progestin compared to placebo. The preliminary results of the Estrogen Replacement and Atherosclerosis (ERA) trial have been reported.

There are several randomized clinical trials underway looking at the effects of HRT on CHD: The Women's Health Initiative (WHI), the Women's Angiographic Vitamin and Estrogen (WAVE) trial, and the Womens Estrogen/Progestin and Lipid Lowering Hormone Atherosclerosis regression (WELL-HART) trial.

The HRT arm in the WHI trial involves 27,500 women with no prior history of CAD. The study will test estrogen alone, as well as estrogen combined with progestin. WAVE, WELL-HART, and ERA involve coronary angiography to study whether HRT has a long-term, positive effect on the progression of atherosclerosis. WAVE is a multicenter trial with 400–450 postmenopausal women taking HRT and/or antioxidant vitamins; it will examine the progression of CAD. WELL-HART will compare the effects of estrogen, estrogen plus progestin, and placebo in 226 postmenopausal women with CAD and moderately elevated LDL. The women will also receive lovastatin.

These studies hope to answer some of the many questions raised by the HERS trial and assist in determining which women may gain cardioprotection from HRT and which women may be susceptible to its potential thrombogenic effects.

Late Breaking Clinical Trials

Previous HRT studies have raised some concern about risks associated with this therapy and the recently reported HERS raised the issue of a potential prothrombotic effect of therapy. These recent findings have been difficult to reconcile with very positive effects associated with HRT in various observational studies.

Most recently, results of the Estrogen Replacement and Atherosclerosis (ERA) trial were presented at the American College of Cardiology, March 2000. In this angiographic trial, 309 postmenopausal women with known CAD (1 or more stenosis of <30%) were received either unopposed estrogen, estrogen plus medroxyprogesterone acetate or placebo. The primary outcome was mean minimum lumen diameter (MLD) as determined by quantitative coronary angiography. After slightly more than 3 yr in 248 women, there was no difference in the mean MLD between treatment arms and placebo. Secondary clinical endpoints were not statistically different. As expected, there was a trend towards and increase incidence of DVT and pulmonary embolus in the treated groups.

SELECTIVE ESTROGEN RECEPTOR MODULATORS

An alternative to classical HRT, the SERMs, such as raloxifene (RAL), are a new class of drugs that exert site specific estrogenic or antiestrogenic effects in different target tissues. The potential benefits of these drugs include protection against four important hormone-dependent diseases: osteoporosis, CHD, and endometrial and breast cancer.

RAL has been shown to produce a reduction in total and LDL-C concentrations similar to that produced by estrogen therapy, but HDL-C and TG concentrations do not increase during RAL therapy. Walsh and colleagues studied 390 healthy postmenopausal women randomized to receive one of four treatments: RAL 60 mg/d, RAL 120 mg/d, HRT (conjugated equine estrogen, 0.625 mg/d and medroxyprogesterone acetate, 2.5 mg/d), or placebo. Lipid levels were obtained at 3 and 6 mo into treatment. Both dosages of RAL significantly lowered LDL-C by 12% ($p < 0.001$), similar to the 14% reduction with HRT

($p < 0.001$). Both dosages lowered significantly lowered Lp(a) by 7% to 8% ($p < 0.001$), less than the 19% decrease with HRT ($p < 0.001$). HDL2-C was increased by 15–17% ($p < 0.05$), which was less than the 33% seen with HRT ($p < 0.001$). RAL was also shown to decrease fibrinogen significantly by 12–14% ($p < 0.001$), whereas HRT had no effect.

Currently the Raloxifene Use for The Heart (RUTH) trial is underway to assess the effects of RAL in postmenopausal women with or at high risk for CHD. About 10,000 women are expected to be recruited, and participants will be randomized to RAL 60 mg/d or placebo. The primary endpoint is nonfatal MI and coronary death.

Conclusion

Cardiovascular disease is the leading cause of morbidity and mortality in women, with the vast majority of cardiovascular events occurring in the postmenopausal years. Most of our knowledge of cardiovascular disease comes from studies in middle-aged men. Recent emphasis on women's health in general, and in cardiovascular health in particular, has lead to increasing evidence that significant gender differences do exist in CAD incidence, in risk factors, and in the modification of cardiovascular risk in women.

Health-care providers must coordinate their efforts to effectively treat and prevent cardiovascular disease in women in such a way as to take into account the unique biology, physiology, and epidemiology of cardiovascular disease in women. There is increasing evidence of the roles of traditional and nontraditional risk factors in the development of cardiovascular disease in women and in developing new strategies to incorporate this evidence into programs of prevention.

KEY POINTS

1. Cardiovascular disease is the leading cause of mortality among women in the US— 500,000 women each year die of CHD.
2. Deaths in women from cardiovascular disease are almost twice that of deaths due to cancer.
3. Approximately one out of every two women in the US will die from some cardiovascular event—most likely, MI, hypertensive heart disease, or stroke.
4. Special emphasis must also be placed on those uniquely female attributes that modify coronary risk; specifically oral contraceptives, pregnancy, menopausal status, and the use of postmenopausal hormone therapy.
5. Most of our knowledge of cardiovascular disease comes from studies in middle-aged men.
6. Recent emphasis on women's health in general, and in cardiovascular health in particular, has lead to increasing evidence that significant gender differences do exist in CAD incidence, in risk factors, and in the modification of cardiovascular risk in women.
7. Health-care providers must coordinate their efforts to effectively treat and prevent cardiovascular disease in women in such a way as to take into account the unique biology, physiology, and epidemiology of cardiovascular disease in women.
8. There is increasing evidence of the roles of traditional and nontraditional risk factors in the development of cardiovascular disease in women and in developing new strategies to incorporate this evidence into programs of prevention.

SUMMARY

Cardiovascular disease is the leading cause of mortality among women in the United States—500,000 women each year die of CHD. Deaths in women from cardiovascular disease are almost twice that of deaths due to cancer. Approximately one out of every two women in the United States will die from some cardiovascular event—most likely myocardial infarction, hypertensive heart disease, or stroke. Although risk factors for CAD are similar in men and women, the impact of individual coronary risk factors and the results of their interventions differ dramatically by gender. Special emphasis must also be placed on those uniquely female attributes that modify coronary risk; specifically oral contraceptives, pregnancy, menopausal status, and the use of postmenopausal hormone therapy. This chapter reviewed the unique characteristics of CAD in women and overview management strategies for the modification of risk in this special population.

REFERENCES

1. 1997 Heart and Stroke Statistical Update. Dallas,TX, American Heart Association, 1996.
2. Wenger NK, Speroff L, Packard B. Cardiovascular health and disease in women [see comments]. N Engl J Med 1993;329:247–256.
3. Barrett-Connor E. Heart disease in women. Fertil Steril 1994;62:127S–132S.
4. Pashkow FJ. The Mona Lisa smiles: impact of risk factors for coronary artery disease in women [editorial; comment]. Cleve Clin J Med 1993;60:411–414.
5. Barrett-Connor E, Bush TL. Estrogen and coronary heart disease in women [see comments]. JAMA 1991;265:1861–1867.
6. Barrett-Connor E. Hypercholesterolemia predicts early death from coronary heart disease in elderly men but not women. The Rancho Bernardo Study. Ann Epidemiol 1992;2:77–83.
7. Kannel WB. Metabolic risk factors for coronary heart disease in women: perspective from the Framingham Study. Am Heart J 1987;114:413–419.
8. Report of the National Cholesterol Education Program Expert Panel on detection, evaluation and treatment of high blood cholesterol in adults. Arch Intern Med 1988;148:36–69.
9. Matthews KA, Meilahn E, Kuller LH, et al. Menopause and risk factors for coronary heart disease [see comments]. N Engl J Med 1989;321:641–646.
10. Castelli WP, Doyle JT, Gordon T. HDL cholesterol and other lipids in coronary heart disease. The cooperative lipoprotein phenotyping study. Circulation 1977;55:767–772.
11. Gordon T, Castelli WP, Hjortland MC, et al. High density lipoprotein as a protective factor against coronary heart disease. The Framingham Study. Am J Med 1977;62:707–714.
12. Kannel WB, Castelli WP, Gordon T. Cholesterol in the prediction of atherosclerotic disease. New perspectives based on the Framingham study. [Review]. Ann Inter Med 1979;90:85–91.
13. Jacobs D Jr, Mebane IL, Bangdiwala SI, et al. High density lipoprotein cholesterol as a predictor of cardiovascular disease mortality in men and women: the follow-up study of the Lipid Research Clinics Prevalence Study. Am J Epidemiol 1990;131:32–47.
14. Bush TL, Fried LP, Barrett-Connor E. Cholesterol, lipoproteins, and coronary heart disease in women. Clin Chem 1988;34.
15. White AD, Hames CG, Tyroler HA. Serum cholesterol and 20-year mortality in black and white men and women aged 65 and older in the Evans County Heart Study. Ann Epidemiol 1992;2:85–91.
16. Knapp RG, Sutherland SE, Keil JE, et al. A comparison of the effects of cholesterol on CHD mortality in black and white women: twenty-eight years of follow-up in the Charleston Heart Study. J Clin Epidemiol 1992;45:1119–1129.
17. Manolio TA, Pearson TA, Wenger NK, et al. Cholesterol and heart disease in older persons and women. Review of an NHLBI workshop. Ann Epidemiol 1992;2:161–176.
18. Brunner D, Weisbort J, Meshulam N, et al. Relation of serum total cholesterol and high-density lipoprotein cholesterol percentage to the incidence of definite coronary events: twenty-year follow-up of the Donolo–Tel Aviv Prospective Coronary Artery Disease Study. Am J Cardiol 1987;59:1271–1276.
19. Rifkind BM, Tamir I, Heiss G, et al. Distribution of high density and other lipoproteins in selected LRC prevalence study populations: a brief survey. Lipids 1979;14:105–112.
20. Khoo JC, Miller E, McLoughlin P, et al. Prevention of low density lipoprotein aggregation by high density lipoprotein or apolipoprotein A-I. J Lipid Res 1990;31:645–652.
21. Van Tol A. Reverse cholesterol transport. In: Steinmetz A, Kaffarnik H, Schneider J, eds. Cholesterol Transport Systems and Their Relation to Atherosclerosis. Springer-Verlag, New York, 1989, pp. 85–91.

22. Miller NE, Hammett F, Saltissi S, et al. Relation of angiographically defined coronary artery disease to plasma lipoprotein subfractions and apolipoproteins. Br Med J (Clin Res Ed) 1981;282:1741–1744.

23. Ballantyne FC, Clark RS, Simpson HS, et al. High density and low density lipoprotein subfractions in survivors of myocardial infarction and in control subjects. Metabolism 1982;31:433–437.

24. Williams PT, Vranizan KM, Austin MA, et al. Familial correlations of HDL subclasses based on gradient gel electrophoresis. Arterioscler Thromb 1992;12:1467–1474.

25. Ohta T, Hattori S, Nishiyama S, et al. Studies on the lipid and apolipoprotein compositions of two species of apoA-I-containing lipoproteins in normolipidemic males and females. J Lipid Res 1988;29:721–728.

26. Jensen J, Nilas L, Christiansen C. Influence of menopause on serum lipids and lipoproteins. Maturitas 1990;12:321–331.

27. Desoye G, Schweditsch MO, Pfeiffer KP, et al. Correlation of hormones with lipid and lipoprotein levels during normal pregnancy and postpartum. J Clin Endocrinol Metab 1987;64:704–712.

28. Stensvold I, Urdal P, Thurmer H, et al. High-density lipoprotein cholesterol and coronary, cardiovascular and all cause mortality among middle-aged Norwegian men and women. Eur Heart J 1992;13:1155–1163.

29. Gordon DJ, Probstfield JL, Garrison RJ, et al. High-density lipoprotein cholesterol and cardiovascular disease. Four prospective American studies. Circulation 1989;79:8–15.

30. Kannel WB. New perspectives on cardiovascular risk factors. Am Heart J 1987;114:213–219.

31. Kannel WB, Wilson PW. Risk factors that attenuate the female coronary disease advantage. Arch Intern Med 1995;155:57–61.

32. Bass KM, Newschaffer CJ, Klag MJ, et al. Plasma lipoprotein levels as predictors of cardiovascular death in women. Arch Intern Med 1993;153:2209–2216.

33. Hong MK, Romm PA, Reagan K, et al. Usefulness of the total cholesterol to high-density lipoprotein cholesterol ratio in predicting angiographic coronary artery disease in women. Am J Cardiol 1991;68:1646–1650.

34. Summary of the second report of the National Cholesterol Education Program (NCEP) Expert Panel on Detection, Evaluation, and Treatment of High Blood Cholesterol in Adults (Adult Treatment Panel II). JAMA 1993;269:3015–3023.

35. Kannel WB. Nutrition and the occurrence and prevention of cardiovascular disease in the elderly. Nutrit Rev 1988;46:68–78.

36. Campos H, McNamara JR, Wilson PW, et al. Differences in low density lipoprotein subfractions and apolipoproteins in premenopausal and postmenopausal women. J Clin Endocrinol Metab 1988;67:30–35.

37. DeGraaf J, Hak LH, Hectors MP, et al. Enhanced susceptibility to in vitro oxidation of the dense low density lipoprotein subfraction in healthy subjects. Arterioscler Thromb 1991;11:298–306.

38. Williams PT, Krauss RM, Vranizan KM, et al. Associations of lipoproteins and apolipoproteins with gradient gel electrophoresis estimates of high density lipoprotein subfractions in men and women. Arterioscler Thromb 1992;12:332–340.

39. Austin MA, Breslow JL, Hennekens CH, et al. Low-density lipoprotein subclass patterns and risk of myocardial infarction. JAMA 1988;260:1917–1921.

40. Slack J. Genetic influences on coronary heart disease in young women. In: Oliver M, ed. Coronary Heart Disease in Young Women. Churchill-Livingstone, Edinburgh, 1978, pp. 24–25.

41. Wagner JD, Clarkson TB, St CR, et al. Estrogen and progesterone replacement therapy reduces low density lipoprotein accumulation in the coronary arteries of surgically postmenopausal cynomolgus monkeys. J Clin Invest 1991;88:1995–2002.

42. Utermann G. The mysteries of lipoprotein(a). Science 1989;246:904–910.

43. Scanu AM. Lipoprotein(a). A potential bridge between the fields of atherosclerosis and thrombosis. [Review]. Arch Pathol Lab Med 1988;112:1045–1047.

44. Genest JJ, Jenner JL, McNamara JR, et al. Prevalence of lipoprotein (a) [Lp(a)] excess in coronary artery disease. Am J Cardiol 1991;67:1039–1145.

45. Bostom AG, Gagnon DR, Cupples LA, et al. A prospective investigation of elevated lipoprotein(a) detected by electrophoresis and cardiovascular disease in women. The Framingham Heart Study. Circulation 1994;90:1688–1695.

46. Maeda S, Abe A, Seishima M, et al. Transient changes of serum lipoprotein(a) as an acute phase protein. Atherosclerosis 1989;78:145–150.

47. Steinmetz J, Tarallo P, Fournier B, et al. Reference values of lipoprotein(a) in a French population. Presse Med 1994;23:1695–1698.

48. Solymoss BC, Marcil M, Wesolowska E, et al. Relation of coronary artery disease in women 60 years of age to the combined elevation of serum lipoprotein(a) and total cholesterol to high-density cholesterol ratio. Am J Cardiol 1993;72:1215–1219.
49. Kuchinskiene Z, Carlson LA. Composition, concentration, and size of low density lipoproteins and of subfractions of very low density lipoproteins from serum of normal men and women. J Lipid Res 1982;23: 762–769.
50. Walden CE, Knopp RH, Wahl PW, et al. Sex differences in the effect of diabetes mellitus on lipoprotein triglyceride and cholesterol concentrations. N Engl J Med 1984;311:953–959.
51. Barrett-Connor E, Wingard DL. Sex differential in ischemic heart disease mortality in diabetics: a prospective population-based study. Am J Epidemiol 1983;118:489–496.
52. Schernthaner G, Kostner GM, Dieplinger H, et al. Apolipoproteins (A-I, A-II, B), Lp(a) lipoprotein and lecithin: cholesterol acyltransferase activity in diabetes mellitus. Atherosclerosis 1983;49:277–293.
53. Cruickshanks KJ, Orchard TJ, Becker DJ. The cardiovascular risk profile of adolescents with insulin-dependent diabetes mellitus. Diabetes Care 1985;8:118–124.
54. Laakso M, Barrett CE. Asymptomatic hyperglycemia is associated with lipid and lipoprotein changes favoring atherosclerosis. Arteriosclerosis 1989;9:665–672.
55. Kannel WB, McGee DL. Diabetes and cardiovascular disease. The Framingham study. JAMA 1979;241: 2035–2038.
56. Ginsberg HN. Lipoprotein physiology in nondiabetic and diabetic states. Relationship to atherogenesis. [Review]. Diabetes Care 1991;14:839–855.
57. Knopp RH, Van AM, McNeely M, et al. Effect of insulin-dependent diabetes on plasma lipoproteins in diabetic pregnancy. J Reprod Med 1993;38:703–710.
58. Anonymous: National Center for Health Statistics: Plan and Operation of the Second National Health and Nurtition Examination Survey, 1976–1980. Washington, DC, US Government Printing Office, 1981.
59. Patterson CC, McCrum E, McMaster D. Factors influencing total cholesterol and high-density lipoprotein cholesterol concentrations in a population at high coronary risk. Acta Medica Scand 1988;728(Suppl): 150–158.
60. Wing RR, Bunker CH, Kuller LH, et al. Insulin, body mass index, and cardiovascular risk factors in premenopausal women. Arteriosclerosis 1989;9:479–484.
61. Van Horn LV, Ballew C, Liu K, et al. Diet, body size, and plasma lipids-lipoproteins in young adults: differences by race and sex. The Coronary Artery Risk Development in Young Adults (CARDIA) study. Am J Epidemiol 1991;133:9–23.
62. Glueck CJ, Taylor HL, Jacobs D, et al. Plasma high-density lipoprotein cholesterol: association with measurements of body mass. The Lipid Research Clinics Program Prevalence Study. Circulation 1980.
63. Hubert HB, Feinleib M, McNamara PM, et al. Obesity as an independent risk factor for cardiovascular disease: a 26-year follow-up of participants in the Framingham Heart Study. Circulation 1983;67:968–977.
64. Despres JP, Allard C, Tremblay A, et al. Evidence for a regional component of body fatness in the association with serum lipids in men and women. Metabolism 1985;34:967–973.
65. Soler JT, Folsom AR, Kushi LH, et al. Association of body fat distribution with plasma lipids, lipoproteins, apolipoproteins AI and B in postmenopausal women. J Clin Epidemiol 1988;41:1075–1081.
66. Dustan HP. Coronary artery disease in women. Can J Cardiol 1990;6:19B–21B.
67. Krauss RM. The tangled web of coronary risk factors. Am J Med 1991;90:36S–41S.
68. Razay G, Heaton KW, Bolton CH. Coronary heart disease risk factors in relation to the menopause. Q J Med 1992;85:889–896.
69. Kaplan NM. The deadly quartet. Upper-body obesity, glucose intolerance, hypertriglyceridemia, and hypertension. [Review]. Arch Intern Med 1989;149:1514–1520.
70. Donahue RP, Orchard TJ, Becker DJ, et al. Physical activity, insulin sensitivity, and the lipoprotein profile in young adults: the Beaver County Study. [Review]. Am J Epidemiol 1988;127:95–103.
71. Thompson CJ, Ryu JE, Craven TE, et al. Central adipose distribution is related to coronary atherosclerosis. Arterioscler Thromb 1991;11:327–333.
72 Martin ML, Jensen MD. Effects of body fat distribution on regional lipolysis in obesity. J Clin Invest 1991;88:609–613.
73. Larsson B, Bengtsson C, Bjorntorp P, et al. Is abdominal body fat distribution a major explanation for the sex difference in the incidence of myocardial infarction? The study of men born in 1913 and the study of women, Goteborg, Sweden. Am J Epidemiol 1992;135:266–273.
74. Lapidus L, Bengtsson C, Larsson B, et al. Distribution of adipose tissue and risk of cardiovascular disease and death: a 12 year follow up of participants in the population study of women in Gothenburg, Sweden. Br Med J 1984;289:1257–1261.

75. Muscat JE, Harris RE, Haley NJ, et al. Cigarette smoking and plasma cholesterol. Am Heart J 1991;121: 141–147.
76. Hellerstein MK, Benowitz NL, Neese RA, et al. Effects of cigarette smoking and its cessation on lipid metabolism and energy expenditure in heavy smokers. J Clin Invest 1994;93:265–272.
77. Facchini FS, Hollenbeck CB, Jeppesen J, et al. Insulin resistance and cigarette smoking [published erratum appears in Lancet 1992 Jun 13;339(8807):1492] [see comments]. Lancet 1992;339:1128–1130.
78. Axelsen M, Eliasson B, Joheim E, et al. Lipid intolerance in smokers [see comments]. J Intern Med 1995; 237:449–455.
79. Morrow JD, Frei B, Longmire AW, et al. Increase in circulating products of lipid peroxidation (F2-isoprostanes) in smokers. Smoking as a cause of oxidative damage. N Engl J Med 1995;332:1198–1203.
80. McCully KS. Vascular pathology of homocysteinemia;implications for pathogenesis of arteriosclerosis. Am J Pathol 1969;56:111–128.
81. Mudd SH, Finkelstein JD, Irreverre F, Laster L. Homocystinuria: an enzymatic defect. Science 1964;143: 1443–1445.
82. Rimm E, et al. Folate and Vitamin B6 from diet and supplements in relation to risk of coronary heart disease among women. JAMA 1997;279:359–364.
83. Kannel WB, Hjortland MC, McNamara PM, et al. Menopause and risk of cardiovascular disease: the Framingham study. Ann Intern Med 1976;85:447–452.
84. Gordon T, Kannel WB, Hjortland MC, et al. Menopause and coronary heart disease. The Framingham Study. Ann Intern Med 1978;89:157–161.
85. Colditz GA, Willett WC, Stampfer MJ, et al. Menopause and the risk of coronary heart disease in women. N Engl J Med 1987;316:1105–1110.
86. Gorodeski GI. Impact of the menopause on the epidemiology and risk factors of coronary artery heart disease in women. [Review]. Exp Gerontol 1994;29:357–375.
87. Downs J, Beere P, Whitney E, et al. Design and rationale of the Air Force/Texas Coronary Atherosclerosis Prevention Study (AFCAPS/TexCAPS). Am J Cardiol 1997;80:287–293.
88. Shepherd J, Cobbe SM, Ford I, et al. and the Group WoSCPS. Prevention of Coronary Heart Disease with Pravastatin in Men with Hypercholesterolemia. N Engl J Med 1995;333:1301–1307.
89. Scandinavian Simvastatin Survival Study Group. Randomised trial of cholesterol lowering in 4444 patients with coronary heart disease: the Scandinavian Simvastatin Survival Study (4S). Lancet 1994; 344:1383–1389.
90. Pfeffer M, Sacks F, Lemuel A, et al., for the CARE Investigators. Cholesterol and Recurrent Events: A Secondary Prevention Trial for Normolipidemic Patients. Am J Cardiol 1995;76:98C–106C.
91. Tonkin A. Management of the Long-Term Intervention with Pravastatin in Ischaemic Disease (LIPID) study after the Scandinavian Simvastatian Survival Study (4S). Am J Cardiol 1995;38:107C–112C.
92. Hussey S, Grady D, Bush T, et al., for the Heart and Estrogen/progestin Replacement Study (HERS) Research Group. Randomized Trial of Estrogen Plus Progestin for Secondary Prevention of Coronary Heart Disease in Post Menopausal Women. JAMA 1998;280:605–613.

A Recognized Risk Factor

Homocysteine and Coronary Artery Disease

Simone Nader, MD *and* Killian Robinson, MD

INTRODUCTION

Homocystinuria, a rare inborn error of metabolism, was originally described in Ireland in 1962 by Carson and Neill in a survey of mentally handicapped children. The most common genetic abnormality that can lead to homocystinuria is cystathionine β-synthase deficiency. This is an autosomal recessive disorder in which complications include ectopia lentis, bone abnormalities, including osteoporosis, mental retardation, atherosclerosis, and thromboembolism. The link between premature atherosclerosis and thromboembolism seen in many patients with homozygous homocystinuria has prompted greater interest in this field. Hyperhomocysteinemia, defined as an elevated level of total homocysteine in blood is emerging as a prevalent and strong risk factor for atherosclerotic vascular disease in the coronary, cerebral, and peripheral vessels, and for arterial and venous thromboembolism. This chapter reviews the mechanism for the possible relationship between high plasma homocysteine and vascular disease.

HOMOCYSTEINE METABOLISM

Homocysteine is formed during the metabolism of methionine *(1,2)*, an essential sulfur-containing amino acid that is supplied from dietary and endogenous proteins (Fig. 1). The first step in the metabolism of methionine is the formation of the intermediate S-adenosylmethionine, which is an essential methyl donor in many methylation reaction. S-adenosylhomocysteine is subsequently formed from the demethylation of adenosylmethionine.

From: *Contemporary Cardiology: Preventive Cardiology:*
Strategies for the Prevention and Treatment of Coronary Artery Disease
Edited by: J Foody © Humana Press Inc., Totowa, NJ

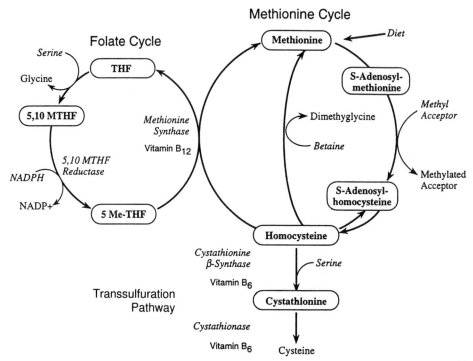

Fig. 1. The metabolism of homocysteine by the remethylation and transsulfuration pathways is shown. Note the dependence of these pathways on folic acid and on vitamins B_{12} and B_6. Key: THF, tetrahydrofolate; 5,10 MTHF-5,10-methylenetetrahydrofolate; NADPH, the reduced form of nicotinamideamideadenine dinucleotide phosphate; NADP, nicotinamide-adenine dinucleotide phosphate; 5 Me-THF, 5 methyltetrahydrofolate.

S-adenosylhomocysteine is then hydrolyzed to adenosine and homocysteine. After homocysteine is formed, it undergoes either remethylation to methionine or transsulfuration to cystathionine. Usually about 50% of intracellular homocysteine is transsulfurated and 50% is reconverted to methionine by one of two remethylation pathways. One pathway requires the presence of the enzyme 5-methyltetrahydrofolate-homocysteine methyltransferase (methionine synthase), which requires vitamin B_{12} as a cofactor. Folic acid is also necessary for this pathway. The second remethylation pathway, which takes place in the liver and the kidney, is catalyzed by the enzyme betaine-homocysteine methyltransferase. The initial step in the transsulfuration pathway, in which homocysteine is first converted to cystathionine, is catalyzed by vitamin B_6 (pyridoxal 5'-phosphate) dependent cystathionine B-synthase. Further reaction lead to the formation of cysteine and other sulfur-containing compounds, including glutathione, and finally to sulfate, which is excreted in the urine.

Normal Plasma Levels

The normal plasma homocysteine levels range from 5–15 μmol/L *(1,2)*. The mean fasting plasma concentration is often in the range of 10–11 μmnol/L in the normal population. A concentration of plasma homocysteine greater than 15 μmol/L is often referred to as hyperhomocysteinemia and is considered to be an independent risk factor for cardiovascular disease *(1,2)*.

Causes of High Plasma Homocysteine

Several mechanisms can cause hyperhomocysteinemia. Genetic deficiency or absence of several key enzymes involved in the homocysteine metabolism, can be an important factor *(1,2)*. Homozygotes for classical homocystinuria have a low or undetectable activity of cystathionine β-synthase. Inherited remethylation cycle abnormalities have also been described, such as derangements of methionine synthase caused by disorders of cobalamin metabolism. On the other hand, a number of mutations of methylenetetrahydrofolate reductase have been reported. Most of these mutations are rare, however, a thermolabile variant caused by a single amino acid substitution (alanine to valine) which occur as a result of a C to T point mutation at position 677 has an allele frequency of 30–40% in the general population. Although not consistently, this variant, which may result in decreased enzyme activity in vivo, is associated with modest elevations in homocysteine concentrations and has been cited as a risk factor for coronary artery disease (CAD) *(3,4)*. Higher plasma levels of homocysteine are seen in the elderly and tend to be higher in men than age-matched women *(5)*. The mechanisms are unknown, however, decreases in cofactor *(6)*, impaired renal function usually seen in the elderly and age-dependent reductions in cystathionine β-synthase activity *(7)*, could all be possible mechanisms. Several nutritional deficiencies can also play an important role. Because folic acid and vitamin B_{12} are essential for the remethylation pathway of homocysteine and vitamin B_6 for transsulfuration, the deficiency or absence of these substances can lead to elevated circulating plasma levels of homocysteine *(1,2)*. Several disease states have also been associated with an increase in homocysteine level, including chronic renal failure, certain cancers, such as acute lymphoblastic leukemia, and severe psoriasis (possible related to lower folate levels). For reasons that are not well understood, homocysteine levels can also rise in hypothyroidism and fall in hyperthyroidism. Hyperhomocysteinemia can also occur as a result of the use of certain medications, including methotrexate, azaribine, nitrous oxide, phenytoin, carbamazepine, and estrogen-containing oral contraceptives by interfering with the normal function of folic acid or vitamins B_6 and B_{12} *(1,2)*.

Homocysteine is known to cause a direct effect on endothelial cells, platelets, clotting factors, and vascular smooth cells. Although several clinical and experimental studies suggest a strong association between high homocysteine concentration and the atherogenic and thrombotic tendencies, the exact mechanism has not been fully elucidated.

Mechanism of Endothelial Damage

The mechanism by which high homocysteine levels are associated with atherosclerosis and thromboembolic diseases remains unclear. The endothelium, instead of platelets or clotting factors, has been the focus of most recent studies. The evidence that homocysteine has a direct toxic effect on endothelial cells is been derived from both in vitro studies in human cell cultures *(8)* and from in vivo animal models (baboons) *(9)*. Short-term intravenous infusion of homocysteine results in desquamation of endothelial cells with subsequent arterial damage resembling premature human atherosclerosis (Fig. 2). Conflicting results have been observed in other animals studies such as pigs *(10)*, rabbits *(11)*, and monkeys *(12)*. The reproducible finding observed in baboons *(9)*, but not in other species, may reflect possible differences in substances infused and species-related responses. In minipigs fed a methionine-rich diet, elevated homocysteine levels were observed after 4 mo on this diet; 2 of 16 animals also developed thromboemboli *(13)*. Besides these

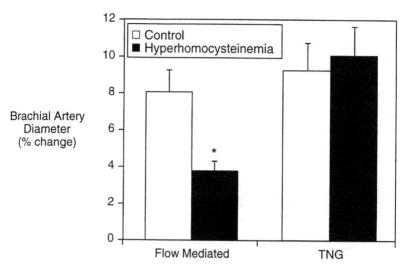

Fig. 2. Relative risks of vascular disease in groups defined by the presence or absence of classic risk factors and elevated plasma homocysteine levels, adjusted for age, sex, and medical center. (From Graham IM, Daly IE, Refsum HM, et al. Plasma homocysteine as a risk factor for vascular disease. The European concerted action project. JAMA 1997;277:1780, with permission.)

observations, pathologic changes were also seen at the elastic lamina of these animals. A recent study performed by Welch and associates *(14)* has demonstrated that homocysteine exposure of endothelial cells leads to a decreased ratio between the concentration of intracellular reduced and oxidized glutathione, known to be an important intracellular buffer. Poddar and colleagues *(15)* recently investigated the expression of the cytokine monocyte chemoattractant protein-1 (MCP-1) in cultured human aortic endothelial cells in the presence of homocysteine (HAEC). Low concentrations of homocysteine are capable of modulating MCP-1 expression in HAEC. This could be attributable to alteration of the transcription process, or to increase the half-life of MCP-1 mRNA. These studies suggested that homocysteine may be atherogenic by promoting recruitment of monocytes to the endothelium by overexpression of MCP-1. Tawakol and coworkers *(16)* recently used high-resolution ultrasonography to study endothelium-dependent and -independent vasodilation in a nonatherosclerotic peripheral conduit artery of 26 elderly hyperhomocysteinemic subjects. They concluded that hyperhomocysteinemia is associated with impaired endothelium-dependent vasodilation in humans and suggested that the bioavailability of nitric oxide (NO) is decreased in hyperhomocysteinemic patients (Fig. 3). Other possible effects of homocysteine on endothelial damage can be expressed by inhibiting the synthesis of prostacyclin, increasing factor V expression, inactivating endothelial anticoagulant protein C, or disrupting the processing and secretion of von Willebrand factor *(1,2)*.

Effects on Platelets

High homocysteine levels may also affect platelet function. Several studies have shown a detrimental effect in platelet function in the presence of high homocysteine concentration such as increased platelet adhesion and aggregation *(1,2)*. In vitro, Graeber and associates *(17)* showed that in vitro D-L-homocysteine alters arachidonic acid metabolism of normal platelets so that 12-hydroxy-5,8,10-heptadecatrienoic acid and thromboxane A$_2$

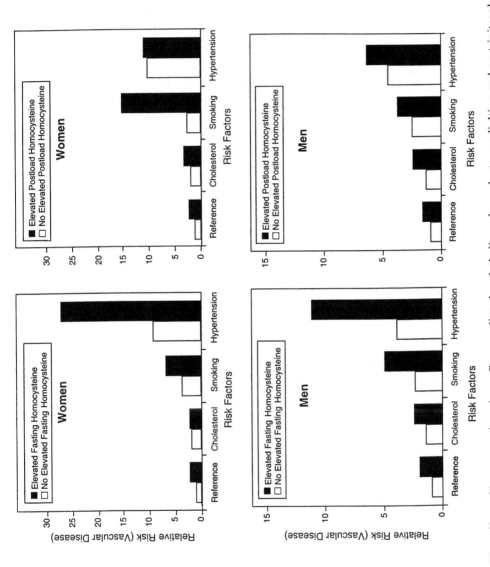

Fig. 3. The effect of homocysteinemia on flow mediated endothelium-dependent vasodialtion and on trinitroglycerine (TNG)-induced endothelium independent vasodilation. (From Tawakol A, Omland T, Gerhard M, et al. Promotion of vascular smooth muscle cell growth by homocysteine: a link to atherosclerosis. Circulation 1997;95:1119, with permission.)

are increased. Di Minno and colleagues *(18)* demonstrated that increased thromboxane A_2 production is seen in patients with homozygous homocystinuria. The mechanism for thrombosis has not been fully elucidated, however. Increased platelet adhesion and aggregation, decreased platelet survival time, increased synthesis of thromboxane B_2, and increased levels of platelet-derived thromboxane A_2 could all represent possible mechanisms.

Effects on Clotting Factors

Several abnormalities of clotting have been demonstrated suggesting the role of homocysteine-promoting prothrombotic activities. Rosenberg and coworkers *(19)* showed that levels of antithrombin activity 50% of normal have been associated with high propensity to intravascular thrombosis. Serum antithrombin activity in seven homocystinuric patients was reduced compared with matched controls subjects *(20)*. Similar results have been showed by others *(2,21)*. Rodgers and Kane *(22)* showed that homocysteine activated endothelial cell factor V in a dose dependent fashion and increased prothrombin activation of Factor Xa.

Effects on Vascular Smooth Muscle Cells

Homocysteine may also adversely affect the vascular smooth smooth cell. Welch and coworkers showed that hydrogen peroxide, which is formed by oxidation of homocysteine, may cause oxidant stress and play an important role in smooth cell damage before definite vascular lesions develop. Recent studies have shown that homocysteine exposure leads to a decrease in the ratio between the intracellular concentrations of reduced and oxidized glutathione, known to be the most important intracellular redox buffer.

DISEASE STATES ASSOCIATED
WITH HIGH PLASMA HOMOCYSTEINE LEVELS

Hyperhomocysteinemia and End-Stage Renal Disease

The causes of hyperhomocysteinemia in renal failure patients are unclear and the major mechanism seen in these patients is thought to be secondary to reduced metabolism. The most important predictors of hyperhomocysteinemia in patients with end-stage renal disease include lower folate and vitamin B_{12} levels, high serum creatinine concentration, and the length of time in dialysis. High homocysteine concentration in a patient with renal failure is an independent risk factor for vascular complications, and this risk increases with increasing plasma homocysteine concentration.

High Homocysteine Levels After Organ Transplantation

High homocysteine levels may be seen after kidney, liver, lung, and heart transplant and transplant recipients have a higher risk of vascular events. Wilcken and colleagues in 1981 first reported elevated, high homocysteine levels in renal transplant patients *(23)*. Berger and associates *(24)* at the Mayo Clinic demonstrated a 70% increased in homocysteine concentration after cardiac transplantation, and levels remain elevated 12 mo later. Gupta and coworkers *(25)* found high homocysteine concentrations in over 60% of transplanted heart recipients, as well as frequent folate and vitamin B_6 deficiency. Higher homocysteine levels were more evident in those patients with vascular complications.

Hyperhomocysteinemia, As an Increased Risk for Deep Venous Thrombosis

Recently, researchers have focused their attention in the relationship of high homocysteine concentration and venous thromboembolism. Mudd and colleagues *(26)* studied 629 patients with homocystinuria and they conclude that deep venous thrombosis was the most frequent thrombotic complication, accounting for approximately 50% of all events. den Heijer and colleagues *(27)* measured the plasma homocysteine concentration in 185 patients with recurrent venous thrombosis before and after a methionine loading test. (This test is used to evaluate the tendency of patients to high homocysteine levels in whom fasting values are normal; patients receive a standard dose of methionine, and homocysteine concentrations are measured at regular intervals afterward). Fasting homocysteine concentrations greater than the 90th percentile for values in normal controls were seen in 25% of cases and conferred an odds ratio (OR) of 3:1 for thrombosis. Similar results were seen following the methionine loading test.

Hyperhomocysteinemia and Coronary Artery Disease

An association between high homocysteine levels and coronary artery disease was first studied by Wilcken and Wilcken *(28)*. They investigated methionine metabolism in patients <50 years old with angiographically documented coronary artery disease. After methionine loading, a higher level of homocysteine mixed disulfide was seen in patients with coronary artery disease than in control subjects. The increased risk of an increased plasma homocysteine levels and the development of vascular disease may begin at levels as low as 10 µmol/L, a level well within the range currently regarded as normal. In the prospective Tromso study from Norway, a total of 21,826 men at ages between 12 and 61yr were evaluated, there was an increased risk of about 40% for myocardial infarction (MI) associated with a 4 µmol/L increase in homocysteine levels.

It was not until 1992 when homocysteine was reported as an independent risk factor for MI in male participants prospectively enrolled in the U.S. Physicians Health Study. Homocysteine levels in the upper 5% of the distribution were associated with a 3.1-fold (1.3–8.8) relative risk of coronary heart disease (CHD) *(29)*. Arnesen and coworkers *(30)* also reported a higher homocysteine concentration in patients who subsequently had MI than in those who did not. Although most case-control and many prospective studies support the strong association between hyperhomocysteinemia and the increased risk for vascular disease, other studies fail to demonstrate this association. For example, a nested case-control study was conducted involving men participating in the Multiple Risk Factor Intervention Trial (MRFIT). Homocysteine samples stored for 20 yr were collected and measured from 712 men. Cases involved nonfatal MI identified through the active phase of the study and deaths due to CHD. There was no association between CAD and the homocysteine concentration. Homocysteine levels were weakly associated with the acute-phase protein (C-reactive protein) *(31)*. Some of the results and discrepancies seen in these studies of patients with CAD may be related to the populations under investigation, their nutritional status, the samples and tests that were used for measurement of homocysteine, and even the sample size of the studied population.

A graded and strong relationship between an increased plasma homocysteine levels and overall mortality has been demonstrated, in patients with CAD, by Nygard and associates *(32)*. They followed these patients for a total of about four years. About 4% of those with homocysteine levels below 9 μmol/L have died as compared with 25% of patients with levels of 15 μmol/L or above. In conclusion, the majority, but not all, studies have shown that homocysteine is an independent risk factor for CAD and that elevated levels may also predispose an adverse outcomes in these patients.

Hyperhomocysteinemia and Peripheral Vascular Disease

Peripheral vascular disease is a common finding among the elderly. The earlier studies conducted by Brattström and colleagues *(33)* and Bores and coworkers *(34)* included patients with peripheral vascular disease and suggested that homocysteine might be a risk factor for this condition. Several large case-control studies have now supported this evidence, and a high homocysteine level is now recognized as an independent risk factor for lower limb atherosclerotic disease. An exemple of this is the study performed by Taylor and colleagues *(35)* They measured the plasma homocysteine levels in 214 patients with symptomatic (claudication, rest pain, gangrene, amputation) lower extremity arterial occlusive disease and/or symptomatic (stroke, transient cerebral ischemic attacks) cerebral vascular disease and compared them with 103 control persons. Mean plasma homocysteine levels were significantly higher in patients than in control subjects. They concluded that elevated plasma homocysteine level is an independent risk factor for symptomatic lower extremity disease or cerebral vascular disease or both. In addition, symptomatic patients with lower extremity disease and with elevated plasma homocysteine levels also appear to have more rapid progression of disease.

Plasma Homocysteine Concentration and Extracranial Carotid Artery Stenosis and Stroke

The risk of carotid-artery atherosclerosis, assesed by carotid ultrasonography, in relation to both plasma homocysteine concentrations and nutritional determinants of hyperhomocysteinemia has been investigated by Selhub and colleagues *(36)*. He performed a cross-sectional study of 418 men and 623 women, aged 67–96 yr, from the Framingham Heart Study. He demonstrated that after adjusting sex, age, plasma high-density lipoprotein cholesterol concentration, systolic blood pressure, and smoking status, the prevalence of carotid stenosis of $\geq25\%$ was 43% in men and 34% in women. The odds ratio for stenosis of $>25\%$ was 2.0 (95% confidence interval, 1.4–2.9) for patients with the highest plasma homocysteine concentrations (≥14.4 μmol/L) as compared with those with the lowest concentrations (≤9.1 μmol). In addition, the plasma concentrations of folate and pyridoxal-5'-phosphate (the coenzyme form of vitamin B_6) and the level of folate intake were inversely associated with carotid-artery stenosis. In the prospective British Regional Heart Study *(37)*, 5661 men were followed for a period of 12.8 yr, and the risk of stroke was directly related to the blood homocysteine concentrations. In the Physicians' Health Study, plasma homocysteine concentration was higher in subjects with stroke, but the difference was not statistically significant. The authors concluded then that, although the sample size was small, the data were compatible with a small but nonsignificant association between elevated homocysteine and risk of stroke *(38)*.

Homocysteine Levels and Risk of Stroke and Thrombosis in Systemic Lupus Erythematous

Petri and colleagues studied the association between homocysteine levels and the risk of stroke and thrombosis in 337 patients with systemic lupus erythematosus (SLE) *(39)*.

Ninety-three percent of the study population were women, 54% African American, and 45% white. There were 29 cases of stroke and 31 arterial thrombotic events. Increased homocysteine concentrations were found in 51 (15%) of the SLE patients. They concluded that homocysteine concentrations were an independent risk factor for both stroke and subsequent thrombotic events.

Treatment of Homocystinuria

Elevated plasma homocysteine can be reduced in normal subjects and, in folate deficient patients, it can be reduced by oral folic acid supplementation. Recently, various combinations of vitamin B_6 and B_{12} and folic acid have reduced homcysteine concentrations in patients with coronary artery disease *(40,41)*. The dose and combination remain unclear; however, evidence suggests that a dose as low as 1 mg or less may be effective in lowering homocysteine levels. At the Cleveland Clinic, a placebo-controlled study of 100 patients with CAD revealed that for those patients treated with folic acid, 0.4, 1.0, and 5 mg daily for 3 mo, homocysteine concentration fell by 30% in all treatment groups compared with no change in the placebo group. For patients with hyperhomocysteinemia due to renal failure, however, extremely high doses of folic acid, such as 15 mg/d, or more, are needed *(42)*.

Although it is now evident that folic acid lowers homocysteine concentration, there is no evidence that it would improve clinical outcomes. Van Den Berg and associates *(43)* have shown that treatment of young patients with vascular disease using vitamin B_6 and folic acid will lower homocysteine levels and improve endothelial function, as assessed by reduction of circulating von Willebrand's factor and thrombomodulin levels. In light of the present data and the consequences of high homocysteine levels, many physicians would therefore consider it reasonable to use vitamin supplementation in hyperhomocysteinemic patients. In these individuals the dosage currently used is 0.4 mg/d of folic acid; homocysteine levels are measured 4–6 wk after initiation of treatment. Pyridoxime may prevent higher homocysteine levels and may also have other beneficial effects on lipids and the clotting process. If folic acid use is long-term, vitamin B_{12} levels may need to be checked both before and during therapy to ensure absence of coexisting vitamin B_{12} deficiency.

Starting in January, 1998, 140 mg of folic acid will be added per 100 g of flour. Even though this is intended to reduce the incidence of neural tube defects, we are hopeful that it would also decrease the risk of atherosclerosis in the general population. Further clinical trials are needed to evaluate the effect of folic acid alone or in combination with vitamin B_6 or B_{12} on clinical outcomes and on the long-term prognosis of patients with atherosclerosis.

REFERENCES

1. Mayer EL, Jacobsen DW, Robinson K. Homocysteine and coronary atherosclerosis. J Am Coll Cardiol 1996;27:517.
2. Ueland PM, Refsum H, Brattstrom L. Plasma homocysteine and cardiovascular disease. In: Francis RB Jr, ed. Atherosclerotic Cardiovascular Disease, Hemostasis, and Endothelial Function. Marcel Dekker, New York, 1992, p. 183.
3. Kang SS, Wong PWK, Susmano A, et al. Thermolabile methylenetetrahydrofolate reductase: An inherited risk factor for coronary artery disease. Am J Hum Genet 1991;48:536.
4. Adams M, Smith PD, Martin D, et al. Genetic analysis of thermolabile methylenetetrahydrofolate reductase as a risk factor for myocardial infarction. Q J Med 1996; 89:437.

5. Kang S-S, Wong PWK, Cook HY, et al. Protein-bound homocysteine. A possible risk factor for coronary artery disease. J Clin Invest 1986;77:1482–1486.
6. Selhub J, Jacques PF, Wilson PWF, et al. Vitamin status and intake as primary determinants of homocysteinemia in an elderly population. JAMA 1993;270:2693–2698.
7. Nordstrom M, Kjellstrom T. Age dependency of cystathionine beta-synthase activity in human fibroblasts in homocysteinemia and atherosclerotic vascular disease. Atherosclerosis 1992;94:213–221.
8. Starkebaum G, Harlan JM. Endothelial cell injury due to copper-catalyzed hydrogen peroxide generation from homocysteine. J Clin Invest 1986;77:1370–1376.
9. Harker LA, Harlan JM, Ross R. Effect of sulfinpyrazone on homocysteine-induced endothelial injury and arteriosclerosis in baboons. Circ Res 1983;53:731–739.
10. Smolin LA, Crenshaw TD, Kurtycz D, Benevenga NJ. Homocysteine accumulation in pigs fed diets deficient in vitamin B_6: relationship to atherosclerosis. J Nutr 1983;113:2122–2133.
11. Donahue S, Sturman JA, Gaull G. Arteriosclerosis due to homocysteinemia: failure to reproduce the model in weaning rabbits. Am J Pathol 1974;77:167–174.
12. Krishnaswamy K, Rao SB. Failure to produce atherosclerosis in macaca radiata on a high-methionine, high fat, pyridoxine-deficient diet. Atherosclerosis 1977;27:253–258.
13. Rolland PH, Friggi A, Barlatier A, et al. Hyperhomocysteinemia induced vascular damage in the minipig. Captopril-hydrochlorothiazide combination prevents elastic alterations. Circulation 1995;91:1161–1174.
14. Welch GN, Upchurch GR Jr, Keaney JF, et al. Homocysteine decreases cell redox potential in vascular smooth muscle cells (abstract). J Am Coll Cardiol 1996;27(Suppl 2a):163A.
15. Poddar R, Sivasubramanian N, Robinson K, et al. Homocysteine modulates the expression of a specific cytokine (monocyte chemoattractant protein-1) in human aortic endothelial cells. Circulation 1997; 96(Suppl, abstr):286.
16. Tawakol A, Omland T, Gerhard M, et al. Hyperhomocyteinemia is associated with impaired endothelium-dependent vasodilation in humans. Circulation 1997;95:1119–1121.
17. Graeber JE, Slott JH, Ulane RE, Schulman JD, et al. Effect of homocysteine and homocystine on platelet and vascular arachidonic acid metabolism. Pediatr Res 1982;16:490–493.
18. Di Minno G, Davi G, Margaglione M, et al. Abnormally high thromboxane biosynthesis in homozygous homocystinuria. Evidence for platelet involvement and probucol-sensitive mechanism. J Clin Invest 1993;92:1400–1406.
19. Rosenberg RD. Actions and interactions of antithrombin and heparin. N Engl J Med 1975;292:146–151.
20. Giannini MJ, Coleman M, Innerfield I. Antithrombin activity in homocystinuria [letter]. Lancet 1975; 1:1094.
21. Palareti G, Coccheri S. Lowered antithrombin III activity and other clotting changes in homocystinuria:effects of a pyridoxine-folate regimen. Haemostasis1989;19(Suppl):24–28.
22. Rodgers GM, Kane WH. Activation of endogenous factor V by homocysteine-induced vascular endothelial cell activator. J Clin Invest 1986;77:1909–1916.
23. Wilcken DEL, Gupta VJ, Betts AK. Homocysteine in the plasma of renal transplant recipients: effects of cofactors for methionine metabolism. Clin Sci 1981;61:743–749.
24. Berger, PB, Jones JD, Olson LJ, et al. Increase in total plasma homocysteine concentration after cardiac transplantation. Mayo Clin Proc 1995;70:125.
25. Gupta A, Moustapha A, Jacobsen DW, et al. High homocysteine, low folate and low vitamin B_6 concentrations: prevalent risk factors for vascular disease in heart transplant recipients. Transplantation 1998; 65:544.
26. Mudd SH, Skovby F, Levy HL, et al. The natural history of homocystinuria due to cystathionine B synthase deficiency. Am J Hum Genet 1985;37:1.
27. Den Heijer M, Blom HJ, Gerrits WBJ, et al. Is hyperhomocysteinemia a risk factor for recurrent venous thrombosis? Lancet 1995;345:882.
28. Wilken DEL, Wilken B. The pathogenesis of coronary artery disease. A possible role for methionine metabolism. J Clin Invest 1976;57:1079.
29. Stampfer MJ, Malinow MR, Willett WC, et al. A prospective study of plasma homocyst(e)ine and risk of myocardial infarction in U.S. physicians. JAMA 1992;268:877.
30. Arnesen E, Refsum H, Bonaa HK, et al. Serum total homocysteine and coronary heart disease. Int J Epidemiol 1995;24:704.
31. Evans RW, Shaten BJ, Hempel JD, et al. Homocyst (e) ine and risk of cardiovascular disease in the Multiple Risk Factor Intervention Trial. Arterioscler Thromb Vasc Biol 1997;17:1947.

32. Nygard O, Vollset SE, Refsum H, et al. Total plasma homocysteine and cardiovascular risk profile: The Hordaland Homocysteine Study. JAMA 1995;274:1526–1533.
33. Brattström LE, Hardebo JE, Hultberg BL. Moderate homocysteinemia—a possible risk factor for arteriosclerotic cerebrovascular disease. Stroke 1984;15:1012.
34. Boers GHJ, Smals AGH, Trijbels FJM, et al. Heterozygosity for homocystinuria in premature peripheral and cerebral occlusive arterial disease. N Engl J Med 1985;313:709.
35. Taylor LM Jr, DeFrang RD, Harris EJ Jr, et al. The association of elevated plasma homocyst(e)ine with progression of symptomatic peripheral arterial disease. J Vasc Surg 1991;13:128.
36. Selhub J, Jacques PF, Bostom AG, et al. Association between plasma homocysteine concentrations and extracranial carotid-artery stenosis. N Engl J Med 1995;332:286.
37. Perry IJ, Refsum H, Morris RW, et al. Prospective study of serum total homocysteine concentration and risk of stroke in middle-aged British men. Lancet 1995;346:1395.
38. Verhoef P, Hennekens CH, Malinow MR, et al. A prospective study of plasma homocyst(e)ine and risk of ischemic stroke. Stroke 1994;25:1924.
39. Petri M, Roubenoff R, Dallal GE, et al. Plasma homocysteine as a risk factor for atherothrombotic events in systemic lupus erythematosus. Lancet 1996;348:1120.
40. Mayer EL, Jacobsen DW, Robinson K. Homocysteine and coronary atherosclerosis. J Am Coll Cardiol 1996;27:517.
41. Ueland PM, Refsum H, Brattström L. Plasma homocysteine and cardiovascular disease. In: Francis RB Jr, ed. Athersclerotic Cardiovascular Disease, Hemostasis and Endothelial Function. Marcel Dekker, New York, 1992, p. 183.
42. Naurath HJ, Joosten E, Riezler R, et al. Effects of vitamin B_{12}, folate, and vitamin B_6 supplements in elderly people with normal serum vitamin concentrations. Lancet 1995;346:85.
43. Van den Berg M, Boers GH, Franken DG, et al. Hyperhomocysteinaemia and endothelial dysfunction in young patients with peripheral arterial occlusoive disease. Eur J Clin Infest 1995;25:176.

III STRATEGIES FOR PREVENTION

13 Pharmacologic Agents in Preventive Cardiology

Michael A. Militello, PHARMD
and Teresa H. Seo, PHARMD

CONTENTS

INTRODUCTION

Cardiovascular disease is the leading cause of death in the United States as well as other developed societies. It has been the leading cause of mortality in men and in women since 1900. According to the 1999 Heart and Stroke Statistical Update, cardiovascular-related deaths in women accounted for more than the next 16 leading causes of death combined (1). Efforts to reduce cardiovascular disease risk remains one of the most important challenges in medicine. Guidance is provided by literature evaluating use of medications for reduction of both primary and secondary cardiovascular events.

Risk factor modification is key in the prevention of coronary artery disease. Patient education on smoking cessation, proper diet, exercise, and maintaining compliance with medications for hypertension, diabetes mellitus, and hypercholesterolemia are essential components in management. Prevention strategies can be viewed as primary or secondary prevention. Primary prevention is defined as treatments or risk factor modification initiated and proven to prevent the first or initial coronary event (e.g., lipid lowering agents used to prevent occurrence of first myocardial infarction). With secondary prevention, treatment modalities are initiated after the first event, such as a myocardial infarction, has taken place in order to prevent subsequent events (e.g., the use of beta blockers after a myocardial infarction to reduce new events) (2). This chapter focuses on clinical trials of pharmacologic therapy in prevention of cardiovascular disease.

From: *Contemporary Cardiology: Preventive Cardiology:*
Strategies for the Prevention and Treatment of Coronary Artery Disease
Edited by: J. Foody © Humana Press Inc., Totowa, NJ

Table 1
Major Trials Evaluating Lipid-Lowering Drugs for Primary Prevention

Trial	Treatment	N =	Primary endpoint	Results
WHO (10–12)	Placebo Clofibrate	5296 5331	Risk of nonfatal MI	Clofibrate-treated patients had a 25% relative risk reduction in primary endpoint. There was a 47% excess mortality in the treated group while they were taking the study drug.
LRC-CPPT (13)	Placebo Cholestyramine	1900 1906	Composite of definite coronary heart disease death and/or nonfatal MI	Cholestyramine-treated patients had a 19% reduction in risk of primary endpoint
HHS (14)	Placebo Gemfibrozil	2030 2050	Composite of fatal or nonfatal MI and cardiac death	Gemfibrozil-treated patients had a 34% reduction in cardiac endpoints
WOSCOPS (7)	Placebo Pravastatin	3293 3302	Composite of nonfatal MI or death from a cardiovascular event	Pravastatin-treated patients had a 30% reduction in the risk of primary event
AFCAPS/ TexCAPS (6)	Placebo Lovastatin	3304 3301	Composite of fatal or nonfatal MI, UA, or SCD	37% decrease in primary endpoint ($p < 0.001$)

MI, myocardial infarction; UA, unstable angina; SCD, sudden cardiac death.

HYPERLIPIDEMIA

Pathophysiology

Atherosclerosis occurs as a result of lipid deposition within the coronary vessel. Cigarette smoking, diabetes, infection, elevated homocysteine levels, hypertension, and hyperlipidemia have all been associated with this multifactorial inflammatory process (3). Coronary atherosclerosis begins early in childhood and progresses throughout life.

It is well known that high levels of total cholesterol and low-density-lipoprotein cholesterol (LDL-C) as well as low levels of high-density-lipoprotein cholesterol (HDL-C) are related to the risk of developing coronary artery disease (2). Inflammatory response is triggered when LDL-C crossing the arterial wall is oxidized, promoting macrophage infiltration and leading to an increase in cholesterol within the arterial wall. Atherosclerotic plaque formation is fostered as a result. Use of lipid-lowering therapy decreases LDL-C levels within the blood and therefore, decreases the coronary artery disease process (4).

Primary Prevention

Lipid-lowering therapy has been shown to decrease cardiovascular events and decrease total mortality in patients with documented coronary artery disease (CAD). It was not until recently that trials have also demonstrated benefits on both cardiovascular and total mortality in treatment of elevated lipid levels in patients without known CAD. Early studies of diet therapy in combination with cholesterol-lowering drugs showed a decrease in cardiovascular event rate; however, they did not decrease total mortality (*see* Table 1) (10–12). These early trials also brought into question whether treating elevated cholesterol levels increased the risk of noncardiovascular death (i.e., violent and cancer related). Yet there was no conclusive data linking the cause of death to the study medications (5).

Another major limitation was that women were excluded from the early studies. Therefore, there was no direct evidence that women benefited from lipid-lowering therapy for primary prevention. Recent trials with 3-hydroxy-3-methylglutaryl-coenzyme A (HMG-CoA) reductase inhibitors or "statins" have shown that treatment can significantly lower coronary events (*see* Table 1), without an excess in total mortality.

The Air Force/Texas Coronary Atherosclerosis Prevention Study (AFCAPS/TexCAPS) study included men and women with average total cholesterol levels (mean 221 mg/dL). Patients treated with lovastatin had a 37% reduction in the composite endpoint of fatal and nonfatal myocardial infarction (MI), unstable angina (UA), and sudden cardiac death (SCD). This benefit was seen within the first year of therapy (mean follow-up 5.2 yr). Noncardiovascular mortality was similar between the treatment and placebo groups *(6)*. The second "statin" trial evaluated pravastatin in men with hypercholesterolemia and no history of myocardial infarction; however, 5% of both the treatment and control group had a history of angina. The primary endpoint was a composite of nonfatal myocardial infarction or death from CAD. Patients were treated with pravastatin 40 mg daily for an average of 4.9 yr. Results of this study show that patients treated with pravastatin had significantly less events than those receiving placebo. Like the AFCAPS/TexCAPS study, the difference in event rate started to diverge within 6 mo and continued to be significant over the follow-up period *(7)*. In both "statin" studies the medications were well tolerated, and there was no difference in noncardiovascular mortality when compared to placebo. The major limitation to the primary prevention trials was the relatively few numbers of women that were studied. Unfortunately, in women, the first cardiovascular event is often fatal; aggressive lipid management should be implemented in high-risk patients *(6,8)*.

Current recommendations for treating hyperlipidemia focus on the level of total cholesterol, LDL-C, and HDL-C and also on risk for future cardiovascular events. Dietary therapy is recommended initially unless multiple risk factors for cardiovascular disease are present (i.e., diabetes mellitus [DM], hypertension, family history of premature heart disease, smoking, HDL-C < 35 mg/dL, age ≥ 45 yr in men or ≥ 55 yr in women or premature menopause without estrogen replacement therapy [ERT]). Drug therapy should be reserved for patients with hypercholesterolemia and multiple risk factors (*see* Table 2). Per the most recent National Cholesterol Education Program (NCEP) guidelines, lipid levels that warrant initial drug therapy are LDL-C levels of ≥ 190 mg/dL with less than two risk factors or LDL-C levels ≥ 160 mg/dL in the presence of two or more risk factors as mentioned earlier (*see* Table 3) *(9)*.

Secondary Prevention

The Coronary Drug Project (CDP) investigated several drug therapies for secondary prevention of coronary events. The dextrothyroxine treatment group was terminated early due to an excess in mortality; the estrogen groups were terminated due to increase in morbidity (nonfatal cardiovascular events and concerns of cancer and thromboembolism). Of the two remaining treatment groups, clofibrate did not demonstrate a reduction in total mortality while there was a 10% lower total mortality in the niacin treatment group over placebo; however, this difference was not statistically significant *(15,16)*. The Stockholm Ischaemic Heart Disease Secondary Prevention Study was the first to demonstrate a reduction in CAD. A 13% reduction in total cholesterol was associated with a 26% reduction in total mortality and 36% reduction in ischemic heart disease mortality *(17)*. Since

Table 2
Comparison of Lipid-Lowering Therapies

Drug	TC	LDL-C	HDL-C	Triglycerides
HMG-CoA reductase inhibitors				
Atorvastatin	↓↓↓↓	↓↓↓↓	↑	↓↓
Cerivaststin	↓↓↓	↓↓↓	↑	↓
Fluvastatin	↓↓	↓↓	↑	↓
Lovastatin	↓↓↓	↓↓↓	↑	↓
Pravastatin	↓↓↓	↓↓↓	↑	↓
Simvastatin	↓↓↓↓	↓↓↓↓	↑	↓
Fibric acid derivatives				
Clofibrate	↓	↓	↑	↓↓↓
Fenofibrate	↓	↓	↑↑	↓↓↓
Gemfibrozil	↓	↓	↑↑	↓↓↓
Bile acid sequestrants				
Cholestyramine	↓	↓	– / ↑	– / ↑
Colestipol	↓	↓	– / ↑	– / ↑
Other				
Niacin	↓↓	↓↓	↑↑	↓↓

↓, decrease; ↑, increase; – / ↑, no effect/minimal increase; TC, total cholesterol; LDL-C, low-density lipoprotein cholesterol; HDL-C, high-density lipoprotein cholesterol.

Table 3
Recommendations for Initial Therapy Based on LDL-C Levels

Patient category	Dietary therapy LDL-C	Drug therapy LDL-C	LDL-C goal
Without CHD and 0–1 risk factors[a]	≥160 mg/dL	≥190 mg/dL	<160 mg/dL
Without CHD and ≥2 risk factors	≥130 mg/dL	≥160 mg/dL	<130 mg/dL
With CHD	>100 mg/dL	≥130 mg/dL	≤100 mg/dL

[a] CHD = coronary heart disease.
Source: Summary of the Second Report of the National Cholesterol Education Program Expert Panel (NCEP) on Detection, Evaluation, and Treatment of High Blood Cholesterol in Adults (Adult Treatment Panel II).

then, several major trials have demonstrated a reduction in CHD death and total mortality using lipid-lowering therapies for secondary prevention (see Table 4) (15–23).

The Scandinavian Simvastatin Survival Study (4S) was a randomized, double-blind, placebo-controlled trial of 4444 patients comparing effects of simvastatin to placebo over a median follow-up period of 5.4 yr. There was a 30% reduction in total mortality and 42% reduction in coronary deaths in the simvastatin group compared to placebo. Unlike earlier studies, the 4S trial did not report an increase in noncardiac deaths (18). The Cholesterol and Recurrent Events (CARE) study included individuals with LDL values between 115 and 174 mg/dL (mean 139 mg/dL) to look at whether benefits could be derived with pravastatin treatment in patients after MI with average baseline cholesterol values. Median follow-up was 5 yr. The pravastatin group had a 24% risk reduction in the combined endpoint of coronary death/nonfatal MI. Also, patients with higher baseline LDL values tended to derive more benefit with pravastatin therapy than those with lower baseline LDL values (e.g., <125 mg/dL) (19). The inclusion of women in these two

Table 4
Major Trials Evaluating Lipid-Lowering Drugs for Secondary Prevention

Trial	Treatment	N =	Primary endpoint	Results
CDP (Coronary Drug Project) (15,16)	Placebo[a] Niacin Clofibrate	1587 616 637	Total mortality	11% lower total mortality with niacin group vs. placebo
SS (Stockholm study) (17)	No intervention Niacin/clofibrate	276 279	Total mortality	26% risk reduction in primary endpoint with niacin/ clofibrate combination ($p < 0.05$)
4S (18)	Placebo Simvastatin	2223 2221	Total mortality	30% risk reduction in total mortality with simvastatin treatment ($p = 0.0003$)
CARE (19)	Placebo Pravastatin	2078 2081	Composite of coronary heart disease death and/or nonfatal MI	24% risk reduction of primary endpoint with pravastatin treatment ($p = 0.003$)
Post-CABG (20)	Moderate Aggressive	675 676	Per-patient percentage of grafts showing progression of atherosclerosis	31% reduction in primary endpoint in aggressive vs. moderate treatment group
LIPID (21)	Placebo Pravastatin	4502 4512	CHD death	24% risk reduction in primary endpoint with pravastatin treatment ($p = <0.001$)

[a]Note: the estrogen and dextrothyroxine groups terminated early. There was no benefit with clofibrate group in total mortality over placebo.

studies helped demonstrate that women benefited as much, if not more, by lipid-lowering therapy (18,19).

Lipid-lowering drugs for secondary prevention are recommended as initial therapy for all patients with CHD and hypercholesterolemia (i.e., LDL-C > 100 mg/dL). In post-menopausal women, lipid-lowering agents such as "statins" are recommended for hyper-cholesterolemia as initial therapy over hormone replacement therapy (HRT). HRT may be an option, but treatment choice should be determined on an individual basis. Lipid-lowering therapy is also recommended for low-risk, premenopausal women with LDL-C levels >220 mg/dL (8).

Patients with DM are at high risk for the development of CAD. In the United States alone, there are approximately 10 million people diagnosed with DM; two thirds of these patients will die from cardiac or vascular disease (1). Current recommendations for treat-ment of dyslipidemia in patients with DM are initiation of appropriate diet therapy, physical activity, and weight loss in overweight individuals. The American Diabetes Association recommends lowering LDL-C to <100 mg/dL in patients with diabetes and without cardiovascular disease, especially in the presence of multiple risk factors (24,25). This differs from NCEP guidelines, which recommend a goal of LDL-C ≤ 160 mg/dL in patients without coronary heart disease (CHD) and ≤1 risk factor (9). For diabetics, LDL-C reduction is a primary goal with secondary goals of increasing HDL-C and lowering tri-glycerides (TGs). Dietary therapy can reduce LDL-C levels by approximately 15–25 mg/dL; therefore, if LDL-C reductions of greater than 25 mg/dL are required, drug therapy may be necessary in addition to initiation of dietary changes (24). It is crucial to maintain optimal glycemic control to help reduce LDL-C and TG levels. Patients unable to meet LDL-C and TG goals may require combination therapy such as a "statin" plus resin binder for patients with inadequate LDL-C control or a "statin" plus a fibric acid derivative in patients with elevated LDL-C and TGs *(25)*. Niacin is relatively contraindicated in patients with diabetes because of potential to worsen glycemic control; however, niacin may be used in select individuals with careful monitoring and initiation at low doses.

HOMOCYSTEINE AND ANTIOXIDANTS

Elevated concentrations of homocysteine, an amino acid necessary for various biochemical processes, may promote atherosclerosis and be a risk factor for cardiovascular disease as well as venous thrombosis. Homocysteine is an intermediate metabolite of methionine metabolism; some individuals have deficiencies in enzymes or cofactors needed for homocysteine metabolism (i.e., folate, vitamin B_6 or B_{12}) *(26,27)*. Although folic acid has been demonstrated to lower homocysteine levels, it is not known yet what the full clinical benefit is from this intervention *(28,29)*.

Antioxidants such as vitamin E have also been evaluated for the prevention of coronary artery disease *(30)*. The primary component in vitamin E believed to prevent oxidation of polyunsaturated fats bound to LDL is alpha-tocopherol. Intake of fruits and vegetables high in vitamin E in conjunction with a low-fat diet should be encouraged. Supplemental vitamin E in dosages of 100–400 IU daily of vitamin E may provide benefit; however, optimal source (i.e., dietary or supplemental), dose, duration, and effects on coronary disease progression of vitamin E are unknown.

SMOKING CESSATION

Cigarette smoking is a well-established risk factor for coronary heart disease *(1,31–33)*. Although the exact mechanism underlying increased cardiovascular morbidity and mortality with smoking is uncertain, nicotine and carbon monoxide are believed to play major roles. Nicotine raises systolic blood pressure and heart rate, and, therefore, increases myocardial oxygen demand, whereas carbon monoxide reduces oxygen availability to body tissues, including the myocardium. Nicotine increases platelet activation and platelet adhesion to the vessel wall. Nicotine, carbon monoxide, and smoke may cause endothelial damage, promoting atherogenic injury. In addition to theses effects, smoking may also have a deleterious effect on lipid profile *(31,32)*.

An estimated 430,700 Americans die each year from smoking-related illness. Smoking has been implicated in nearly 1 out of 5 deaths from cardiovascular diseases *(1)*. Current estimates are that 26.7% of men and 22.8% of women in the United States are active smokers, placing them at a two- to fourfold increased risk of CAD, a greater than 70% increased risk of death from CAD, and an increased risk for sudden death compared to nonsmokers *(1,31)*. Smoking cessation confers significant health benefits, with a reduction in mortality by 50% from CHD within the first year and reaching levels comparable to nonsmokers after 10 yr *(31)*.

Tobacco addiction is a complex process composed of physiologic, behavioral, and psychological components. Although a coronary event such as myocardial infarction may be sufficient impetus to quit smoking for some individuals, in general, several quit attempts are often required before success is achieved *(34,35)*. Various guidelines support use of nonpharmacologic therapies (e.g., behavior modification programs, support groups) and pharmacologic therapies to assist nicotine-dependent patients quit the smoking habit *(36,37)*. In general, success rates are doubled compared to no intervention *(35–37)*.

Withdrawal symptoms from nicotine can occur in several hours with peak intensity within a few days after smoking cessation *(38)*. Nicotine replacement therapy or bupropion may alleviate physical withdrawal symptoms and reduce cravings to smoke; however, nicotine replacement therapy should be used with caution in patients with cardiovascular disease *(34,35,38–41)*. Nicotine replacement therapy is relatively contraindicated in unstable CAD due to concern that nicotine could cause platelet activation and catecholamine release *(39)*. Risk-to-benefit ratio should be assessed for each patient.

HYPERTENSION

Hypertension is defined as an elevation in systolic blood pressure (SBP) of $\geq$140 mmHg, diastolic blood pressure (DBP) of $\geq$90 mmHg, or both. This is based on an average of two or more readings taken at two or more office visits after an initial screening *(42)*. In more than 90% of individuals, the cause of hypertension is unknown (i.e., primary or essential hypertension). Although there are fewer individuals with a known etiology for hypertension (i.e., secondary hypertension), identification is important since these are often correctable conditions *(43)*.

According to 1988–1991 data from the National Health and Nutrition Examination Survey (NHANES), an estimated 50 million Americans or 24% of the adult American population have high blood pressure *(42)*. Major complications of untreated hypertension are stroke, renal insufficiency, congestive heart failure (CHF), MI, and CHD *(43–45)*. Cardiovascular risk is known to increase with rise in blood pressure. Since publication of earlier NHANES data, there has been a decrease in morbidity and mortality associated with hypertension; however, number of patients with blood pressure controlled to <140/90 mmHg remains suboptimal at 29% *(42)*.

The Sixth Joint National Committee on the Detection, Evaluation, and Treatment of Hypertension has stratified patients on basis of blood pressure measurements, presence of target-organ damage, and risk factors for cardiovascular disease (CVD). Based on blood pressure measurements, individuals are placed into one of several categories (*see* Table 5). Those with high-normal blood pressure or stage 1–3 hypertension can be risk stratified to assist clinicians in decision for initial therapy (*see* Table 6). For example, individuals with high-normal blood pressure without target-organ damage or clinical CVD may first try lifestyle modifications, whereas drug therapy would be recommended initially for those at higher risk *(42)*.

Lifestyle modifications have been recommended to lower blood pressure, prevent hypertension, and reduce other cardiovascular risk factors *(42,46)*. Reduction of excess weight and sodium restriction appear effective in reducing blood pressure. Other lifestyle changes consist of regular aerobic exercise, relaxation/biofeedback for stress-related situations, dietary considerations (e.g., reduced alcohol, saturated fat, and cholesterol intake), and smoking cessation to improve overall cardiovascular health *(42,43,46)*.

Diuretics and beta blockers remain the preferred initial therapy unless there are specific indications for other medications (*see* Table 7) *(42,44)*. These two drug classes reduce morbidity and mortality as demonstrated in large-scale trials. Patients treated with antihypertensive agents have approximately a 40% reduction in stroke and 14–16% reduction in CHD *(47–51)*. Earlier observational studies suggested a greater reduction in CHD of about 20–25% *(47)*. Proposed explanations for the smaller risk reduction seen in trials are (1) stroke benefits may be more immediate and closely related to BP lowering, whereas

Table 5
Blood Pressure Categories for Adults Ages 18 Yr or Older[a]

	SBP (mmHg)		DBP (mmHg)
Optimal[b]	<120	AND	<80
Normal	<130	AND	<85
High-normal	130–139	OR	85–89
Stage 1 hypertension	140–159	OR	90–99
Stage 2 hypertension	160–179	OR	100–109
Stage 3 hypertension	≥180	OR	≥110

[a]For individuals not taking antihypertensive agents and not acutely ill. When SBP and DBP fall into different categories, use the higher category to classify the individual's BP status. In addition to classifying stages of hypertension on basis of average BP measurements, clinicians should specify the presence or absence of target organ damage and additional risk factors.

Evidence of target organ damage (TOD) or clinical cardiovascular disease (CCD) include presence of stroke or transient ischemic attack, nephropathy, peripheral arterial disease, retinopathy, or heart diseases (left ventricular hypertrophy, angina or prior MI, prior coronary revascularization, or heart failure). Major factors associated with increased cardiovascular risk include smoking, dyslipidemia, diabetes, age >60 yr, gender (men and postmenopausal women), and family history of cardiovascular disease.

[b]Optimal BP with respect to cardiovascular risk is <120/80 mmHg; however, unusually low readings should be further evaluated.

Source: Joint National Committee on Prevention, Detection, Evaluation, and Treatment of High Blood Pressure, 1997.

SBP = systolic blood pressure, DBP = diastolic blood pressure.

Table 6
Risk Stratification and Treatment Recommendations

Blood pressure category (mmHg)	Risk group A (No risk factors; No TOD/CCD[a])	Risk group B (at least 1 risk factor not including diabetes; no TOD/CCD	Risk group C (TOD/CCD and/or diabetes ± other risk factors)
High-normal (130–139/85–89)	Lifestyle change	Lifestyle change	Drug therapy[c]
Stage 1 (140–159/90–99)	Lifestyle change (up to 12 mo)	Lifestyle change (up to 6 mo)[b]	Drug therapy
Stage 2 and 3 hypertension (≥160/≥100)	Drug therapy	Drug therapy	Drug therapy

[a]TOD/CCD indicates target organ damage/clinical cardiovascular disease (see Table 5).

[b]For multiple risk factors, should consider initial drug therapy plus lifestyle changes.

[c]For those with heart failure, renal insufficiency, or diabetes.

Source: Joint National Committee on Prevention, Detection, Evaluation, and Treatment of High Blood Pressure, 1997.

maximal effects on CHD may be delayed (e.g., chronic atherosclerosis), (2) metabolic changes (i.e., glucose, insulin, and lipoprotein abnormalities) may independently increase CHD risk, and (3) discrepancy may be due to chance and diminish with more data (47,52). Other classes of drugs are being investigated to address whether they are more effective in reducing cardiovascular morbidity and mortality (53).

Table 7
Special Indications for Antihypertensive Agents

Condition or comorbidity	Therapy
Compelling indication	**Preferred initial therapy**
Uncomplicated Hypertension	Diuretics
	Beta blockers
DM (type 1) with proteinuria	ACE inhibitors
Heart failure	ACE inhibitors
	Diuretics
Isolated systolic hypertension (older persons)	Diuretics
	Long-acting dihydropyridine calcium antagonists
MI	Beta blockers without intrinsic sympathomimetic activity (ISA)
	ACE inhibitors (patients with systolic dysfunction)
Relative contraindications	**Agents to use cautiously or avoid**
Bronchospastic disease	Beta blockers (contraindicated)
Depression	Beta blockers
	Centrally acting alpha agonists
	Reserpine (contraindicated)
DM (type 1 and 2)	Beta blockers
	Diuretics (high doses)
Gout	Diuretics
Heart block (2nd or 3rd degree)	Beta blockers (contraindicated)
	Nondihydropyridine calcium antagonists (contraindicated)
Heart failure	Beta blockers (except carvedilol)
	Calcium antagonists (except felodipine, amlodipine)
Liver disease	Labetalol
	Methyldopa
Peripheral vascular disease	Beta blockers
Pregnancy	ACE inhibitors (contraindicated)
	Angiotensin II receptor blockers (contraindicated)
Renal insufficiency	Potassium-sparing agents
Renovascular disease	ACE inhibitors
	Angiotensin II receptor blockers

Source: Joint National Committee on Prevention, Detection, Evaluation, and Treatment of High Blood Pressure, 1997.

ISCHEMIC HEART DISEASE

New or recurrent MI or fatal cardiovascular events occur in an estimated 1.1 million Americans each year, resulting in approximately 330,000 deaths (1).

Acute MI will occur when lack of blood flow to an area of myocardium produces heart muscle cell death. This is in contrast to myocardial ischemia, where there is lack of blood flow without resultant necrosis. The initiating event in MI is typically coronary artery plaque rupture and thrombus formation. We know from thrombolytic trials that the sooner coronary artery blood flow is restored, the more myocardium is saved (54). We also know that medications can be utilized to help limit infarction size. Therapies that improve survival include thrombolytics, aspirin, beta blockers, and angiotensin-converting enzyme inhibitors (ACEI). Alternative therapies that may have limited usefulness in improving survival or may worsen survival include nitroglycerin, calcium channel blockers, and vasodilators.

Antiplatelet Medications

PRIMARY PREVENTION

Aspirin has been a cornerstone of therapy since the early 1980s, when it was proven to be as efficacious as thrombolytics in decreasing mortality and was found to be synergistic with thrombolytics *(55)*. The Physicians' Health study evaluated the effects of aspirin 325 mg every other day in decreasing the risk of first coronary event *(56)*. In this trial, there was a 44% reduction in first myocardial infarction, primarily in subjects greater than 50 yr of age. However, there was no reduction in cardiovascular mortality. Also, there was a nonsignificant increase in hemorrhagic stroke observed in subjects receiving aspirin. A study of British male doctors evaluated aspirin 500 mg daily in a randomized trial of 5139 patients. They found no significant improvement in those treated with aspirin *(57)*. Hennekens and associates evaluated the two trials and found that there was a 32% reduction in non-fatal myocardial infarction; however, there was not a significant reduction in cardiovascular or total mortality with a trend toward an increase in nonfatal stroke *(58)*. The Thrombosis Prevention Trial evaluated the effects of aspirin with or without warfarin. The aspirin alone trial did not demonstrate a significant benefit; therefore, at this time data are inconclusive that aspirin use for primary prevention reduces cardiovascular mortality.

A 1997 statement by the American Heart Association suggests routine use of aspirin in primary prevention is not universally warranted and that its use should be determined individually for patients at risk for MI *(59)*. This statement is reiterated by the 1998 American College of Chest Physicians (ACCP) Consensus Conference, which recommends primary prevention in those individuals >50 yr of age who have at least one major risk factor for CAD and are without contraindications to aspirin therapy *(60)*.

Whether women will experience the same benefits from aspirin therapy as men remains unanswered, as earlier trials excluded women. The only trial to evaluate women was a cohort study of US nurses, which found there were fewer initial MIs in women greater than 50 yr old *(61)*. The issue of aspirin in women is being addressed in the Women's Health Study.

SECONDARY PREVENTION

It is well established that aspirin therapy after an MI reduces further events *(55)*. In 1994, the Antiplatelet Trialist's Collaboration study was published. This collaboration is an overview of 145 randomized trials of antiplatelet therapy in patients at high and low risk for coronary events. They found a significant reduction (approx 25%) in nonfatal MI, nonfatal stroke, and vascular events. The dosing range for aspirin was 75–1300 mg/d. They found that low-dose aspirin was as efficacious as high-dose aspirin in reducing MI and stroke *(62)*. The current recommendations are for all patients with stable angina or evidence of CAD to receive a daily aspirin dose of 160–325 mg indefinitely *(60)*. Alternatively, the recommendations from the American Heart Association suggest that doses of 75–325 mg daily are also effective *(59)*.

Table 8
ACE Inhibitors for Prevention after MI

Trial	Treatment	N =	Duration of therapy	Primary endpoint	Results
Selective trials					
SAVE *(66)*	Captopril	1115	42 mo	All-cause mortality	19% risk reduction in
	Placebo	1116			the treatment group
AIRE *(67)*	Ramipril	1014	15 mo	All-cause mortality	The treatment group
	Placebo	992			had a 27% risk
					reduction in all
					cause mortality
TRACE *(69)*	Trandolapril	876	24–50 mo	All-cause mortality	22% reduction in
	Placebo	873			mortality in the
					treatment group
SMILE *(68)*	Zofenopril	772	6 wk	Combined endpoint	34% reduction in
	Placebo	784		of death and severe	primary endpoint
				CHF	at 6 wk and 29%
					reduction at 1 yr
Nonselective trials					
CONSENSUS-II	Enalapril	3044	6 mo	All-cause mortality	No survival benefit
(70)	Placebo	3046		during the 6-mo	and trend toward
				trial	worsening survival in
					the treatment group
GISSI-3 *(71)*	Lisinopril	9435	6 wk	All-cause mortality	Lisinopril-treated
	Placebo	9460		and combined	patients had a 11%
				mortality, CHF, LV	lower risk of death
				damage w/o CHF	than controls
ISIS-4 *(72)*	Captopril	2088	5 wk	Total mortality	7% risk reduction
	Placebo	2231			in the captopril-
					treated-group

For patients unable to tolerate aspirin or those with a true aspirin allergy, clopidogrel 75 mg daily is recommended *(60)*. Clopidogrel was evaluated in a large randomized trial of patients at risk of ischemic events. The primary endpoint was a composite of myocardial infarction, ischemic stroke, or vascular death. In this trial of 19,185 patients, those treated with clopidogrel had a relative risk reduction in primary endpoint of 8.7%. The majority of the benefit was from a reduction in death associated with peripheral arterial disease. There was no difference in outcome among the clopidogrel- and aspirin (325 mg/d)-treated groups in composite endpoints of ischemic stroke and MI. Clopidogrel should be considered as a second-line therapy for prevention after aspirin *(60)*.

Angiotensin-Converting Enzyme Inhibitors

Angiotensin-converting enzyme inhibitors (ACEI or ACE inhibitors) have been well studied in patients after an acute MI. Following an acute myocardial injury, the ventricle undergoes a remolding process that includes left ventricular dilation, myocyte growth, interstitial collagen deposition, and fibrosis *(63)*. ACE inhibition improves hemodynamics, reduces angiotensin II-mediated vasoconstriction, and reduces myocardial oxygen demand. Another potential beneficial effect is that ACEIs may reduce ischemic events by improving endothelial dysfunction *(64–66)*. There have been seven major trials evaluating the use of ACE inhibitors in patients post-MI (*see* Table 8). The trials have different criteria for inclusion and can be separated into selective and nonselective patient populations.

Table 9
ACE Inhibitors for Prevention in Patients with Heart Failure

Trial	Treatment	N =	Mean follow-up	Primary endpoint	Results
CONSENSUS (77)	Enalapril Placebo	127 126	6 mo	Total mortality	40% reduction in mortality at 6 mo in the treatment group and 31% reduction at 1 yr
SOLVD- Treatment (78)	Enalapril Placebo	1285 1284	41 mo	Total mortality	16% reduction in risk of death in the treatment group
SOLVD- Prevention (79)	Enalapril Placebo	2111 2117	37.4 mo	Total mortality	No reduction in total mortality
VHeFT-II (76)	Enalapril Hydralazine/ Isosorbide dinitrate	403 401	30 mo	Total mortality	28% reduction in mortality in the treatment group

The selective trials evaluated patients with poor left ventricular function (i.e., low ejection fraction, anterior location of the myocardial infarction, presence of symptomatic heart failure). The nonselective trials had less specific inclusion criteria based on ventricular function and symptomatology.

Several selective trials evaluating the use of ACEIs post myocardial infarction are shown in Table 9. The trials varied in time to ACEI initiation, ranging from the first 24 h to 16 d (66–69). The studies also varied with regards to overt heart failure and/or ejection fractions and follow-up period. The selective trials demonstrated significant reductions in mortality in patients with anterior wall myocardial infarction, ejection fractions less than 40%, or clinical signs of heart failure treated with ACEIs. The non-selective trials included all patients regardless of ejection fraction, overt heart failure, and location of myocardial infarction (70–72). ACEIs were initiated within the first 24 h, and there were shorter follow up periods, ranging from 5 wk–6 mo (70–72).

An overview of trials evaluating post-MI ACEI therapy showed a 6.5% reduction in 1 mo mortality ($p = 0.006$) or about 5 lives saved per 1000 treated (72). An exception to the studies demonstrating benefits of ACEIs post-MI was the Cooperative New Scandinavian Enalapril Survival Study II (CONSENSUS II). In this trial, intravenous enalaprilat was given within the first 24 h with transition to oral therapy. The ACEI treatment group had excessive mortality compared to placebo, and the trial was terminated early (70). Excessive hypotension in the treatment group may have contributed to or caused these negative effects.

The beneficial effects of ACEIs have been demonstrated in patients treated early (within 24–48 h) as well as late (within 16 d), and initiation should be considered in patients post-MI, specifically in patients with anterior wall MIs with or without symptoms of heart failure or ejection fractions less than 40%. ACEI therapy should be considered in all patients post-MI unless they have hypotension or other contraindications to ACEI therapy (70–72). Difficulty in determining appropriate time to start ACEI therapy may be eased by considering patient-specific factors for each individual.

Anticoagulation

The American College of Chest Physicians (ACCP) Consensus Conference recommends anticoagulation be reserved for patients intolerant to aspirin or clopidogrel and postinfarction at high risk for embolic complications (e.g., anterior Q-wave infarction, severe left ventricular dysfunction, CHF, history of embolic complications, echocardiographic evidence of mural thrombus, or atrial fibrillation). Anticoagulation should be considered for up to 3 mo. For patients with continued atrial fibrillation, anticoagulation duration is indefinite *(60)*. Anticoagulation with or without aspirin as primary prevention should be considered in men at high risk for cardiovascular events *(60)*.

Beta Blockers

Beta blockers have many pharmacologic effects including lowering heart rate and blood pressure, decreasing contractility, and increasing the fibrillation threshold of the ventricles *(73)*. The benefits of beta-blocker use in CAD patients are related to the fact that they decrease myocardial oxygen demand by decreasing both blood pressure and heart rate *(74)*. Beta-blocker therapy reduces the risk of both sudden and nonsudden cardiac death *(54)*. Benefits of beta blockers are seen when given long term; timolol improved 6-yr survival when given to patients post-acute MI *(75)*. The protective effects of beta blockers are likely a class effect with the exception of agents with intrinsic sympathomimetic activity (ISA). Beta blockers with ISA prevent slowing of resting heart rate and provide blockade when there is an increase in sympathetic output.

Current recommendations from the American Heart Association and American College of Cardiology are to initiate beta-blocker therapy in all high-risk patients *(54)*. High-risk patients include those with large or anterior wall myocardial infarctions, previous infarction, ventricular arrhythmias, or elderly. There is still debate as to whether lower-risk patients derive as much benefit. Even though most of the trials evaluating use of beta-blocker therapy were conducted in the prethrombolytic era, recommendations remain the same for patients undergoing revascularization *(54)*.

Nitrates

Large-scale randomized trials have failed to demonstrate that long-term nitrate administration reduces mortality after acute MI *(71,72)*. However, because nitrates do reduce preload of the heart and cause coronary vascular vasodilatation, nitrates will remain a widely used adjunctive therapy *(54)*.

HEART FAILURE

ACEIs

Trials evaluating the effectiveness of ACEIs have included both symptomatic and asymptomatic patients with heart failure. The Veterans Administration Cooperative Study II (VHeFT-II) evaluated enalapril vs. the combination of hydralazine and isosorbide dinitrate in the treatment of the congestive heart in 804 patients *(76)*. Those treated with enalapril had a reduction in mortality, mostly attributed to a reduction in sudden death. Other treatment trials (CONSENSUS and SOLVD-Treatment [Studies of Left Ventricular Dysfunction]) and prevention trials (SAVE [Survival and Ventricular Enlargement], AIRE [Acute Infarction Ramipril Efficacy], and SOLVD-Prevention) have also found reduction in mortality in the ACEI-treated groups (*see* Table 9) *(66,67,77–79)*.

ACEIs should be initiated in all patients with ejection fractions less than 40% regardless of signs and symptoms of heart failure unless they have demonstrated intolerance to ACEIs or have contraindications to ACEIs (e.g., bilateral renal artery stenosis, unilateral renal artery stenosis with solitary kidney, or pregnancy).

Beta Blockers

Considerable interest has been dedicated over the years to effects of beta-adrenergic blockade in patients with left ventricular systolic dysfunction. Our increased understanding of pathophysiology has led to a shift from the belief that beta blockers are contraindicated in heart failure to a belief that beta blockade may provide significant benefit in these individuals.

Patients with decreased left ventricular systolic function initially have a reduction in cardiac output. In response, compensatory mechanisms are activated via stimulation of the renin–angiotensin–aldosterone system (RAAS) and sympathetic nervous system as well as alterations in other neurohumoral mechanisms. Although initially these processes provide support to the failing heart, long-term they are deleterious and lead eventually to a worsening of heart failure.

An early response to decrease in cardiac output is an increase in plasma norepinephrine levels. Norepinephrine stimulates both beta- and alpha-adrenergic receptors. Stimulation of $beta_1$ receptors augments heart rate and contractility, whereas stimulation of $alpha_1$ receptors causes vasoconstriction. These compensatory responses are essential for maintaining adequate tissue perfusion by increasing both blood pressure and cardiac output. Prognosis in patients with heart failure is related to resting plasma level of norepinephrine: the higher the level, the worse the prognosis for the individual (80,81).

Elevated levels of norepinephrine also increase the risk of development of ventricular arrhythmias (82). Continuous stimulation of beta receptors by norepinephrine eventually leads to downregulation of the receptors and ultimately results in loss of contractility mediated by these receptors (83). Inhibiting the sympathetic nervous system potentially could decrease the direct cardiotoxic effects of norepinephrine and limit downregulation or desensitization of the beta-adrenergic receptors (82). A better understanding of neurohormonal mechanisms of heart failure has lead to the utilization of ACE inhibitors and now beta blockers to alter the long-term adverse effects of these systems.

Beta blockers were initially evaluated for the treatment of heart failure in the 1970s. These early studies were conducted in patients with idiopathic cardiomyopathy, and improvements were noted in both hemodynamic measurements and symptoms of heart failure (83,84). Later studies evaluating beta blockers have failed to demonstrate similar findings. Many of the later studies used agents with intrinsic sympathomimetic activity and had relatively short follow-up periods (86).

In 1993, Waagstein and associates evaluated metoprolol versus placebo in 383 patients with idiopathic dilated cardiomyopathy in the Metoprolol in Dilated Cardiomyopathy study (MDC) (87). Patients were considered for entry into the trial if they were on a stable heart failure regimen including ACEIs, diuretics, digitalis, and nitrates and had symptomatic dilated cardiomyopathy with an ejection fraction of less than 40%. Metoprolol was initiated at 5 mg twice daily and titrated up to a maximum dose of 100–150 mg/d over a 7-wk period. In this 12-mo trial, the primary endpoint of death or heart transplantation was not significantly different between the two groups. However, patients receiving metoprolol had a lower incidence of heart transplantation when compared with placebo

(1% vs. 10%, respectively; $p = 0.0001$). Improvement in myocardial function was independent of ACEI usage, suggesting different mechanisms for improvement (87).

The Cardiac Insufficiency Bisoprolol Study (CIBIS) evaluated the effects of bisoprolol in patients with various etiologies of heart failure. This was a randomized, placebo-controlled, blinded study in 641 patients with ejection fractions less than 40%. This study was designed to evaluate the effects of bisoprolol on mortality over a 2-yr follow up period. Patients were randomized to receive either placebo or bisoprolol 1.25 mg/d titrated up to 5 mg/d over a 4-wk period. All patients were on diuretics and vasodilator therapy with encouragement to utilize ACE inhibitors (91% in the placebo group and 89% in the bisoprolol group). Digitalis, amiodarone, and calcium channel blockers were allowed; however, calcium channel blocker use was discouraged. Most patients were considered to be in New York Heart Association Class (NYHA) III failure, and 5% were considered functional class IV. Baseline characteristics were similar between the two groups, although there was a higher incidence of MI in the bisoprolol group and a lower diastolic blood pressure in the placebo group. Fewer patients in the bisoprolol-treated group had decompensated heart failure and more patients had improvement in functional class. There was no difference in withdrawal rates between the two groups, suggesting that bisoprolol was well tolerated in the study population. Analysis of results showed no difference in mortality between the bisoprolol (16.6%) and placebo (20.9%) groups (88).

The MDC and CIBIS studies evaluated use of second-generation beta blockers (or cardioselective agents) in the treatment of heart failure of various etiologies. Survival was not significantly improved in patients treated with beta-blocker therapy; however, patients treated with metoprolol had fewer transplantations, and both metoprolol- and bisoprolol-treated patients had fewer heart failure decompensations leading to fewer hospital admissions.

Carvedilol, a non-selective β-adrenergic receptor blocker with α_1-receptor antagonism, was approved by the Food and Drug Administration for the treatment of mild to moderate heart failure (NYHA Classes II and III). There have been eight placebo-controlled trials evaluating carvedilol therapy in patients with mild to severe heart failure. Initial small, short-term studies of patients with heart failure demonstrated improvements in hemodynamic parameters, ejection fraction, and functional class (89–91).

Carvedilol was evaluated by the US Carvedilol Heart Failure Trials Program and consisted of 1094 patients with mild to severe heart failure stratified on the basis of a 6-min corridor walk. Based on this exercise test, patients were randomized to one of four placebo-controlled study arms. The morbidity and mortality data were compiled for final analysis. Inclusion criteria were ejection fractions of ≤35%, symptoms of heart failure for 3 mo, and at least 2 mo of treatment with ACEIs and diuretics. Use of digoxin, hydralazine, and nitrates was allowed. All patients enrolled in the study received 6.25 mg of carvedilol twice daily for 2 wk. Patients unable to tolerate this regimen had dosage reduction to 3.125 mg twice daily. Dosages were titrated upward to a target dose of 25 mg or 50 mg twice daily or maximum tolerated dose. All patients were followed for 6 mo, and patients in the mild heart failure study were followed for a total of 12 mo (92). The US Carvedilol Heart Failure Program was terminated early based on recommendations from the Data and Safety Monitoring Board secondary to dramatic survival benefits seen in the carvedilol-treated patients. There was a 65% reduction in the risk of death in the carvedilol-treated patients (CI 39–80%; $p < 0.001$). Patients treated with carvedilol had a reduction in progressive heart failure and sudden death. Hospital admissions and length of hospital stay were also reduced in the carvedilol-treated patients. Only one of the four treatment arms, the dose-ranging study in moderate heart failure, showed significant reductions in mortality (92).

The Australia/New Zealand Heart Failure Research Collaborative Group was a randomized, placebo-controlled trial in 415 patients with ischemic cardiomyopathy evaluating carvedilol treatment. The Group found a reduction in the risk of death and hospitalization by 26% in the carvedilol group. However, in this study there was no significant effect on reducing symptoms, episodes of decompensation, or ability to exercise (93).

Two recently published trials, CIBIS II and Metoprolol CR/XL Randomised Intervention Trial in Congestive Heart Failure (MERIT-HF) of beta blockers in heart failure have supported previous studies. The findings in the CIBIS II trial were quite significant. This trial was stopped early after the second interim analysis secondary to a significant reduction in all-cause mortality, hazard ratio 0.66 (95% CI 0.54–0.81) in the bisoprolol-treated group. There were also fewer hospitalizations secondary to heart failure and a reduction in sudden death in those patients on bisoprolol (94).

In the MERIT-HF trial, patients with NYHA Class II-IV were treated with extended-release metoprolol. This trial was also stopped early secondary to a significant reduction in all-cause mortality in the metoprolol-treated group with a relative risk of 0.67 (95% CI 0.53–0.81). As in the CIBIS-II trial there were fewer cases of sudden death. Also there were fewer deaths associated with worsening heart failure (95).

Which patients should receive beta-blocker therapy? Although carvedilol is the only beta blocker approved for adjunctive therapy in heart failure, other agents in this class have demonstrated significant benefits as well. Beta blockers should be initiated in all patients with systolic dysfunction who fall into NYHA Classes II and III (96). Patients should be stabilized on ACEIs and diuretics with or without digoxin prior to initiation of beta-blocker therapy: ACEIs dose should be stable for at least 4 wk, with no diuretic changes for 2 wk, and no recent inotropic support for at least 4 wk (86,97). Patients may initially experience worsening of symptoms during the titration period, which can be minimized by starting with low doses and advancing to target doses or maximally tolerated doses slowly. Full benefits may not be observed for weeks to months. Beta blockers should not be used in patients with decompensated heart failure, hypotension, fluid-overloaded states, bronchospastic airway disease, or in other conditions in which beta blockers should be avoided (e.g. complete heart block, symptomatic bradycardia).

Hydralazine/Nitrates

The gold standard for the treatment of heart failure prior to ACEIs was the combination of hydralazine and nitrate therapy. The VHeFT I trial showed a trend in reduction of mortality after a mean follow-up of 28 mo in the hydralazine/isosorbide dinitrate treatment group. There was a significantly higher rate of side effects such as gastrointestinal intolerance in the treatment group as compared to placebo. A second arm of the study using prazosin found no effect on mortality (98). This combination of hydralazine and isosorbide dinitrate is considered to be second-line therapy in patients with heart failure not able to tolerate ACEIs, or in some cases in addition to ACEIs.

Digoxin

Although digoxin therapy has been used for over 200 yr, there are still questions regarding its benefits in heart failure. Two trials that evaluated withdrawal of digoxin in patients with heart failure demonstrated worsening heart failure in the withdrawal patients as compared to those who continued therapy *(99,100)*. These trials were not powered to detect a difference in mortality. The Digitalis Investigation Group (DIG) conducted a landmark trial of 6800 patients with CHF *(101)*. This study did not show a reduction in the primary endpoint of mortality; however, the trial showed a decrease in overall hospitalizations and in hospitalizations associated with worsening heart failure.

Diuretics

It is not known whether standard diuretics (i.e., loop and thiazide) affect mortality in heart failure patients, as they have not been formally evaluated in long-term trials. However, because diuretics increase sodium and water excretion, decrease pulmonary congestion and jugular venous distension, improve symptoms, and improve exercise tolerance, they do improve morbidity *(102,103)*. Most major heart failure studies have included these standard diuretics as part of treatment.

Recently the Randomized Aldactone Evaluation Study (RALES), found that patients with severe heart failure and ejection fractions less than 35% had a significant decrease in mortality (30%) when treated with spironolactone 25 mg daily. The findings in this study were so striking that the trial was terminated early. The authors also found that there was a decrease in hospitalizations and significant improvement in symptoms. The most common side effect in the study group was gynecomastia (10%). Significant hyperkalemia was low in the treatment group *(104)*. Based on this trial, patients with severe heart failure stage III or IV, with serum creatinine <2.5 mg/dL and normal potassium levels, on standard therapy for heart failure, should significantly benefit from an inexpensive modality of spironolactone 25 mg daily.

Currently, recommendations for treatment of heart failure are to utilize ACEIs in maximally tolerated doses to reduce mortality and improve symptoms. Diuretics are needed to control fluid-overloaded states, and in the case of spironolactone, reduce mortality. Beta blockers should be initiated in all patients with NYHA Class II and III heart failure to help reduce mortality and improve long-term symptoms of heart failure. The use of digoxin is useful to decrease hospitalizations and symptoms of heart failure; however, it has not demonstrated improved mortality. Patients unable to tolerate ACEIs should be on the combination of hydralazine and nitrates or on an angiotensin II receptor blocker (trials are currently ongoing) *(96)*.

SUMMARY

Patient education, medication compliance, and risk factor modification are crucial elements for the prevention of CAD. In addition, various pharmacologic modalities have demonstrated benefits in reducing cardiovascular morbidity and mortality. Recommendations include the following:

Lipids

Lipid-lowering therapy should be considered in all individuals with hypercholesterolemia and established CAD. In individuals without CAD but with risk factors, dietary with or without lipid-lowering therapies should be considered.

Lipid-lowering agents are recommended as first-line agents for hypercholesterolemia in postmenopausal women; however, HRT may be considered in select individuals.

Choice of drug therapy should be based upon lipid profile, comorbidities, and other patient-specific factors.

Use of folic acid and antioxidants such as vitamin E may be considered for prevention; however, full benefits and adverse effects are unknown at this time.

Smoking Cessation

All smokers should be encouraged to quit, as smoking is a known risk factor for CHD. Behavioral and pharmacologic therapies are available to assist nicotine-dependent individuals quit successfully.

Hypertension

Diuretics and beta blockers remain the preferred initial therapy for treatment of hypertension. Other medication classes may be considered as first-line therapies in patients, depending on disease-state and patient-specific factors.

CAD

Aspirin should be standard therapy for all patients with CAD, and aspirin use may be considered in patients without CAD but with multiple risk factors. Patients intolerant or allergic to aspirin should receive clopidogrel or warfarin.

Beta blockers are useful in reducing ischemia and sudden death in patients with a history of myocardial infarction.

ACEIs reduce mortality in patients with myocardial infarction, especially in the presence of left ventricular dysfunction with or without symptomatic heart failure.

Nitrates are useful as adjunctive therapy in patients with chronic ischemia to reduce episodes of chest pain; however, large trials have not shown reduced mortality with chronic therapy.

Anticoagulation with warfarin may be considered in patients post-anterior-wall MI with evidence of anterior wall akinesis, dyskinesis, aneurysm formation, or mural thrombus formation.

Heart Failure

Patients with systolic dysfunction, with or without heart failure symptoms, should be on ACEIs unless intolerant or contraindicated. Those unable to tolerate ACEIs should be taking the combination of hydralazine and nitrates or may be considered for angiotensin receptor blockers.

Beta blockers should be initiated in all patients with NYHA Classes II and III heart failure. At this time there are little data in patients with Class IV heart failure.

Diuretics are used to prevent and treat symptoms of heart failure secondary to fluid-overloaded states.

Digoxin is useful in preventing hospitalizations in patients with CHF and also to improve symptoms of heart failure.

Spironolactone has recently been shown to reduce mortality in patients with Class III heart failure with minimal side effects.

REFERENCES

1. American Heart Association. 1999 Heart and Stroke Statistical Update. American Heart Association, Dallas, TX, 1998.
2. Grundy SM, Balady GJ, Criqui MH, et al. Primary prevention of coronary heart disease: guidance from Framingham. Circulation 1998;97:1876–1887.

3. Ross R. Atherosclerosis—An inflammatory disease. N Engl J Med 1999;340:115–126.

4. DiPiro JT, Talbert RL, Yee GC, et al., eds. Pharmacotherapy: A Pathophysiologic Approach, 3rd ed. Appleton & Lange, Stamford, CT, 1997.

5. Gotto AM. Lipid-lowering therapy for the primary prevention of coronary heart disease (review). J Am Coll Cardiol 1999;33(7):2078–2082.

6. Downs JR, Clearfield M, Weis S, et al. Primary prevention of acute coronary events with lovastatin in men and women with average cholesterol levels: results of AFCAPS/TexCAPS. JAMA 1998;279: 1615–1622.

7. Shepherd J, Cobbe SM, Ford I, et al. Prevention of coronary heart disease with pravastatin in men with hypercholesterolemia. N Engl J Med 1995;333:1301–1307.

8. Mosca L, Grundy SM, Judelson D, et al. Guide to preventive cardiology for women. Circulation 1999; 99:2480–2484.

9. Expert Panel on Detection, Evaluation, and Treatment of High Blood Cholesterol in Adults. Summary of the Second Report of the National Cholesterol Education Program (NCEP) Expert Panel on Detection, Evaluation, and Treatment of High Blood Cholesterol in Adults (Adult Treatment Panel II). JAMA 1993;269:3015–3023.

10. WHO Cooperative Trial Committee of Principal Investigator. A co-operative trial in the primary prevention of ischaemic heart disease using clofibrate. Br Heart J 1978;40:1069–1118.

11. WHO Cooperative Trial Committee of Principal Investigator. WHO cooperative trial on primary prevention of ischaemic heart disease with clofibrate to lower serum cholesterol: mortality follow-up. Lancet 1980;2:379–385.

12. WHO Cooperative Trial Committee of Principal Investigator. WHO cooperative trial on primary prevention of ischaemic heart disease with clofibrate to lower serum cholesterol: final mortality follow-up. Lancet 1984;2:600–604.

13. Lipid Research Clinics Program. The Lipid Research Clinics Coronary Primary Prevention Trial results. I. Reduction in incidence of coronary heart disease. JAMA 1984;251:351–364.

14. Frick MH, Elo O, Haapa K, et al. Helsinki Heart Study: primary prevention trial with gemfibrozil in middle-aged men with dyslipidemia. Safety of treatment, changes in risk factors, and incidence of coronary heart disease. N Engl J Med 1987;317:1237–245.

15. Canner PL, Berge KG, Wenger NK, et al. Fifteen year mortality in coronary drug project patients: long-term benefit with niacin. J Am Coll Cardiol 1986;8:1245–1255.

16. The Coronary Drug Project Research Group. Clofibrate and niacin in coronary heart disease. JAMA 1975;231:360–381.

17. Carlson LA, Rosenhamer G. Reduction of mortality in the Stockholm Ischaemic Heart Disease Secondary Prevention Study by combined treatment with clofibrate and nicotinic acid. Acta Med Scand 1988;223:405–418.

18. Scandinavian Simvastatin Survival Study Group. Randomised trial of cholesterol lowering in 4444 patients with coronary heart disease: the Scandanavian Survival Study (4S). Lancet 1994;344:1383–1389.

19. Sacks FM, Pfeffer MA, Moye LA, et al. The effect of pravastatin on coronary events after myocardial infarction in patients with average cholesterol levels. N Engl J Med 1996;335:1001–1009.

20. The Post Coronary Artery Bypass Graft Trial Investigators. The effect of aggressive lowering of low-density lipoprotein cholesterol levels and low-dose anticoagulation on obstructive changes in saphenous vein coronary-artery bypass grafts. N Engl J Med 1997;336:153–162.

21. The Long-term Intervention with Pravastatin in Ischaemic Disease (LIPID) Study Group. Prevention of cardiovascular events and death with pravastatin in patients with coronary heart disease and a broad range of initial cholesterol levels. N Engl J Med 1998;339:1349–1357.

22. Buchwald H, Varco RL, Matts JP, et al. Effect of partial ileal bypass surgery on mortality and morbidity from coronary heart disease in patients with hypercholesterolemia: report of the program on the surgical control of the hyperlipidemias (POSCH). N Engl J Med 1990;323:946–955.

23. Williamson DR, Pharand C. Statins in the prevention of coronary heart disease. Pharmacotherapy 1998;18:242–254.

24. American Diabetes Association: Standards of medical care for patients with diabetes mellitus (position statement). Diabetes Care 1999;22(Suppl 1):s32–s41.

25. Grundy SM, Benjamin IJ, Burke GL, et al. Diabetes and cardiovascular disease: a statement for healthcare professionals from the American Heart Association. Circulation 1999;100:1134–1146.

26. Stein JH, McBride PE. Hyperhomocysteinemia and atherosclerotic vascular disease: pathophysiology, screening and treatment. Arch Intern Med 1998;158:1301–1306.

27. Malinow MR, Bostom AG, Krauss RM. Homocyst(e)ine, diet, and cardiovascular diseases: a statement for healthcare professionals from the nutrition committee, American Heart Association. Circulation 1999;99:178–182.

28. Ballal RS, Jacobsen DW, Robinson K. Homocysteine: update on a new risk factor. Cleveland Clin J Med 1997;64:543–549.

29. Bostom AG, Selhub J. Homocysteine and arteriosclerosis: subclinical and clinical disease associations. Circulation 1999;99:2361–2363.

30. Spencer AP, Carson DS, Crouch MA. Vitamin E and coronary artery disease. Arch Intern Med 1999; 159:1313–1320.

31. Lakier JB. Smoking and cardiovascular disease. Am J Med 1992;93(Suppl):8–12.

32. Rigotti NA, Pasternak RC. Cigarette smoking and coronary heart disease: risks and management. Cardiol Clin 1996;14:51–68.

33. Jacobs DR, Adachi H, Mulder I, et al., for the Seven Countries Study Group. Cigarette smoking and mortality risk: twenty-five-year follow-up of the seven countries study. Arch Intern Med 1999;159: 733–740.

34. Rose JE. Nicotine addiction and treatment. Annu Rev Med 1996;47:493–507.

35. Hughes JR, Goldstein MG, Hurt RD, Shiffman S. Recent advances in the pharmacotherapy of smoking. JAMA 1999;281:72–76.

36. Agency for Health Care Policy and Research Smoking Cessation Clinical Practice Guideline. JAMA 1996;275:1270–1280.

37. Hughes JR, Fiester S, Goldstein MG, et al. American Psychiatric Association practice guideline for the treatment of patients with nicotine dependence. Am J Psychiatry 1996;153(Suppl):S1–S13.

38. Henningfield JE. Nicotine medications for smoking cessation. N Engl J Med 1995;333:1196–1203.

39. Thompson GH, Hunter DA. Nicotine replacement therapy. Ann Pharmacother 1998;32:1067–1075.

40. Hurt RD, Sach DP, Glover ED, et al. A comparison of sustained-release bupropion and placebo for smoking cessation. N Engl J Med 1997;337:1195–1202.

41. Jorenby DE, Leischow SJ, Nides MA, et al. A controlled-trial of sustained-release bupropion, a nicotine patch, or both for controlled smoking cessation. N Engl J Med 1999;340:685–691.

42. Joint National Committee on Prevention, Detection, Evaluation, and Treatment of High Blood Pressure: The Sixth Report of the Joint National Committee on Prevention, Detection, Evaluation, and Treatment of High Blood Pressure. Arch Intern Med 1997;157:2413–2446.

43. Kaplan NM. Clinical Hypertension, 6th ed. Williams & Wilkins, Baltimore, MD, 1994.

44. Houston MC. New insights and new approaches for the treatment of essential hypertension: selection of therapy based on coronary heart disease risk factor analysis, hemodynamic profiles, quality of life, and subsets of hypertension. Am Heart J 1989;117:911–951.

45. Pepine CJ. Systemic hypertension and coronary artery disease. Am J Cardiol 1998;82:21H–24H.

46. The Trials of Hypertension Prevention Collaborative Research Group. The effects of nonpharmacologic interventions on blood pressure of persons with high normal levels: results of the trials of hypertension prevention, Phase I. JAMA 1992;267:1213–1220.

47. Hebert PR, Moser M, Mayer J, Hennekens CH. Recent evidence on drug therapy of mild to moderate hypertension and decreased risk of coronary heart disease. Arch Intern Med 1993;153: 578–581.

48. Moser M. National recommendations for the pharmacologic treatment of hypertension: should they be revised? Arch Intern Med 1999;159:1403–1406.

49. SHEP Cooperative Research Group. Prevention of stroke by antihypertensive drug treatment in older persons with isolated systolic hypertension: final results of the Systolic Hypertension in the Elderly Program (SHEP). JAMA 1991;265:3255–3264.

50. Dahlof B, Lindholm LH, Hansson L, et al. Morbidity and mortality in the Swedish trial in old patients with hypertension. Lancet 1991;338:1281–1285.

51. MRC Working Party. Medical Research Council trial of treatment of hypertension in older adults: principal results. Br Med J 1992;304:405–412.

52. Reaven GM, Lithell H, Landsberg L. Hypertension and associated metabolic abnormalities—the role of insulin resistance and the sympathoadrenal system. N Engl J Med 1996;334:374–381.

53. Pickering TG. Advances in the treatment of hypertension. JAMA 1999;281:114–116.

54. Ryan TJ, Anderson JL, Antman EM, et al. ACC/AHA guidelines for the management of patients with acute myocardial infarction: executive summary: a report of the American College of Cardiology/American Heart Association Task Force on Practice Guidelines (Committee Management of Acute Myocardial Infarction). Circulation 1996;94:2341–2350.

55. ISIS-2 Collaborative Group. International study of infarct survival 2. Lancet 1988;II:349–360.
56. Steering Committee of the Physician's Health Study Research Group. Final report on the aspirin component of the ongoing Physician's Health Study. N Engl J Med 1989;321:129–135.
57. Peto R, Gray R, Collins R, et al. Randomised trial of prophylactic daily aspirin in British male doctors. Br Med J 1988;296:313–316.
58. Hennekens CH, Buring JE, Sandercock P, et al. Aspirin and other anti-platelet agents in the secondary and primary prevention of cardiovascular disease. Circulation 1989;80:749–756.
59. Hennekens CH, Dyken ML, Fuster V. Aspirin as a therapeutic agent in cardiovascular disease. a statement for healthcare professionals from the American Heart Association. Circulation 1997;96:2751–2753.
60. Cairns JA, Theroux P, Lewis HD Jr, et al. Antithrombotic agents in coronary artery disease. Chest 1998;114:611s–633s.
61. Manson JE, Stampfer J, Colditz GA, et al. A prospective study of aspirin use and primary prevention in cardiovascular disease in women. JAMA 1991;266:521–527.
62. Antiplatelet Trialists' Collaboration. Collaborative overview of randomised trials of anti-platelet therapy I: prevention of death, myocardial infarction, and stroke by prolonged anti-platelet therapy in various categories of patients. Br Med J 1994;308:81–106.
63. Francis GS. Changing the remodeling process in heart failure: basic mechanisms and laboratory results. Curr Opin Cardiol 1998;13:156–161.
64. van den Heuvel AF, van Gilst WH, van Veldhuisen DJ, et al. Long term anti-ischemic effects of angiotensin-converting inhibition in patients after myocardial infarction. J Am Coll Cardiol 1997;30:400–405.
65. van Gilst W. Quinapril on vascular ACE and determinants of ischemia (abstract). American Heart Association 71st Scientific Session, November 1998.
66. Pfeffer MA, Braunwald E, Moyer LA, et al. Effect of captopril on mortality and morbidity in patients with left ventricular dysfunction after myocardial infarction: results of the Survival and Ventricular Enlargement Trial. N Engl J Med 1992;327:669–677.
67. The Acute Infarction Ramipril Efficacy (AIRE) Study Investigators. Effect of ramipril on mortality and morbidity of survivors of acute myocardial infarction with clinical evidence of heart failure. Lancet 1993;342:821–828.
68. Ambrosioni E, Borghi C, Magnani B. The effect of angiotensin converting enzyme inhibitor zofenopril on mortality and morbidity after anterior myocardial infarction. N Engl J Med 1995;332:80–85.
69. Kober L, Torp Pedersen C, Carlsen JE, et al. A clinical trial of the angiotensin converting enzyme inhibitor trandolapril in patients with left ventricular dysfunction after myocardial infarction. N Engl J Med 1995;333:1670–1676.
70. Swedberg K, Held P, Kjekhus J, et al. Effects of the early administration of enalapril on mortality in patients with acute myocardial infarction. Results of the Cooperative New Scandinavian Enalapril Survival Study II. N Engl J Med 1992;327:678–684.
71. Gruppo Italiano per lo Studio della Sopravvivenza nell'Infarto Miocardico. GISSI-3: effects of lisinopril and transdermal glyceryl trinitrate singly and together on 6-week mortality and ventricular function after acute myocardial infarction. Lancet 1994;343:1115–22.
72. ISIS-4 Collaborative Group. ISIS-4: A randomised factorial trial assessing early oral captopril, oral mononitrate, and intravenous magnesium sulphate in 58,050 patients with suspected acute myocardial infarction. Lancet 1995;345:669–85.
73. Mehta RH, Eagle KA. Secondary prevention in acute myocardial infarction. Br Med J 1998;316:838–842.
74. Yusuf S, Peto R, Lewis J, Collins, Sleight P. Beta blockade during and after myocardial infarction: an overview of randomized trials. Prog Cardiovasc Dis 1985;27:335–371.
75. Pederson TR, Six-year follow-up of the Norwegian Multicenter Study on timolol after acute myocardial infarction. N Engl J Med 1985;313:1055–1058.
76. Cohn JN, Johnson G, Ziescher S, et al. A comparison of enalapril with hydralazine-isosorbide dinitrate in the treatment of chronic congestive heart failure. N Engl J Med 1991;325:303–310.
77. The CONSENSUS Trial Study Group. Effects of enalapril on mortality in severe congestive heart failure: results of the Cooperative North Scandinavian Enalapril Survival Study (CONSENSUS). N Engl J Med 1987;316:1429–1435.
78. The SOLVD Investigators. Effect of enalapril on survival in patients with reduced left ventricular ejection fractions and congestive heart failure. N Engl J Med 1991;325:293–302.
79. The SOLVD Investigators. Effect of enalapril on mortality and the development of heart failure in asymptomatic patients with reduced left ventricular ejection fractions. N Engl J Med 1992;327:685–691.

80. Cohn JN, et al. Plasma norepinephrine as a guide to prognosis in patients with chronic congestive heart failure. N Engl J Med 1984;311:819–823.

81. Thomas JA, Marks BH. Plasma norepinephrine in congestive heart failure. Am J Cardiol 1978;41: 233–243.

82. Esler M, Kaye D, Lambert G, et al. Adrenergic nervous system in heart failure. Am J Cardiol 1997; 80(11a):7L–14L.

83. Bristow MR. Pathophysiologic and pharmacologic rationales for clinical management of chronic heart failure with β-blocking agents. Am J Cardiol 1993;71:12C–22C.

84. Doughty RN, MacMahon S, Sharpe N. Beta blockers in heart failure: promising or proved. J Am Coll Cardiol 1994;23:814–821.

85. Waagstein F, Hjalmarson A, Varnauskas E, Wallentin I. Effect of chronic β-adrenergic receptor blockade in congestive cardiomyopathy. B Heart J 1975;37:1022–1036.

86. Young JB. Carvedilol for heart failure: renewed interest in β-blockers. Cleveland Clin J Med 1997; 64(8):415–422.

87. Waagstein F, Bristow MR, Swedberg K, et al. Beneficial effects of metoprolol in idiopathic dilated cardiomyopathy. Lancet 1993;342:1441–1446.

88. CIBIS Investigators and Committees. A randomized trial of β-blockade in heart failure. The Cardiac Insufficiency Bisoprolol Study (CIBIS). Circulation 1994;90:1765–1773.

89. Krum H, Sackner-Bernstein JD, Goldsmith RL, et al. Double-blind, placebo-controlled study of the long-term efficacy of carvedilol in patients with severe chronic heart failure. Circulation 1995;92:1499–1506.

90. Metra M, Nardi M, Giubbini R, et al. Effects of short and long-term carvedilol administration on rest and exercise hemodynamic variables, exercise capacity and clinical conditions in patients with idiopathic dilated cardiomyopathy. J Am Coll Cardiol 1994;24:1678–1687.

91. Olsen SL, Gilbert EM, Renlund DG, et al. Carvedilol improves left ventricular function and symptoms in chronic heart failure: a double-blind randomized study. J Am Coll Cardiol 1995;25:1225–1231.

92. Packer M, Bristow MR, Cohn JN, et al. The effect of carvedilol on morbidity and mortality in patients with chronic heart failure. N Engl J Med 1996;334:1349–1355.

93. Australia/New Zealand Heart Failure Research Collaborative Group. Randomised, placebo-controlled trial of carvedilol in patients with congestive heart failure due to ischaemic heart disease. Lancet 1997; 349:375–380.

94. CIBIS-II Investigators and Committees. The Cardiac Insufficiency Bisoprolol Study II (CIBIS-II): a randomised trial. Lancet 1999;353:9–13.

95. MERIT-HF Study Group. Effect of metoprolol CR/XL in chronic heart failure: Metoprolol CR/XL Randomised Intervention Trial in Congestive Heart Failure (MERIT-HF). Lancet 1999;353:2001-2007.

96. Consensus recommendations for the management of chronic heart failure. On behalf of the membership of the advisory council to improve outcomes nationwide in heart failure. Am J Cardiol 1999 Jan 21;83(2A):1A–38A.

97. Bleske BE, Gilbert EM, Munger MA. Carvedilol: therapeutic application and practice guidelines. Pharmacotherapy 1998;18(4):729–737.

98. Cohn JN, Johnson G, Ziesche S, et al. Effect of vasodilator therapy on mortality in chronic congestive heart failure: results of a Veterans Administration Cooperative Study. N Engl J Med 1986;314: 1547–1552.

99. Uretsky BF, Young JB, Shahidi FE, et al. Randomized study assessing the effect of digoxin withdrawal in patients with mild to moderate chronic congestive heart failure: results of the PROVED trial. J Am Coll Cardiol 1993;22:955–962.

100. Packer M, Gheorghiade M, Young JB, et al. Withdrawal of digoxin from patients with chronic heart failure treated with angiotensin-converting-enzyme inhibitors. N Engl J Med 1993;329:1–7.

101. The Digitalis Investigation Group. The effect of digoxin on mortality and morbidity in patients with heart failure. N Engl J Med 1997;336:525–533.

102. Wilson JR, Reichek N, Dunkman WB, Goldberg S. Effect of diuresis on the performance of the failing left ventricular in man. Am J Med 1981;70:234–239.

103. Brater DC. Diuretic therapy. N Engl J Med 1998;339:387–395.

104. Pitt B, Zannad F, Remme WJ, Cody R, et al. The effect of spironolactone on morbidity and mortality in patients with severe heart failure. N Engl J Med 1999;341:709–717.

14

Aspirin and Antiplatelet Agents in the Prevention of Complications of Coronary Artery Disease

Scott A. Moore, MD
and Steven R. Steinhubl, MD

CONTENTS

INTRODUCTION

If not for the arterial thrombus, atherosclerosis—the principal cause of mortality in industrialized nations—might be an essentially benign disease. Even though the relationship between atherosclerosis and thrombosis was recognized as early as 1852 by von Rokitansky *(1)*, not until recently has its fundamental role been appreciated. Today, the disruption of an atherosclerotic plaque with resultant intracoronary thrombus formation has been consistently demonstrated to be central to the pathophysiological process underlying unstable angina (UA), acute myocardial infarction (MI), and sudden cardiac death *(2–5)*. There is also increasing evidence that asymptomatic plaque fissuring with associated nonocclusive thrombus is the etiology of atherosclerotic plaque progression *(6–9)*.

From: *Contemporary Cardiology: Preventive Cardiology:*
Strategies for the Prevention and Treatment of Coronary Artery Disease
Edited by: J. Foody © Humana Press Inc., Totowa, NJ

Furthermore, the level of platelet activity has been shown to be associated with the risk of future cardiac events *(10–12)*. These findings suggest that antithrombotic therapy, and in particular antiplatelet therapy, is central to the prevention of intracoronary thrombosis and the prevention of the complications of coronary artery disease (CAD).

The formation of a thrombus on injured arterial endothelium involves a complex interaction between platelets and a cascade of coagulation proteins that results in the production of fibrin. First, the normally thrombosis-resistant endothelium is rendered prothrombotic by atherosclerosis. Disruption of the endothelial monolayer, as well as high shear flow that is characteristic of stenosed coronary arteries, induce platelet adhesion. The initial binding of platelets to the vessel wall (adhesion) is strongly reliant on binding of specific platelet-membrane glycoprotein binding to adhesive proteins such as the von Willebrand factor and collagen *(13)*. Platelet activation can be initiated by any of over 100 known agonists including thromboxane A_2, thrombin, norepinephrine, collagen, and adenosine diphosphate (ADP). Activation leads to platelet degranulation and the release of serotonin, ADP, and thromboxane A_2, which triggers the recruitment and activation of neighboring platelets *(14)*. These platelets ultimately become aggregated into a hemostatic plug by the binding of primarily fibrinogen and von Willebrand factor to glycoprotein IIb/IIIa integrins on adjacent platelets. The membrane surface of the activated platelets also serves to accelerate the conversion of prothrombin to thrombin, thereby promoting the development of an occlusive, stabilized thrombus containing platelets, thrombin, and fibrin.

Many antiplatelet agents have been studied in the primary and secondary prevention of CAD to prevent adhesion, activation, aggregation, and thrombus formation. Because platelet function is multifaceted and antagonists function via different mechanisms, platelet inhibitors are likely to have variable effects. A number of antiplatelet agents are currently available or undergoing evaluation. This chapter reviews the available data regarding the use of antiplatelet agents in the prevention of complications of CAD.

KEY POINTS

1. Antithrombotic therapy, as it is currently used, prevents heart attacks and saves lives.
2. For every 1000 individuals free of diagnosed atherosclerotic disease treated with aspirin over a 5-yr period, up to seven important cardiac events will be prevented.
3. When aspirin is used in patients following MI or with UA, an almost one-fourth reduction in mortality can be realized.
4. For patients in whom aspirin is not a therapeutic option, data support the use of the thienopyridine derivatives as an effective aspirin alternative.
5. The role of more aggressive long-term antiplatelet protection, in the form of either the combination of a thienopyridine and aspirin, oral GPIIb/IIIa inhibition with or without aspirin, or other agents, in secondary prevention is currently being investigated and holds great promise.

ASPIRIN

The benefits of willow bark as an antipyretic were first reported by Reverend Edmund Stone in 1763 *(15)*. The potential for aspirin to cause a bleeding tendency was recognized as early as 1891 *(16)*, but its inhibitory effect on platelets specifically was not discovered until the late 1960s *(17)*. Aspirin's first described use in CAD was in 1953 in a preventative role *(18)*. Even though this nonrandomized observational study of daily

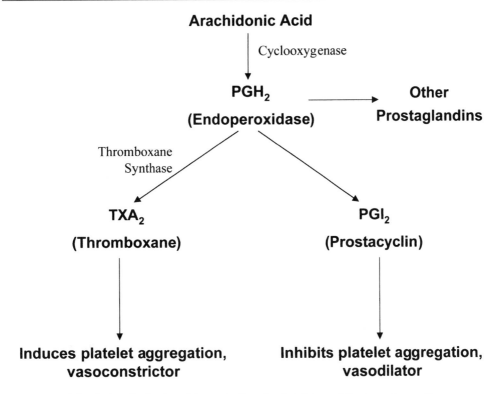

Fig. 1. Arachadonic acid metabolism in platelets and the vascular wall.

aspirin use demonstrated 100% successful prevention of "coronary occlusion" among 1465 asymptomatic male patients, aspirin therapy has only recently become a cornerstone of therapy in CAD.

The mechanism by which aspirin induces a functional defect in platelets is through the inhibition of thromboxane A_2 production *(19,20)*. During platelet activation, the hydrolysis of membrane phospholipids yields arachidonic acid, which is converted to prostaglandin H_2 (PH_2) by the catalytic activity of the cyclooxygenase enzyme prostaglandin G/H synthase *(21)* (Fig. 1). PGH_2 is then converted via thromboxane synthase to thromboxane A_2. By the selective and irreversible acetylation of a single serine residue within prostaglandin G/H synthase, aspirin causes the permanent inactivation of cyclooxygenase activity. Because the nonnucleated platelets lack the biosynthetic capabilities necessary to synthesize new protein, the aspirin-induced defect cannot be repaired for the 8–10 d life span of the platelet.

The ability of aspirin to inhibit cyclooxygenase activity also accounts for its variety of pharmacologic effects in other tissues. This effect is of particular importance with respect to aspirin's use in the prevention of intraarterial thrombosis as it inhibits the production of endothelial-produced prostacyclin, a vasodilator and inhibitor of platelet aggregation. This counterbalancing effect has raised the concern of a possible prothrombotic effect of aspirin therapy. Unlike platelets, endothelial cells possess the biosynthetic machinery necessary to produce new enzyme, and therefore recover their ability to synthesize prostacyclin within a few hours. Currently there is no direct evidence that prostacyclin inhibition of aspirin is clinically relevant, although a recent study showing improved

Table 1
Relative Mean Percentage Decrease in Events
with Aspirin Compared with Placebo in Primary Prevention Trials

	US Physicians Health Study	British Doctors' Trial	Hypertension Optimal Treatment Trial	Thrombosis Prevention Trial
All MI	44%	3%	36%	20%
All stroke	(22%)	(17%)	2%	3%
Total vascular morality	0%	6%	5%	(12.5%)

Data are presented as mean % reduction. Data in parenthesis represent a negative value (or increased % of events). MI = myocardial infarction.

outcomes in patients randomized to low-dose compared to high-dose aspirin is consistent with this hypothesis *(22)*.

Aspirin for Primary Prevention

The efficacy of aspirin to prevent a first ischemic event has been evaluated in four large randomized trials involving over 51,000 participants *(23–27)* (Table 1). The first of these, the British Doctors' Trial, enrolled 5139 male British physicians between the ages of 50 and 78. Two thirds were randomized to take 500 mg of aspirin daily and the remaining third were instructed to "avoid" aspirin and products containing aspirin. By the end of the 6-yr study there was no significant difference between groups in the occurrence of myocardial infarction, stroke, the combined endpoint of adverse vascular events, or total vascular mortality, but the 95% confidence intervals were very wide. A second trial, the US Physicians Health Study was a double-blind, placebo-controlled trial that utilized a 2×2 factorial design to test simultaneously the effects of aspirin in reducing cardiovascular disease and beta carotene in the prevention of cancer. A total of 22,071 US male physicians ranging in age from 40–84 yr were randomized to receive 325 mg of aspirin every other day, or placebo. The aspirin/placebo component of the study was prematurely terminated due to a marked reduction in the occurrence of a MI (relative risk [RR]: 0.56; 95% confidence interval [CI]: 0.45–0.70; $p < 0.00001$) among those receiving aspirin. This reduction in risk was apparent only among those over 50 yr of age. A trend toward an increased risk of any stroke (RR: 1.22; 95% CI: 0.93–1.60; $p = 0.15$) was observed, influenced primarily by the subgroup with hemorrhagic stroke (RR: 2.14; 95% CI: 0.96–4.77; $p = 0.06$). There was a significant decrease in the rate of fatal MI ($p = 0.004$) in the aspirin group, but this benefit was offset by an apparent increased risk for sudden death ($p = 0.09$), resulting in no reduction in total cardiovascular mortality (81 in the aspirin group vs. 83 in the placebo group, $p = 0.87$).

When these two groups were evaluated together, due to the much larger size of the US study, a highly significant 32% reduction in the risk of a nonfatal MI was demonstrated *(28)*. Despite the trend toward an increased risk of stroke in the aspirin arm of both of these studies, the combined data still provided too few endpoints on which any firm conclusions could be made. Before generalizing the findings of these trials to the entire male population, it is important to note that the participants in these studies represented a very health conscious group of individuals. This likely explains the unusually low cardiovascular mortality rate among the participants—approximately 15% of that expected for an age-matched group of white American males.

The Hypertension Optimal Treatment (HOT) study has helped to clarify aspirin's role in primary prevention in a more representative population *(27)*. The HOT study was the first large-scale, randomized trial to examine the role of aspirin for primary prevention in patients with hypertension, a population with a higher cardiovascular event rate than described in the earlier primary prevention trials. Over 19,000 patients were randomized to one of three target blood pressure goals to determine if there are additional benefits in lowering blood pressure of hypertensive patients to fully normotensive levels. Patients were also randomized to either low-dose aspirin (75 mg daily) or placebo to examine aspirin's efficacy in primary prevention in this group at higher risk for vascular events. After 3.8 yr of follow-up, major cardiovascular events (fatal and nonfatal MI, fatal and nonfatal stroke, all other cardiovascular deaths) were reduced by 15% in the aspirin group ($p = 0.03$). This benefit was largely due to a 36% reduction in the rate of MI ($p = 0.002$). There was no significant difference in the rates of stroke, cardiovascular mortality, or total mortality. Importantly, aspirin did not increase the rates of fatal bleeding (including cerebral), but nonfatal major and minor bleeding, primarily gastrointestinal and nasal, were 1.8 times more frequent with aspirin ($p < 0.001$). In contrast to the small benefit previously described in healthy populations *(28)*, in patients at higher risk for CAD, aspirin prevented 7.5 MIs per 1000 patients treated for 5 yr without increasing the risk of hemorrhagic stroke. This is in contrast to the 4 events per 1000 patients treated for 5 yr in the Physicians' Health Study and British Doctors' Trial.

The most recent study of aspirin in primary prevention is the Thrombosis Prevention Trial *(26)*. This trial confirmed the protective effect of aspirin and further evaluated the role of warfarin with or without aspirin in this population of males at risk for ischemic heart disease. These investigators found that although the addition of low-dose warfarin (target international normalized ratio [INR] of 1.5) to daily low-dose aspirin (75 mg) did demonstrate a trend towards decreased cardiac events, its use was associated with a significant increase in the risk of major hemorrhage.

There are several ongoing studies to evaluate further the role of aspirin in primary prevention. The largest of these, The Women's Health Study, began in 1992 and randomized approx 40,000 women >45 yr of age to alternate-day 100 mg aspirin or placebo *(29)*. The additional insight provided by trials such as these should help resolve remaining uncertainty for the role of aspirin in the primary prevention of ischemic heart disease. Until these results are available, current data suggest that aspirin should be considered for primary prevention in at risk patients. A greater benefit-to-risk ratio should be expected if therapy targets patients over age 50 or with risk factors for CAD.

Aspirin for Secondary Prevention

Patients with an established history of a cardiovascular event are at particular risk for subsequent cardiac events as well as a cardiovascular death. A large number of randomized trials have been carried out in order to determine whether aspirin therapy can modify the clinical course of these patients. An overview of 25 of the earliest antiplatelet trials involving approximately 29,000 patients was reported in 1988 by the Antiplatelet Trialists' Collaboration *(30)*. They concluded that antiplatelet therapy decreased vascular mortality by 15% and nonfatal vascular events (stroke or MI) by 30%. A second overview was reported by this same group in 1994 *(31)*. The updated study included over 145 randomized trials and involved over 100,000 patients. Overall, the results confirmed the earlier findings with a one-third reduction in nonfatal vascular events, as well as a one-sixth decrease in vascular deaths in high-risk patients receiving antiplatelet therapy. The larger number of pooled studies and patients allowed the potential benefit in specific subgroups to be discerned.

Stable Angina

Three prospective studies evaluated aspirin in patients with chronic stable angina. A subgroup analysis of the Physician's Health Study *(24)* evaluated 333 patients who had stable angina at enrollment *(32)*. Even though aspirin therapy did not influence the frequency or severity of angina episodes during 4 yr of study, it was associated with a 50% reduction in nonfatal first MIs ($p < 0.019$). All fatal MIs occurred in the placebo group (0 vs. 4), whereas of the 13 strokes that occurred, 11 were among patients taking aspirin. A double-blind, randomized trial by Chesebro and colleagues involved 370 patients with stable CAD and evaluated the impact of combined aspirin and dipyridamole therapy versus placebo over a 5-yr period *(33)*. There was a two-thirds reduction in the incidence of MI ($p = 0.007$) in treated patients as well as a trend for a reduction in new angiographic lesion formation (30% placebo vs. 21% treated, $p = 0.06$). Finally, the largest trial evaluating aspirin therapy in patients with stable angina was a Swedish trial of 2035 patients *(34)*. All patients received sotalol, aspirin, or aspirin-placebo, and were followed for over 4 yr. Patients receiving aspirin demonstrated a 34% reduction (95%, CI = 24–49%, $p = 0.003$) in MI and sudden death. In aggregate, these studies suggest that aspirin therapy in 1000 patients with stable angina would prevent 51 important cardiovascular events over a 4-yr period—a benefit approx 10 times greater than that seen in primary prevention trials.

Unstable Angina and Non-Q Wave MI

The 1-yr mortality of patients with unstable angina (UA) ranges from 5–14% with the majority of deaths occurring within several weeks of diagnosis *(35)*. The benefit of aspirin therapy alone or in combination with heparin in the acute treatment of UA has been proved in several randomized trials. In the landmark study "Heparin, Aspirin or Both to Treat Acute Unstable Angina," Theroux and colleagues *(36)* demonstrated a >70% reduction in cardiac death or MI from 11.9% in the placebo group to 3.3% with aspirin alone and 1.6% with the combination of aspirin and heparin ($p = 0.0042$). The Research Group on Instability in Coronary Artery Disease in Southeast Sweden (RISC) *(37)* demonstrated a 57% ($p = 0.033$) reduction in MI and death with aspirin compared with placebo, whereas intermittent intravenous heparin showed no significant influence on these endpoints. One-year follow-up of these patients continued to show an almost 50% reduction ($p < 0.0001$) in death and MI in aspirin-treated patients compared with placebo *(38)*. The results of these studies and others *(39,40)* suggest that aspirin therapy can reduce the occurrence of death and MI by approximately 50% in patients with UA or non-Q-wave MI.

Evolving MI and Post-MI

The ability of aspirin to reduce the risk of recurrent cardiovascular complications compared with placebo in patients who have survived a MI has been studied in eight trials involving nearly 16,000 patients *(31)*. When considered collectively, these studies demonstrate a one-third reduction in the risk of nonfatal MI and a one-fourth decrease in the occurrence of MI, stroke, or vascular death. In terms of absolute risk reduction, treatment of 1000 patients with a prior MI for 2 yr will prevent 36 major cardiovascular events.

The role of aspirin in the treatment of an evolving MI has been well established. The Second International Study of Infarct Survival (ISIS-2) *(41)* randomized 17,187 patients to receive streptokinase, aspirin daily for 1 mo, neither or both beginning within 24 h of a suspected MI. Aspirin alone and streptokinase alone decreased 35-d vascular mortality similarly (23% and 25%, respectively), whereas the combination decreased mortality by 42% compared with placebo.

Adverse Effects

As with most medical therapies, but in particular with therapies designed to be preventive in nature, the physician must optimize the benefits while minimizing the risks. Patients who regularly take nonsteroidal anti-inflammatory drugs have an increased risk of gastrointestinal bleeding or other events that result in hospitalization or death *(42)*. The gastrointestinal side effects of aspirin are clearly dose related with doses as low as 75 mg/d causing peptic ulcer disease *(43)*. A dose-related risk of hemorrhagic stroke has also been suggested by several trials evaluating high- and low-dose aspirin *(44,45)*. Buffered aspirin preparations as well as enteric-coated aspirin are better tolerated and have been associated with fewer gastrointestinal side effects than plain aspirin but are still associated with peptic ulcers *(46,47)*. There is some suggestion that controlled-release preparations currently being evaluated may limit side effects. An interim analysis of the safety results in the first 3667 patients enrolled of the Thrombosis Prevention Trial (TPT) demonstrated no excess of gastrointestinal symptoms after an average follow-up of 1.1 yr in those treated with 75 mg of enteric-coated, controlled-release aspirin daily compared with placebo *(48)*. Regardless, to minimize side effects the lowest effective dose should be used.

In order for aspirin therapy to be effective it must be prescribed to the patient. Despite the overwhelming evidence supporting its use, as well as its incomparably low cost, studies have shown that up to one-third of elderly patients do not receive aspirin at the time of an acute MI *(49)*, and that a quarter do not receive it chronically following a MI *(50)*. With over 1 million patients admitted to US hospitals each year with an acute MI, by increasing the use of aspirin to include essentially all patients, nearly 8000 premature deaths each year would be prevented *(51)*.

THIENOPYRIDINE DERIVATIVES— TICLOPIDINE AND CLOPIDOGREL

Ticlopidine was first introduced as an antiplatelet agent in the early 1980s. Its analog, clopidogrel, was approved for clinical use by the FDA in 1998. The thienopyridines have now emerged as important agents in the prevention of complications in CAD. Ticlopidine and clopidogrel interfere with ADP-mediated platelet activation and cause an irreversible, noncompetitive inhibition of platelet function by preventing ADP from producing the conformational changes in the glycoprotein IIb/IIIa receptor needed for high-affinity ligand binding *(52)*. Ticlopidine is usually administered orally in doses of 250 mg twice daily and clopidogrel in a dose of 75 mg once daily. Inhibition of platelet aggregation is both dose and time related, with onset of activity 24–48 h following oral administration, and near maximal activity at 3–5 d *(53)*. Unique to clopidogrel is the capacity to achieve maximal activity within several hours following the administration of a single loading dose of 375 mg *(54)*. Within an hour of administration, there is significant inhibition of platelet aggregation, with maximal inhibition by 5 h. Because their action is irreversible like aspirin, the duration of effect persists for 7–10 d (55). Thienopyridines are inactive in vitro and require hepatic metabolism for the development of their antiplatelet activity (53). When considering the relative mechanisms of action of aspirin and the thieno-pyridines, there are theoretical advantages associated with the ADP receptor antagonists. The thienopyridines do not affect platelet arachidonic acid metabolism and therefore are not expected to interfere with platelet-dependent synthesis of prostacyclin, an important vasodilatory prostaglandin (56,57). It has also been observed that thienopyridines, par-ticularly clopidogrel, are significantly more effective in preventing platelet aggregation evoked by shear stress, as may be seen at sites of atherosclerotic plaque or vessel bifur-cations (58–61). These potential advantages are at a cost of $1–$3 per tablet compared to <$0.01 for aspirin (62).

Thienopyridines for Primary Prevention

Unlike aspirin, there have been no large, prospective trials of thienopyridines in the primary prevention of acute coronary syndromes. However, in several large secondary prevention trials for stroke and peripheral vascular disease, there have been significant reductions in rates of MI. This suggests that in patients at risk for CAD, particularly those with peripheral and cerebrovascular disease and those who are intolerant of aspirin, thienopyridines may have a role in the primary prevention of MI. In the Canadian Ameri-can Ticlopidine Study (CATS) (63), patients with a recent thromboembolic stroke were randomized to either ticlopidine or placebo. At 2 yr of follow-up, there was a 30.2% relative risk reduction compared to placebo (95% CI 7.5–48.3%, $p = 0.006$) in stroke, MI, or vascular death with ticlopidine. A similar reduction in vascular events was demon-strated in the Swedish Ticlopidine Multicentre Study (64). In patients with a history of intermittent claudication treated with ticlopidine there was a significant reduction in the rate of MI, stroke, or transient ischemic attack (TIA) compared with placebo (13.8% vs. 22.4%, $p = 0.017$). Other trials of secondary prevention in peripheral vascular disease have confirmed ticlopidine's efficacy with 75% reductions in 6-mo vascular event rates compared with placebo (65,66). These data suggest that thienopyridines have a role in the primary prevention of complications of CAD and are acceptable alternatives for patients who cannot tolerate aspirin.

Thienopyridines for Secondary Prevention

The thienopyridines have been compared with aspirin in controlled trials for the secon-dary prevention of stroke, peripheral arterial occlusive disease, and MI (63,64,67–69). Each of these studies demonstrated a benefit with ticlopidine compared with aspirin. The Ticlopidine Aspirin Stroke Study (TASS) (67) was the first to suggest that in the second-ary prevention of stroke, ticlopidine may be more effective than aspirin. The 3-yr event rate for nonfatal stroke or death from any cause was 17% with ticlopidine and 19% for aspirin, a 12% risk reduction with ticlopidine ($p = 0.048$). The largest trial addressing the role of thienopyridines in secondary prevention is the Clopidogrel versus Aspirin in Patients at Risk for Further Ischemic Events (CAPRIE) trial (70). This was a prospective, random-ized, blinded study involving over 19,000 patients with atherosclerotic vascular disease. Patients with a recent ischemic stroke, MI, or symptomatic peripheral vascular disease were randomized to either daily aspirin or clopidogrel therapy. After a mean follow-up of approx 2 yr, those receiving clopidogrel had an annual risk of ischemic stroke, MI, or vascular death of 5.3% compared with 5.8% for those receiving aspirin ($p = 0.043$). These results suggest that for every 1000 patients with manifestations of atherosclerotic vascular disease receiving antiplatelet therapy for secondary prevention, clopidogrel would be expected to prevent five more major clinical events per year than aspirin with a decreased incidence of side effects.

There have been no large-scale trials of thienopyridines in secondary prevention with chronic stable angina. However, there are experimental data demonstrating that ticlopidine does achieve significantly greater degrees of platelet inhibition as compared with dipyridamole in patients with chronic stable angina (71). In patients admitted with unstable angina, treatment with ticlopidine has demonstrated efficacy in the reduction of subsequent cardiac events (72). The addition of ticlopidine to conventional treatment (beta blockers, calcium-channel blockers, and nitrates) in patients admitted with unstable angina resulted in a 46.3% reduction (7.3% vs. 13.6%, $p = 0.009$) in the relative risk of nonfatal MI or vascular death at 6 mo follow-up. Of note, there was no aspirin arm in this study so the relative efficacy of ticlopidine compared with aspirin in secondary prevention after unstable angina cannot be assessed.

Ticlopidine has also been investigated in surgical revascularization. Platelets play an important role in early graft occlusion from thrombosis and may contribute to the process of intimal proliferation and late graft occlusion (73). A trial of 77 patients randomized to ticlopidine or placebo 3 d before CABG failed to show a benefit for ticlopidine over placebo at the 3-mo angiographic follow-up of saphenous vein graft patency (74). However, on-treatment analysis demonstrated a 67% reduction in the rate of occlusion (7.1% vs. 21.8%, $p < 0.02$). In a subsequent study, ticlopidine's efficacy relative to placebo was demonstrated with statistically significant reductions in graft occlusion at 1-yr follow-up (15.9% vs. 26.1%, $p < 0.01$) (75). Ticlopidine's efficacy in maintaining saphenous graft patency also applies to grafts used in peripheral arterial revascularization with 2-yr graft patency of 82% compared to 51.2% for placebo ($p = 0.002$) (76).

Ticlopidine and clopidogrel share similar long-term antiplatelet efficacy, but differ primarily in their side-effect profile. Risk of hemorrhage for both agents is low and similar to aspirin. A 9.3% rate of any bleeding and 1.38% rate of major bleeding were reported for clopidogrel in the CAPRIE study (70), both rates comparable to aspirin. The most frequently reported complaints for both agents are gastrointestinal—more commonly with ticlopidine than clopidogrel. Diarrhea is reported by as many as 20% of patients treated with ticlopidine, and nausea, dyspepsia, and anorexia are also frequent (62). In general, clopidogrel is better tolerated, but gastrointestinal complaints were still the most frequent adverse reaction reported in CAPRIE with diarrheas occurring in 4.5% of clopidogrel patients vs. 3.36% with aspirin ($p < 0.05$) and indigestion/nausea/vomiting developing in 15% with clopidogrel and 17.6% with aspirin ($p < 0.05$) (70). Rash is the other major side effect shared by these agents occurring in 3–11% with ticlopidine (77,78) and in up to 6% of clopidogrel patients (70).

Unique to ticlopidine is the occurrence of potentially life-threatening hematologic complications. A review of an estimated 10 million patient-years of ticlopidine treatment identified 645 cases of agranulocytosis, pancytopenia, aplastic anemia, and bone marrow suppression with an associated mortality of 16% (79). The most frequently recognized hematologic complication associated with ticlopidine is neutropenia, which occurs in 2–3% of patients and is severe in 0.85%. This typically occurs within the first 3 mo of treatment and appears to be reversible when the drug is discontinued (80). Close monitoring of the white blood cell count is therefore mandatory during the first 3 mo of therapy.

Clopidogrel does not appear to share ticlopidine's marrow-suppressive effects. In CAPRIE *(70)*, the rate of neutropenia (0.1%) was not significantly different from that observed with aspirin (0.17%).

A less common, but potentially more devastating, complication associated with ticlopidine is thrombotic thrombocytopenic purpura (TTP). Ticlopidine's association with TTP was first described in 1991 in a report of 4 patients *(81)*. A recent summary of 60 cases suggested the incidence might be higher than previously believed *(82)*. Two groups have evaluated the incidence of TTP in patients receiving short-term ticlopidine following stenting *(83,84)*. These results suggest an incidence of 1 in 1500 to 1 in 4500 patients treated. The clinical presentation of ticlopidine-associated TTP is similar to that of TTP in general and there is a comparable mortality rate of 21–33%. Early recognition and management with plasmapheresis have consistently been shown to be the most important determinants of survival *(82,83)*. Clopidogrel has not been reported to cause this syndrome.

Despite the disadvantages of increased cost relative to aspirin and a greater delay in onset of maximal antiplatelet activity, the thienopyridine derivatives (ticlopidine and clopidogrel) provide an effective antiplatelet alternative in aspirin-intolerant patients and play a major role in combination antiplatelet therapy after percutaneous coronary interventions. With its more favorable side effect profile and potential for a more rapid onset of action, clopidogrel is emerging as the preferred thienopyridine.

COMBINATION THERAPY WITH ASPIRIN AND THIENOPYRIDINES

The recurrence of ischemic events despite aspirin therapy in some patients suggests the need for more complete inhibition of the platelet and the coagulation cascade. A clear rationale exists for combination antiplatelet therapy as there are multiple pathways of platelet activation independent of aspirin's target, cyclooxygenase. Experimentally, it has been shown in normal volunteers that the combination of ticlopidine and aspirin is more effective than either alone in inhibiting collagen-induced platelet aggregation *(85)*. This synergistic effect is a consequence of the combination of the different antiplatelet activities of these agents. In patients with a history of stroke or TIA, aspirin alone markedly inhibited platelet aggregation induced by arachidonic acid, but not by ADP or platelet activating factor (PAF) *(86)*. Ticlopidine inhibited ADP- and PAF-induced platelet aggregation, but not arachidonic acid. The combination, by virtue of the complimentary mechanisms of action, markedly inhibited platelet aggregation in response to all three agonists. Similar results have been demonstrated in patients who have been treated with intracoronary stents with significantly greater degrees of platelet inhibition with combination therapy than with monotherapy utilizing either agent *(87)*.

Clinically, the effect of combination therapy has been most clearly demonstrated in percutaneous coronary intervention. Combination antiplatelet therapy compared with aggressive anticoagulant therapy plus aspirin has dramatically reduced the risk of subacute thrombosis after coronary stent implantation. The Intracoronary Stenting and Antithrombotic Regimen (ISAR) trial was the first randomized trial of antiplatelet vs. anticoagulant therapy after coronary stenting *(88)*. At 30-d, treatment with ticlopidine and aspirin was associated with a 1.6% rate of cardiac death, MI, coronary artery bypass grafting (CABG), or repeat percutaneous revascularization in contrast to the 6.2% rate with warfarin and aspirin (RR = 0.25; 95% CI 0.06–0.77; p = 0.01). There were no major bleeding complications with the antiplatelet regimen, whereas 6.5% of patients in the warfarin arm experienced a major hemorrhagic event ($p < 0.001$). These results were confirmed in the Stent Anticoagulation Regimen Study (STARS) *(89)*, the first large, multicenter trial comparing combined antiplatelet therapy and anticoagulant therapy. The combination of ticlopidine and aspirin was shown to be more effective than aspirin alone (0.5% vs. 3.6% event rate) or aspirin and warfarin (2.7%, $p = 0.001$ for the comparison of all three groups). The efficacy of combined antiplatelet therapy in the prevention of subacute thrombosis has now been extended to the entire spectrum of acute coronary syndromes *(78,90)*.

In addition to its efficacy in reducing subacute thrombosis, combination therapy with aspirin and thienopyridines has shown promise in reducing the rates of periprocedural non-Q-wave MIs. Non-Q-wave MIs complicate up to one-third of percutaneous coronary interventions *(91)* and have been shown to have long-term prognostic significance *(92–95)*. Pretreatment with ticlopidine among patients undergoing intracoronary stent implantation has been shown to significantly reduce the risk of procedural non-Q-wave MI *(96)*. For patients treated for ≥3 d before the procedure, there was an almost 80% reduction in the rate of non-Q wave MI compared to those pre-treated for <3 d (odds ratio 0.18; 95% CI 0.04–0.78; $p = 0.01$). Because of the potential for near maximal activity within 8 h of a 375mg loading dose *(54)*, clopidogrel may be able to achieve a similar effect with therapy initiated the day of the procedure.

Two currently ongoing trials, CREDO (Clopidogrel for the Reduction of Events During Extended Observation) and CURE (Clopidogrel in Unstable Angina to Prevent Recurrent Ischemic Events), will evaluate the acute benefit of the rapid onset of dual antiplatelet protection with aspirin and clopidogrel, as well as the long-term benefit of continued combination therapy. In the CREDO trial, 2000 patients undergoing, or at high likelihood for, a planned coronary intervention will be randomized to either pretreatment with 300 mg of clopidogrel beginning 6–24 h prior the intervention or aspirin alone. At the time of the intervention all patients will receive 75 mg and 325 mg clopidogrel, continued daily for 28 d. Patients who randomized to clopidogrel pretreatment will then be maintained on this regimen for 1 yr, whereas the other group will continue on daily aspirin alone. In the CURE trial 9000 patients with UA or non-Q MI will be randomized at presentation to either aspirin alone or a loading dose (300 mg) of clopidogrel plus aspirin. Patients randomized to dual therapy will continue clopidogrel 75 mg daily plus aspirin up to 1 yr. The results of both of these studies will substantially expand our understanding of the acute and long-term efficacy and safety of combined antiplatelet therapy with clopidogrel and aspirin.

PLATELET GLYCOPROTEIN IIB/IIIA RECEPTOR INHIBITORS

The newest, most potent, and one of the most promising family of antiplatelet agents currently evolving are the glycoprotein IIb/IIIa receptor inhibitors. As already noted, platelet aggregation can be initiated by a number of pathways. However, the final common pathway of aggregation, regardless of how it is initiated, involves the binding of the IIb/IIIa receptors of adjacent platelets. By blocking these platelet receptors, aggregation can be essentially eliminated. Coller and colleagues were the first to demonstrate that a murine monoclonal antibody (7E3) directed against the IIb/IIIa receptor, could inhibit binding of fibrinogen to platelets, thereby inhibiting platelet aggregation *(97)*. This monoclonal antibody was later redesigned as a half-murine, half-human chimeric Fab fragment (c7E3 Fab, abciximab) using recombinant techniques. Subsequently, a number of other parenteral glycoprotein IIb/IIIa receptor antagonists have been developed and clinically evaluated, including the peptide inhibitor, eptifibatide, and nonpeptide inhibitors, tirofiban and lamifiban (98). Over 10 large-scale, placebo-controlled, randomized trials involving over 35,000 patients have been carried out to evaluate the short-term, intravenous use of these agents in the setting of percutaneous coronary interventions or acute coronary syndromes. When the data are considered collectively, there is a 13% reduction in the 30-d rate of death and MI when IIb/IIIa inhibitors are added to standard therapy with aspirin and heparin (99).

The trials of IIb/IIIa inhibitors to date have largely been treatment trials of acute coronary syndromes and percutaneous revascularization. However, a number of oral agents have been developed and are undergoing extensive clinical testing. In the realm of secondary prevention, a need clearly exists for longer-term inhibition of this receptor complex as the favorable short-term benefits of parenteral IIb/IIIa inhibitors, particularly target vessel revascularization, have not been maintained with longer follow-up in some trials (100–102). With acute coronary syndromes, activation of the hemostatic system persists for months after the acute event (103), supporting a potential role for oral GPIIb/IIIa agonists in long-term secondary prevention.

There are a number of oral GPIIb/IIIa antagonists undergoing evaluation, with several agents recently completing, or still undergoing phase 3 testing. The results of phase 2 trials with these agents suggested that bleeding complications were frequent, with minor hemorrhagic events occurring in 30% of patients receiving certain dosing regimens (104). Of patients with bleeding events, the drug was discontinued in over one half. Therefore, successful treatment with these agents will require a careful balance between clinical efficacy and safety.

Preliminary results currently available from two phase 3 trials of oral agents have been disappointing. The OPUS/TIMI-16 (Orbofiban in Patients with Unstable Coronary Syndromes/Thrombolysis in Myocardial Infarction) had trial enrollment halted by the Data Safety Monitoring Board at 8000 of a planned 12,000 patients due to safety concerns. Preliminary efficacy and safety results were recently presented at the 1999 American College of Cardiology meeting. Surprisingly, both at 30 d, and over the long term (median of 7 mo), treatment with orbofiban was associated with a trend toward increased adverse cardiac events. The higher dosing regimen of orbofiban was also associated with a significant increase in major bleeding compared with placebo (3.7% vs. 1.9%). A second trial, the EXCITE (Evaluation of Oral Xemilofiban in Controlling Thrombotic Events) trial was a double-blind, placebo-controlled study of the efficacy and safety of xemilofiban when administered prior to, and for up to 6 months after a percutaneous coronary revascularization procedure. Preliminary results from this trial, also presented at the 1999 American College of Cardiology meeting, did not show a benefit of treatment with the oral GPIIb/IIIa inhibitor xemilofiban in this population. The third Phase 3 trial of oral GPIIb/IIIa inhibitors to announce disappointing results was the SYMPHONY (Sibrafiban vs. Aspirin to Yield Maximum Protection from Ischemic Heart Events Post-Acute Coronary Syndromes). This study involving approx 6000 patients presenting with an acute coronary syndrome and randomized patients to one of 2 doses of sibrafiban without aspirin, or aspirin only. Preliminary results were just announced at the 1999 meeting of the European Society of Cardiology and, as in the previous two phase 3 trials, showed no benefit of prolonged GPIIb/IIIa inhibition.

These disappointing, yet intriguing, results in light of the success of short-term use of these agents suggest that there is much more that needs to be learned about these agents. Full analysis of the completed trials may identify subgroups that did obtain significant benefit through prolonged GPIIb/IIIa inhibition and may help focus future therapies. Also, substantial interpatient variability in response to these agents may be overcome through the use of recently developed point-of-care platelet function monitors and individual titration of therapy.

DIPYRIDAMOLE

Dipyridamole, a primidopyrimidine derivative with vasodilator properties, was introduced for the treatment of angina in 1961. Its antithrombotic properties were first reported in 1965 *(105)*. The basis for any antiplatelet and antithrombotic properties is not clear, but may be related to (1) inhibition of platelet phosphodiesterase resulting in an increase in intraplatelet cyclic adenosine monophosphate (cAMP), (2) stimulation of endogenous prostaglandin release from the endothelium, or (3) inhibition of adenosine uptake with subsequent degradation by the vasculature. Dipyridamole alone is a weak inhibitor of platelet aggregation in vitro. The potential antithrombotic effect of dipyridamole has been assessed in a large number of studies, but typically in combination with aspirin rather than compared directly with a placebo. Doses from 75–400 mg daily in divided doses have been investigated. In early clinical trials of stroke and CAD in which aspirin alone has been compared with the combination of aspirin and dipyridamole, dipyridamole contributed no benefit *(106)*. However, the recent European Stroke Prevention Study 2 evaluating a long-acting formulation of dipyridamole in stroke patients demonstrated a significant benefit of dipyridamole alone compared with placebo and an even greater benefit when used in combination with aspirin *(107)*. Based on the results of this trial a combination formulation of aspirin and a long-acting preparation of dipyridamole has recently received FDA approval.

SULFINPYRAZONE

Sulfinpyrazone was discovered in 1957 as a metabolite of the anti-inflammatory phenylbutazone and was first used for the treatment of gout. Its effect on platelets were reported in 1965 *(108)* when it was noted that it normalized the shortened platelet survival associated with gout. Further investigation determined that sulfinpyrazone (or a metabolite) is a weak inhibitor of platelet cyclooxygenase *(109)*. Two randomized, placebo-controlled trials completed in the mid-1970s evaluated the impact of sulfinpyrazone therapy in survivors of acute MI *(110,111)*. Even though both trials demonstrated an improvement in outcome compared with placebo, inconsistent findings between the studies leave the results in doubt. At best, sulfinpyrazone provides no greater benefit than aspirin, and it is not recommended for routine antiplatelet therapy.

INHIBITORS OF THROMBOXANE FORMATION AND/OR BINDING

Due to aspirin's theoretical disadvantage of endothelial cyclooxygenase inhibition as well as its side effects, specific inhibitors of thromboxane A_2 synthase were created to induce greater and more focused platelet inhibition than aspirin. When thromboxane A_2

synthase is inhibited, arachidonic acid metabolism in platelets leads to the accumulation of prostaglandin endoperoxides, which are then shunted to endothelial prostacyclin production. In fact, it is this enhanced generation of the platelet-inhibitory prostacyclins (and not the blockade of thromboxane A_2 production) that appears to determine the antiplatelet effects of thromboxane A_2 synthase inhibitors (112). However, because accumulating prostaglandin endoperoxides can also activate platelets via the thromboxane A_2 receptor (113), agents that inhibit both thromboxane synthase and block thromboxane receptors would theoretically provide the greatest antiplatelet effect.

Clinical trials have been carried out evaluating the thromboxane synthase inhibitor, sulotroban (114); the thromboxane receptor antagonist, vapiprost (115); and the combined-mode agent, ridogrel (116). The first two trials demonstrated no benefit of these agents on restenosis following percutaneous transluminal coronary angioplasty (PTCA). The third study compared ridogrel with aspirin in acute MI patients being treated with streptokinase. Although ridogrel was not superior to aspirin in terms of its adjunct impact on fibrinolytic efficacy, a post hoc analysis demonstrated a significantly lower incidence of new ischemic events (reinfarction, recurrent angina, and ischemic stroke) in the ridogrel group.

CILOSTAZOL

Cilostazol is a new antiplatelet agent with vasodilator properties recently approved for the treatment of intermittent claudication (117). Cilostazol selectively inhibits platelet phosphodiesterase type III, thereby increasing intracellular concentrations of cAMP and inhibiting platelet aggregation (118). Antiplatelet activity is detected within six hours of oral ingestion and persists for 48 h after drug withdrawal (119). In a cAMP-dependent mechanism, it also acts as an arterial vasodilator (120). The drug is well tolerated with the most commonly reported side effects being headache, diarrhea, and dizziness (121).

In the setting of peripheral vascular disease, cilostazol has been shown to significantly improve symptoms of intermittent claudication with up to 40% increases in maximal walking distance (122). This benefit is assumed to be primarily due to its vasodilatory effects, but may also be related to its antiplatelet properties. Based on animal models of carotid artery balloon injury demonstrating significantly decreased rates of neointimal proliferation (123), the role of cilostazol in percutaneous coronary intervention has also been investigated. In a preliminary study of 36 patients undergoing Palmaz–Schatz coronary stent implantation, randomization to cilostazol was associated with a significantly greater minimal luminal diameter at 6 mo compared with aspirin (124). In a larger study of 211 patients undergoing PTCA, angiographic follow-up was performed 3 mo after randomization to either cilostazol or aspirin (125). Angiographic restenosis was significantly less frequent with cilostazol compared with aspirin (17.9% vs. 39.5%, $p < 0.001$) and target lesion revascularization was also less frequent with cilostazol (11.4% vs. 28.7%, $p < 0.001$). When compared with ticlopidine in aspirin-treated patients after coronary stent implantation, cilostazol has similar efficacy in preventing subacute thrombosis and may confer an advantage in reducing 6-mo angiographic restenosis (126). Cilostazol is thought to decrease neointimal proliferation after balloon angioplasty by way of its antiplatelet actions and subsequent decreases in platelet-derived growth factors (127). By a mechanism that is not yet understood, cilostazol is also thought to be capable of direct inhibition of smooth muscle cell proliferation (128). This may be the primary mechanism of reduction of late lumen loss after PTCA with this agent.

Table 2
Studies Evaluating Interindividual Variations in Response to Aspirin

Study	N	Test	Percent of patients considered partial- or nonresponders to aspirin
Hurlen (164)	93	Platelet Aggregate Ratio	15%
Grotemeyer (136)	180	Platelet Aggregate Ratio	33%
Mueller (139)	100	Whole Blood Aggregometry	60%
Buchanan (129)	40	Bleeding Time	42%
Pappas (130)	31	Whole Blood Adherence	Change after aspirin normally distributed
Helgason (137)	306	Platelet-Rich-Plasma Aggregometry	26%
Valles (148)	82	Platelet Recruitment	61%
Valettas (132)	30	Flow Cytometry	57%
Poggio (165)	113	Platelet-Rich Plasma Aggregometry	8%
		PFA-100®	12%
			(4% by both methods)
Total	975		Corrected mean 32%

SPECIAL TOPICS:
ASPIRIN RESISTANCE

While aspirin therapy has been shown to reduce the risk of stroke, MI, or vascular death by as much as 25% in patients at high risk for vascular events (31), there remains a subset of patients treated with aspirin who continue to experience complications of atherosclerotic vascular disease. An incomplete response to aspirin is a major challenge facing cardiologists in the primary and secondary prevention of complications of CAD. To date, there is no consensus definition of aspirin resistance, but a variety of clinical and experimental definitions exists. In clinical terms, aspirin resistance is defined as the occurrence of vascular thrombotic events despite aspirin therapy. Experimentally, failure to prolong the bleeding time, failure to inhibit platelet aggregation (129–131), and detection of surface markers of activated platelets by flow cytometry have been used to define aspirin responsiveness (132,133).

The prevalence of aspirin resistance is variable depending on the definitions used, but ranges from 8–45% (129,132–137) (Table 2). This heterogeneity of aspirin responsiveness is observed in healthy controls (129,130,132,133), patients with CAD (129,138), cerebrovascular disease (134–137), and peripheral vascular disease (139). It appears that individual responsiveness to aspirin remains constant over the short term (130), but when patients are followed long term, one study has suggested that changes in aspirin responsiveness can occur (134). Therefore, there may be not only intersubject variability, but also time-dependent intrasubject variability in aspirin responsiveness.

The exact etiology of aspirin resistance is not known, but it is likely that a variety of mechanisms contribute to the occurrence of vascular events despite treatment with aspirin. Historically, variability in the rates of hydrolysis of aspirin presystemically in the gut and liver and systemically in the circulation has been used to explain the variation in individual responses to aspirin (140,141). However, there have been no studies to determine if this truly results in a qualitative difference in platelet function (130).

Although it has been suggested that higher doses of aspirin may be required to achieve adequate platelet inhibition in some individuals *(137)*, when clinical endpoints are examined, there is no significant difference in clinical outcomes in high-risk patients treated with high (500–1500 mg daily) vs. lower dose (75–325 mg daily) aspirin based on the meta-analysis conducted by the Antiplatelet Trialists' Collaboration *(31)*. Similarly, there are experimental data suggesting an advantage of low-dose aspirin. It has been shown that low-dose aspirin causes less inhibition of endothelial synthesis of prostacyclin, a vasodilatory prostaglandin capable of inhibiting platelet aggregation while maintaining inhibition of thromboxane-A_2 synthesis by platelets *(142)*. This theoretical benefit of low-dose aspirin is supported by the recent Aspirin and Carotid Endarterectomy (ACE) trial comparing low-dose aspirin (81 mg or 325 mg) and high-dose aspirin (650 mg or 1300 mg) in patients under-going carotid endarterectomy *(143)*. At 3 mo, the combined endpoint of stroke, MI, and death was significantly lower in the lower-dose aspirin group (6.2% vs. 8.4%, $p = 0.03$).

Gender variations in platelet responsiveness to inhibition by aspirin may exist. Aspirin has been suggested to be more efficacious in males *(132,144)* in a testosterone-dependent mechanism *(131)*, possibly through increased activity and/or slower acetylation of platelet cyclooxygenase *(145)*. In recent years, attention has focused on genetic variations in glycoproteins expressed on the surface of platelets and one investigation has suggested the platelet integrin polymorphisms may be associated with significant variability in platelet inhibition by aspirin *(146)*. Cell-to-cell interactions between platelets and erythrocytes have also been shown to be important thromboxane-A_2 independent pathways of platelet activation and recruitment *(147–149)*. Finally, aspirin resistance may be mediated by the biosynthesis of thromboxane-A_2 by sources other than the platelet. Endothelial cyclooxygenase, COX-2, is an inducible enzyme that recovers expression within hours of administration of aspirin and may therefore provide an extraplatelet mechanism of thromboxane-A_2 synthesis that is resistant to aspirin *(150–153)*. COX-2 is also expressed by platelets *(154)* and aspirin is about 170-fold less potent in inhibiting COX-2 compared to COX-1 *(155)*. Consequently, the relative extent of platelet COX-2 expression may be a determinant of aspirin responsiveness.

The clinical consequences of aspirin resistance are demonstrated along the entire spectrum of atherosclerotic vascular disease. There are reports of increased synthesis of thromboxane-A_2 despite aspirin therapy in patients with unstable angina *(138,156)* and this appears to be due to increased extraplatelet synthesis of thromboxane-A_2 *(138)*. In a study of 100 patients with peripheral vascular disease treated with aspirin (100 mg daily) for 1 yr after peripheral angioplasty, 60% of patients were either partial or nonresponders to aspirin as defined by the degree of inhibition of platelet aggregation *(139)*. Clinically, this translated into limb reocclusion in 8 of 60 aspirin nonresponders, whereas none of the aspirin responders experienced limb reocclusion ($p = 0.0093$). Among patients who have recently suffered an ischemic stroke, aspirin responsiveness was observed in only 67% of patients *(136)*. After 2 yr of follow-up, aspirin responders had an almost 10-fold lower rate of stroke, MI, or vascular death compared to aspirin nonresponders (4.4% vs. 40.1%, $p < 0.0001$).

In summary, aspirin resistance appears to be a real entity of significant clinical relevance that is likely a multifactorial process involving individual variations in the response to aspirin, alternative pathways of platelet activation, and nonplatelet mechanisms of thromboxane-A_2 synthesis. Aspirin has remained the cornerstone of primary and secondary prevention of complications of CAD. It is clear that this foundation requires reexamination and future research must be directed at the important challenge of aspirin resistance.

COMBINATION THERAPY
WITH ANTICOAGULANT AND ANTIPLATELET AGENTS

Because both platelets and the coagulation cascade are integral in the pathophysiology of intracoronary thrombosis, therapy using a combination of antiplatelet and anticoagulant agents may offer an additive benefit. This hypothesis is supported by studies among patients with prosthetic heart valves that have demonstrated a decreased risk of thromboembolic complications with combination therapy (157). The TPT study was initiated to evaluate primary prevention with either low-dose aspirin (75 mg daily), low-dose warfarin (INR target of 1.5), both, or neither in 5493 men at "greater than average risk" for ischemic heart disease (26). Overall, warfarin use, either alone or in combination with aspirin, was associated with a 21% reduction ($p = 0.003$) in all events (coronary death and fatal and nonfatal MI), with the benefit largely due to a 39% reduction in fatal events. Aspirin therapy, either alone or in combination with coumadin, was associated with a 20% reduction in events ($p = 0.004$), with most of the benefit due to a 32% reduction in nonfatal events. Combination therapy with warfarin and aspirin was associated with 15% relative reduction in the event rate compared to aspirin alone. This small effect must be considered in light of the increased rates of hemorrhagic (0.9%) and fatal (1.5%) stroke with the warfarin and aspirin combination, as well as significantly higher rates of intermediate (6.2%) and minor bleeding (48%). These results suggest a small potential benefit for combining warfarin and aspirin for primary prevention. Whether the increased risk of adverse events and the requirement for close monitoring of the INR outweigh these benefits is left up to the individual provider.

The role of combined antiplatelet and anticoagulant therapy in secondary prevention has been addressed in several trials. The CARS compared the efficacy of fixed, low-dose warfarin and aspirin with aspirin alone for secondary prevention in patients with clinically stable CAD (158). The trial was prematurely terminated due to a lack of efficacy in the combination arms vs. aspirin alone. The combination arms of this study employed rather low, set doses (1 or 3 mg) of warfarin that may have limited efficacy. The ATACS Research Group studied the combination of aspirin and anticoagulant therapy (heparin followed by warfarin) vs. aspirin alone in 214 nonprior aspirin users with either unstable angina or non-Q-wave MI (159). Those randomized to receive warfarin had a target INR of 2–3, and active treatment was maintained for 12 wk. Although combination therapy significantly reduced the incidence of primary ischemic events within the first 14 d (27% aspirin alone, 10% combination therapy, $p = 0.004$), by 12 wk there was only a trend favoring combination therapy (28% aspirin alone, 19% combination therapy, $p = 0.09$). These results are consistent with the benefit demonstrated by some studies of the acute treatment of UA with a combination of aspirin and heparin (36,160), but they do not offer strong support for prolonged oral anticoagulant therapy for these patients.

The OASIS pilot study also addressed the role of combination therapy after unstable angina or non-Q-wave MI (161). Phase 1 of this study randomized 309 patients to either fixed, low-dose warfarin (3 mg/d) or standard therapy with 87% of patients receiving aspirin in each group. This portion of OASIS confirmed the findings of the CARS trial–there was no significant reduction in events at 6 mo of follow-up with the combination of fixed, low-dose warfarin and aspirin. In phase 2, 197 patients were randomized to

Table 3
Current Trials of Combined Antiplatelet and Anticoagulant Therapy

	OASIS-2	CHAMP	WARIS-2	ASPECT-2	APRICOT-2
No. of patients	500	5000	6000	9000	300
Aspirin alone dose	NR	160 mg	75 mg	80 mg	80 mg
Combination therapies					
Aspirin Dose	NR	80 mg	75 mg	80 mg	80 mg
Warfarin Dose or Target INR	INR < 1.5 or 2.0–2.5	INR 1.5–2.5	INR 2.0–2.5 or 2.8–4.2	INR 2.0–2.5 or 2.8–4.8	INR 2.0–2.5
Follow-Up	3 mo	4 yr	2 yr	3 yr	3 mo

OASIS = Organization to Assess Strategies for Ischemic Syndromes
CHAMP = Combination Hemotherapy and Mortality Prevention
WARIS = Warfarin Re-infarction Study
ASPECT = Anticoagulants in the Secondary Prevention of Events in Coronary Thrombosis
APRICOT = Antithrombotics in the Prevention of Reocclusion in Coronary Thrombolysis
INR = International Normalized Ratio
NR = Not reported

either adjusted-dose warfarin with a target INR of 2–2.5 or standard therapy with 85% of patients in each group receiving aspirin. At 3 mo, there was a trend favoring combination therapy with a 58% relative reduction in the risk of the primary endpoint of cardiovascular death, new MI, and refractory angina (5.8% vs. 12.1%; RR = 0.42, 95% CI 0.15–1.15, $p = 0.08$). The substantially higher event rate in the aspirin arm compared with the event rate of the phase 1 study suggests a higher risk population and a potential bias favoring combination therapy. The event rates for major bleeding were too small for statistical comparison, but again, minor bleeding was significantly more frequent with combination therapy. These data suggest that adjusted-dose warfarin, unlike fixed, low-dose warfarin, in combination with aspirin may have a role in secondary prevention. Because of the consistently higher rates of minor bleeding as well as the unclear efficacy, the relative benefit of combination therapy requires further study. There are currently five ongoing trials, involving over 23,000 patients, designed to evaluate the combination of aspirin and anticoagulant therapies in patients following an acute coronary syndrome *(161,162)* (Table 3). The results of these ongoing investigations should aid considerably in determining the optimal antithrombotic regimen for secondary prevention.

Combination anticoagulant and antiplatelet therapy has also been investigated in surgical revascularization. The Post Coronary Artery Bypass Graft Trial Investigators addressed the role of low-dose warfarin and aspirin for the prevention of the progression of saphenous vein graft disease *(163)*. In this study, 1351 patients who had undergone bypass surgery 1–11 yr prior were randomized using a 2 × 2 factorial design to either aggressive or moderate cholesterol-lowering therapy, and either warfarin or placebo. All patients were encouraged to take 81 mg of aspirin daily. The warfarin dose was regulated to maintain the INR less than 2 (mean INR 1.4). After a mean follow-up of 4.3 yr, those randomized to warfarin showed no significant difference in angiographic outcomes or the combined clinical endpoint of death, nonfatal MI, stroke, CABG, or PTCA compared with placebo. Although these results cannot exclude a benefit of more aggressive long-term anticoagulation, they do not support low-dose combination therapy over aspirin alone.

CONCLUSION

Antithrombotic therapy, as it is currently used, prevents heart attacks and saves lives. For every 1000 individuals free of diagnosed atherosclerotic disease treated with aspirin over a 5-yr period, up to seven important cardiac events will be prevented. More importantly, by targeting preventative therapy to those at higher risk, a 10 times greater benefit can be achieved. In fact, when aspirin is used in patients following MI or with UA, an almost one-fourth reduction in mortality can be realized. Even though aspirin is extremely inexpensive, generally well tolerated, and at least as effective as all other currently studied antithrombotic preventative regimens, there are those individuals in whom it is not a viable therapeutic option. For these patients, data support the use of the thienopyridine derivatives as an effective aspirin alternative. The role of more aggressive long-term antiplatelet protection, in the form of either the combination of a thienopyridine and aspirin, oral GPIIb/IIIa inhibition with or without aspirin, or other agents, in secondary prevention is currently being investigated and holds great promise.

Undoubtedly, the results of numerous current trials should help better define the optimal preventative antithrombotic therapy in many patient groups. Just as the last 50 yr of antithrombotic therapy in CAD has allowed for some dramatic changes in treatment philosophy, as our understanding of the pathophysiology of all aspects of CAD continues to grow, further innovations in antithrombotic therapy will undoubtedly lead to even more dramatic results in the prevention of ischemic heart disease.

REFERENCES

1. von Rokitansky C. A Manual of Pathologic Anatomy. The Sydenham Society, London, 1852.
2. Falk E. Unstable angina with fatal outcome: dynamic coronary thrombosis leading to infarction and/ or sudden death. Autopsy evidence of recurrent mural thrombosis with peripheral embolization culminating in total vascular occlusion. Circulation 1989;71:699–708.
3. DeWood MA, Spores J, Notske R, et al. Prevalence of total coronary occlusion during the early hours of transmural myocardial infarction. N Engl J Med 1980;303:897–902.
4. Davies MJ, Thomas AC. Plaque fissuring—the cause of acute myocardial infarction, sudden ischaemic death, and crescendo angina. Br Heart J 1985;53:363–373.
5. Buja LM, Willerson JT. Clinicopathologic correlates of acute ischemic heart disease syndromes. Am J Cardiol 1981;47:343–356.
6. Bini A, Fenoglio JJJ, Mesa-Tejada R, et al. Identification and distribution of fibrinogen, fibrin and fibrin(ogen) degradation products in atherosclerosis. Arteriosclerosis 1989;9:109–121.
7. MacIsaac AI, Thomas JD, Topol EJ. Toward the quiescent plaque. J Am Coll Cardiol 1993;22:1228–1241.
8. Fuster V, Badimon L, Badimon JJ, Chesebro JH. The pathogenesis of coronary artery disease and the acute coronary syndromes. N Engl J Med 1992;326:242–250:310–318.
9. Davies MJ, Bland MJ, Hangartner WR, et al. Factors influencing the presence or absence of acute coronary thrombi in sudden ischemic death. Eur Heart J 1989;10:203–208.
10. Thaulow E, Erikssen J, Sandvik L, et al. Blood platelet count and function are related to total and cardiovascular death in apparently healthy men. Circulation 1991;84:613–617.
11. Trip MD, Cats VM, van Capelle FJL, Vreeken J. Platelet hyperactivity and prognosis in survivors of myocardial infarction. N Engl J Med 1990;322:1549–1554.
12. Tschoepe D, Schultheiss HP, Kolarov P, et al. Platelet membrane activation markers are predictive for increased risk of acute ischemic events after PTCA. Circulation 1993;88:37–42.
13. Kaplan AV, Leung LL-K, Leng W-H, et al. Roles of thrombin and platelet membrane glycoprotein IIb/IIIa in platelet-subendothelial deposition after angioplasty in an ex vivo whole artery model. Circulation 1991;84:1279–1288.
14. Holmsen H, Weiss HJ. Secretable storage pools in platelets. Ann Rev Med 1979;30:119–134.
15. Stone E. An account of the success of the bark of the willow in the cure of agues. Philos Trans R Soc Lond [Biol] 1763;53:195–200.

16. Binz C. Vorlesungen Ueber Pharmakologie, 2nd ed. Berlin, 1891.
17. Weiss HJ, Aledort LM. Impaired platelet-connective-tissue reaction in man after aspirin ingestion. Lancet 1967;2:495–497.
18. Craven LL. Experiences with aspirin (acetylsalicylic acid) in the nonspecific prophylaxis of coronary thrombosis. Mississippi Valley Med J 1953;75:38–44.
19. Vane JR. Inhibition of prostaglandin synthesis as a mechanism of action for aspirin-like drugs. Nature 1971;231:231–235.
20. Smith JB, Willis AL. Aspirin selectively inhibits prostaglandin production in human platelets. Nature 1971;231:235–237.
21. Patrono C. Aspirin as an antiplatelet drug. N Engl J Med 1994;330(18):1287–1294.
22. Taylor D, Barnett H, Haynes R. Low-dose and high-dose acetylsalicylic acid for patients undergoing carotid endarterectomy: a randomised controlled trial. Lancet 1999;353:2179–2184.
23. Steering Committee of the Physicians' Health Study Research Group. Preliminary report: findings from the aspirin component of the ongoing physicians' health study. N Engl J Med 1988;318(4): 262–264.
24. Steering Committee of the Physicians' Health Study Research Group. Final report on the aspirin component of the ongoing physicians' health study. N Engl J Med 1989;321(3):129–135.
25. Peto R, Gray R, Collins R, et al. Randomised trial of prophylactic aspirin in British male doctors. Br Med J 1988;296:313–316.
26. The Medical Research Council's General Practice Research Framework. Thrombosis prevention trial: randomised trial of low-intensity oral anticoagulation with warfarin and low-dose aspirin in the primary prevention of ischaemc heart disease in men at increased risk. Lancet 1998;351:323–341.
27. Hansson L, Zanchetti A, Carruthers S. Effects of intensive blood pressure lowering and low-dose aspirin in patients with hypertension: results of the Hypertension Optimal Treatment (HOT) randomised trial. Lancet 1998;351:1755–1762.
28. Hennekens CH, Peto R, Hutchison GB, Doll R. An overview of the British and American aspirin studies. N Engl J Med 1988;318:923–924.
29. Buring JE, Hennekens CH, for the Women's Health Study Research Group. The Women's Health Study: Summary of the study design. J Myocardial Ischemia 1992;4:27–29.
30. Antiplatelet Trialists' Collaboration. Secondary prevention of vascular disease by prolonged antiplatelet therapy. Br Med J 1988;296:320–331.
31. Antiplatelet Trialists' Collaboration. Collaborative overview of randomised trials of antiplatelet therapy—II: maintenance of vascular graft or arterial patency by antiplatelet therapy. Br Med J 1994; 308:159–168.
32. Ridker PM, Manson JE, Gaziano JM, et al. Low-dose aspirin therapy for chronic stable angina. A randomised, placebo-controlled clinical trial. Ann Intern Med 1991;114:835–839.
33. Chesebro JH, Webster MWI, Zoldhelyi P, et al. Antithrombotic therapy and progression of coronary artery disease. Antiplatelet versus antithrombins. Circulation 1992;86(Suppl III):III-100-III–111.
34. Juul-Moller S, Edvardsson N, Johnmatz B, et al., for the Swedish Angina Pectoris Aspirin Trial (SAPAT) group. Double-blind trial of aspirin in primary prevention of myocardial infarction in patients with stable chronic angina pectoris. Lancet 1992;340:1421–1425.
35. Rahimtoola SH. Coronary bypass surgery for unstable angina. Circulation 1984;69:842–848.
36. Theroux P, Ouimet H, McCans J, et al. Aspirin, heparin or both to treat acute unstable angina. N Engl J Med 1988;319:1105–1111.
37. The RISC Group. Risk of myocardial infarction and death during treatment with low dose aspirin and intravenous heparin in men with unstable coronary artery disease. Lancet 1990;336:827–830.
38. Wallentin LC, and the RISC Group. Aspirin (75 mg/day) after an episode of unstable coronary artery disease: long-term effects on the risk of myocardial infarction, occurrence of severe angina and the need for revascularization. J Am Coll Cardiol 1991;18:1587–1593.
39. Lewis Jr HD, Davis JW, Archibald DG, et al. Protective effects of aspirin against acute myocardial infarction and death in men with unstable angina: results of a Veterans Administration Cooperative Study. N Engl J Med 1983;309:396–403.
40. Holdright D, Patel D, Cunningham D, et al. Comparison of the effect of heparin and aspirin versus aspirin alone on transient myocardial ischemia and in-hospital prognosis in patients with unstable angina. J Am Coll Cardiol 1994;24:39–45.
41. ISIS-2 Collaborative Group. Randomised trial of intravenous streptokinase, oral aspirin, both, or neither among 17,187 cases of suspected acute myocardial infarction: ISIS-2. Lancet 1988;2:349–360.

42. Gabriel SE, Jaakkimainen L, Bombardier C. Risk of serious gastrointestinal complications related to nonsteroidal anti-inflammatory drugs: a meta-analysis. Ann Intern Med 1991;115:787–796.
43. Weil J, Colin-Jones D, Langman M, et al. Prophylactic aspirin and risk of peptic ulcer bleeding. Br Med J 1995;310:827–830.
44. The Dutch TIA Study Group. A comparison of two doses of aspirin (30 mg vs. 283 mg a day) in patients after transient ischemic attack or minor ischemic stroke. N Engl J Med 1991;325:1261–1266.
45. Farrell B, Godwin J, Richards S, Warlow C. The United Kingdom transient ischemic attack (UK-TIA) aspirin trial: final results. J Neurol Neurosurg Psychiatry 1991;54:1044–1054.
46. Hofteizer JW, Silvoso GR, Burks M, Ivey K. Comparison of the effects of regular and enteric coated aspirin on gastroduodenal mucosa of man. Lancet 1980;2:609–612.
47. Leonards JR, Levy G. Effect of pharmaceutical formulation on gastrointestinal bleeding from aspirin tablets. Arch Intern Med 1972;129:457–460.
48. Meade TW, Roderick PJ, Brennan PJ, et al. Extracranial bleeding and other symp-toms due to low dose aspirin and low intensity oral anticoagulation. Thromb Haemost 1992;68:1–6.
49. Krumholz HM, Radford MJ, Ellerbeck EF, et al. Aspirin in the treatment of acute myocardial in elderly medicare beneficiaries. Patterns of use and outcomes. Circulation 1995;92:2841–2847.
50. Krumholz HM, Radford MJ, Ellerbeck EF, et al. Aspirin for secondary prevention after acute myo-cardial infarction in the elderly: prescribed use and outcomes. Ann Intern Med 1996;124:292–298.
51. Hennekens CH, Jonas MA, Buring JE. The benefits of aspirin in acute myocardial infarction: still a well kept secret in the U.S. Arch Intern Med 1994;154:37–39.
52. Hardisty R, Powling M, Nokes T. The action of ticlopidine on human platelets: studies on aggregation, secretion, calcium mobilization and membrane glycoproteins. Thromb Haemost 1990;64:150–155.
53. Defreyn G, Bernat A, Delebasse D, Maffrand J-P. Pharmacology of ticlopidine: a review. Semin Thromb Hemost 1989;15:159–166.
54. Bachman F, Savcic M, Hauert J, et al. Rapid onset of inhibition of ADP-induced platelet aggregation by a loading dose of clopidogrel [abs]. Eur Heart J 1996;17:263.
55. McTavish D, Faulds D, Goa K. Ticlopidine: an updated review of its pharmacology and therapeutic use in platelet-dependent disorders. Drugs 1990;40:238–259.
56. Pengo V, Boschello M, Marzari A. Adenosine diphosphate induces alpha-granules release from plate-lets of native whole blood is reduced by ticlopidine but not by aspirin or dipyridamole. Thromb Hae-most 1986;56:147–150.
57. Rotondo S, Tascione E, Cerletti C. Ticlopidine does not reduce in vivo platelet thromboxane biosyn-thesis and metabolism in diabetic patients. Platelets 1990;4:97–100.
58. Makkar R, Litvack F, Kaul S. High shear overrides the antithrombotic effects of aspirin on stent throm-bosis. J Am Coll Cardiol 1997;29(Suppl A):354A.
59. Cattaneo M, Lombardi R, Bettega D. Shear-induced platelet aggregation is potentiated by desmopressin and inhibited by ticlopidine. Arterioscler Thromb 1993;13:393–397.
60. Makkar R, Eigler NSK. Clopidogrel, a novel platelet ADP-receptor antagonist inhibits aspirin and ticlopidine resistant stent thrombosis. J Am Coll Cardiol 1997;29(Suppl A):353A.
61. Roald H, Barstad R, Kierulf P. Clopidogrel—a platelet inhibitor which inhibits thrombogensis in nonanti-coagulated human blood independently of blood flow conditions. Thromb Haemost 1994;71:655–662.
62. Sharis P, Cannon C, Loscalzo J. The antiplatelet effects of ticlopidine and clopidogrel. Ann Intern Med 1998;129:394–405.
63. Gents M, Blakely J, Easton J. The Canadian American Ticlopidine Study (CATS) in thromboembolic stroke. Lancet 1989;1:1215–1220.
64. Janzon L, Bergqvist D, Boberg J, et al. Prevention of myocardial infarction and stroke in patients with intermittent claudication; effects of ticlopidine. Results from STIMS, the Swedish Ticlopidine Multi-centre Study. J Intern Med 1990;227:301–308.
65. Arcan J, Blanchard J, Boissel J. Multi-center double-blind study of ticlopidine in the treatment of intermittent claudication and prevention of its complications. Angiology 1988;39:802–811.
66. Blanchard J, Carreras L, Kindermans M. Results of EMATAP: a double-blind placebo-controlled multicentre trial of ticlopidine in patients with peripheral arterial disease. Nouv Rev Fr Hematol 1993; 35:523–528.
67. Hass W, Easton J, Adams JH, et al. A randomized trial comparing ticlopidine hydrochloride with aspirin for the prevention of stroke in high risk patients. N Engl J Med 1989;321:501–507.
68. Knudsen JB, Kjoller E, Skagen K, Gormsen J. The effect of ticlopidine on platelet functions in acute myocardial infarction. A double blind controlled trial. Thromb Haemost 1985;53(3):332–336.

69. Sadowski Z, Luczak D, Dyduszynski A, et al. Comparison of ticlopidine and aspirin in unstable angina [abstract]. Eur Heart J 1995;16(Suppl):259.
70. CAPRIE SC. A randomised, blinded, trial of clopidogrel versus aspirin in patients at risk of ischaemic events. Lancet 1996;348:1329–1339.
71. Ramirez J, Mansur A, Martins J. Effect of ticlopidine and dipyridamole on platelet aggregation and count in patients with chronic stable angina pectoris. Arg Bras Cardiol 1991;56:323–327.
72. Balsano F, Rizzon P, Violi F, et al. Antiplatelet treatment with ticlopidine in unstable angina. A controlled multicenter clinical trial. Circulation 1990;82:17–26.
73. Fuster V, Chesebro JH. Role of platelets and platelet inhibitors in aorto-coronary vein graft disease. Circulation 1986;73:227–232.
74. Chevigne M, David J, Rigo P. Effect of ticlopidine on saphenous vein patency rates: a double-blind study. Ann Thorac Surg 1984;37:371–378.
75. Limet R, David J, Rigo P. Prevention of aorta-coronary bypass graft occlusion. Beneficial effect of ticlopidine on early and late patency rates of venous coronary bypass grafts: a double-blind study. J Thorac Cardiovasc Surg 1987;94:773–783.
76. Becquemin J. Effect of ticlopidine on the long-term patency of saphenous-vein bypass grafts in the legs. N Engl J Med 1997;337:1726–1731.
77. Bellavance A. Efficacy of ticlopidine and aspirin for prevention of reversible cerebrovascular ischemic events: the ticlopidine and aspirin stroke study. Stroke 1993;24:1452–1457.
78. Bertrand M, Legrand V, Boland J. Randomized multicenter comparison of conventional anticoagulation versus antiplatelet therapy in unplanned and elective coronary stenting: the Full Anticoagulation Versus Aspirin and Ticlopidine (FANTASTIC) study. Circulation 1998;98:1597–1603.
79. Wysowksi DK, Bacsanyi J. Blood dyscrasias and hematologic reactions in ticlopidine users. JAMA 1996;276(12):952.
80. Schror K. Antiplatelet drugs: a comparative review. Drugs 1995;50:7–28.
81. Page Y, Tardy B, Zeni F, et al. Thrombotic thrombocytopenic purpura related to ticlopidine. Lancet 1991;337:774–776.
82. Bennet CL, Weinberg PD, Rozenberg-Ben-Dror K, et al. Thrombotic thrombocytopenic purpura associated with ticlopidine. A review of 60 cases. Ann Intern Med 1998;128:541–544.
83. Steinhubl S, Tan W, Foody J. TTP due to ticlopidine following coronary stenting. JAMA 1999;281:806–810.
84. Bennett C, Kiss J, Weinberg P, et al. Thrombotic thrombocytopenic purpura after stenting and ticlopidine. Lancet 1998;352:1036–1037.
85. Splawinska B, Kuzniar J, Malinga K, et al. The efficacy of and potency of antiplatelet activity of ticlopidine is increased by aspirin. Int J Clin Pharmacol Ther 1996;34:352–356.
86. Uchiyama S, Sone R, Nagayama T, et al. Combination therapy with low-dose aspirin and ticlopidine in cerebral ischemia. Stroke 1989;20:1643–1647.
87. Rupprecht H-J, Darius H, Borkowski U, et al. Comparison of antiplatelet effects of aspirin, ticlopidine, or their combination after stent implantation. Circulation 1998;97:1046–1052.
88. Schomig A, Neumann F, Kastrati A, et al. A randomized comparison of antiplatelet and anticoagulant therapy after placement of coronary-artery stents. N Engl J Med 1996;334:1084–1089.
89. Leon MB, Baim DS, Popma JJ, et al. A clinical trial comparing three anti-thrombotic regimens following coronary artery stenting. N Engl J Med 1998;339:1665–1671.
90. Morice M, Aubry P, Benveniste E. The MUST trial: acute results and six-month clinical follow-up. J Invas Cardiol 1998;10:457–463.
91. Simonton CA, Leon MB, Baim DS, et al. "Optimal" directional coronary atherectomy. Final results of the Optimal Atherectomy Restenosis Study (OARS). Circulation 1998;97:332–339.
92. Califf RM, Abdelmeguid AE, Kuntz RE, et al. Myonecrosis after revascularization procedures. J Am Coll Cardiol 1998;31:241–251.
93. Abdelmeguid AE, Topol EJ. The myth of the myocardial "Infarctlet" during percutaneous coronary revascularization procedures. Circulation 1997;94:3369–3375.
94. Kong TQ, Davidson CJ, Meyers SN, et al. Prognostic implication of creatine kinase elevation following elective coronary artery interventions. JAMA 1997;277:461–466.
95. Topol E, Ferguson J, Weisman H. Long-term protection from myocardial ischemic events in a randomized trial of brief integrin b_3-blockade with percutaneous coronary intervention. JAMA 1997;278:479–484.

96. Steinhubl SR, Lauer MS, Mukerjee DP, et al. The duration of pretreatment with ticlopidine prior to stenting is associated with the risk of procedure-related non-Q-wave myocardial infarctions. J Am Coll Cardiol 1998;32:1366–1370.
97. Coller B, Peerschke E, Scudder L. A murine monoclonal antibody that completely blocks the binding of fibrinogen to platelets produces a thrombasthenic-like state in normal platelets and binds to glycoproteins IIb and/or IIIa. J Clin Invest 1983;72:325–338.
98. Lefkovits J, Plow E, Topol E. Platelet glycoprotein IIb/IIIa receptors in cardiovascular medicine. N Engl J Med 1995;332:1553–1559.
99. Madan M, Berkowitz S, Tcheng J. Glycoprotein IIb/IIIa integrin blockade. Circulation 1998;98: 2629–2635.
100. The Platelet Receptor Inhibition in Ischemic Syndrome Management (PRISM) study investigators. A comparison of aspirin plus tirofiban with aspirin plus heparin for unstable angina. N Engl J Med 1998; 338:1498–1505.
101. The EPILOG Investigators. Platelet glycoprotein IIb/IIIa receptor blockade and low-dose heparin during percutaneous coronary revascularization. N Engl J Med 1997;336:1689–1696.
102. The RESTORE investigators. Effects of platelet glycoprotein IIb/IIIa blockade with tirofiban on advers cardiac events in patients with unstable angina or acute myocardial infarction undergoing coronary angioplasty. Circulation 1997;1997:1445–1453.
103. Merlini PA, Bauer KA, Oltrona L, et al. Persistant activation of the coagulation system in unstable angina and myocardial infarction. Circulation 1994;90:61–68.
104. Cannon C, McCabe C, Borzak S. Randomized trial of oral platelet glycoprotein IIb/IIIa receptor antagonist, sibrafin, in patients after an acute coronary syndrome. Circulation 1998;97:340–349.
105. Emmons PR, Harrison MJG, Honour AJ, Mitchell JRA. Effect of dipyridamole on human platelet behaviour. Lancet 1965;2:603–606.
106. FitzGerald GA. Dipyridamole. N Engl J Med 1987;316(20):1247–1257.
107. Diener H, Cunha L, Forbes C, Sivenius J, Smets P, lowenthal A. European Stroke Prevention Study 2. Dipyridamole and acetylsalicylic acid in the secondary prevention of stroke. J Neuro Sci 1996;143:1–13.
108. Smythe HA, Orgryzlo MA, Murphy EA, Mustard JF. The effect of sulfinpyrazone (Anturane) on platelet economy and blood coagulation in man. Can Med Assoc J 1965;92:818.
109. Ali M, McDonald JWD. Effects of sulfinpyrazone on platelet prostoglandin synthesis and platelet release of serotonin. J Lab Clin Med 1977;89:868–875.
110. Anturane Reinfarction Italian Study. Sulphinpyrazone in post-myocardial infarction. Lancet 1982;1: 237–242.
111. Anturane Reinfarction Trial Group. Sulfinpyrazone in the prevention of sudden death after myocardial infarction. N Engl J Med 1980;302:250–256.
112. Sills T, Heptinstall S. Effects of a thromboxane synthase inhibitor and a cAMP phosphodiesterase inhibitor, singly and in combination, on platelet behaviour. Thromb Haemost 1986;55:305–308.
113. Mayeux PR, Morton HE, Gillard J, et al. The affinities of prostaglandin H2 and thromboxane A2 for their receptors are similar in washed human platelets. Biochem Biophys Res Commun 1988;157:733–739.
114. Savage MP, Goldberg S, Bove AA, et al. Effect of thromboxane A2 blockade on clinical outcome and restenosis after successful coronary angioplasty. Multi-Hospital Eastern Atlantic Restenosis Trial (M-HEART II). Circulation 1995;92:3194–3200.
115. Serruys PW, Rutsch W, Heyndrickx GR, et al. Prevention of restenosis after percutaneous transluminal coronary angioplasty with thromboxane A2 receptor blockade: a randomized, double-blind placebo-controlled trial. Circulation 1991;84:1568–1580.
116. The RAPT Investigators. Randomized trial of ridogrel, a combined thromboxane A2 synthase inhibitor and thromboxane A2/prostaglandin endoperoxide receptor antagonist, versus aspirin as adjunct to thrombolysis in patients with acute myocardial infarction. The Ridogrel versus Aspirin Patency Trial (RAPT). Circulation 1994;89:588–595.
117. Anonymous. Cilostazol. Med Lett Drugs Ther 1999;7:44.
118. Kimura Y, Tani T, Kanbe T, Wantanabe K. Effect of cilostazol on platelet agregation and experimental thrombosis. Arzneimittelforschung/Drug Res 1985;35:1144–1449.
119. Yasunaga K, Mase K. Antiaggregatory effect of oral cilostazol and recovery of platelet aggregability in patients with cerebrovascular disease. Arzneimittelforschung/Drug Res 1985;35:1189–1192.
120. Tanaka T, Ishikawa T, Hagiwara M, et al. Effect of cilostazol, a selective cAMP phosphodiesterase inhibitor on the contraction of vascular smooth muscle. Pharmacology 1988;36:313–320.

121. Sarkin E, Markham A. Cilostazol. Drugs Aging 1999;14:63–71.
122. Dawson D, Cutler B, Strandness D. Cilostazol has beneficial effects in treatment of intermitent claudi-cation: results from a multicenter, randomized, prospective, double-blinded trial. Circulation 1998;98: 678–686.
123. Ishizaka N, Taguchi J, Kimura Y, et al. Effects of a single local administration of cliostazol on neointima formation in balloon injured rat carotid arteries. Atherosclerosis 1999;142:41–46.
124. Yamasaki M, Hara K, Ikari Y, et al. Effect of cilostazol on late lumen loss after Palmaz-Schatz stent implantation. Cathet Cardiovasc Diagn 1998;44:387–391.
125. Tsuchikane E, Fukuhara A, Kobayashi T, et al. Impact of cilostazol on restenosis after percutaneous balloon angioplasty. Circulation 1999;100:21–26.
126. Yoon Y, Lee D, Pyun W, Kim I. Comparison of cilostazol and ticlopidine after coronary artery stenting: immediate and long-term results. J Am Coll Cardiol 1999;33(Suppl A):40A.
127. Matsumoto Y, Tani T, Watanabe K, Kimura Y. Effects of cilostazol, an antiplatelet drug, on smooth muscle cell proliferation after endothelial cell denudation in rats. Jpn J Pharmacol 1992;58:284.
128. Takahashi S, Oida K, Fujiwara R, Maeda H. Effect of cilostazol, a cyclic AMP phosphodiesterase inhibitor, on the proliferation of rat aortic smooth muscle cells in culture. J Cardiovasc Pharmacol 1992;20:900–906.
129. Buchanan M, Brister S. Individual variation in the effects of ASA on platelet function: implications for the use of ASA clinically. Can J Cardiol 1995;11:221–227.
130. Pappas J, Westengard J, Bull B. Population variability in the effect of aspirin on platelet function. Arch Pathol Lab Med 1994;118:801–804.
131. Spranger M, Aspey B, Harrison D. Sex differences in antithrombotic effect of aspirin. Stroke 1988; 20:34–37.
132. Valettas N, Morgan C, Reis M. Aspirin resistance using flow cytometry. Blood 1997;90(Suppl I):124b.
133. Farrell T, Hayes P, Tracey B. Unexpected, discordant effects of aspirin on platelet reactivity. J Am Coll Cadiol 1998;31(Suppl A):352A.
134. Helgason CM, Bolin KM, Hoff JA, et al. Development of aspirin resistance in persons with previous ischemic stroke. Stroke 1994;25:2331–2336.
135. Helgason C, Hoff J, Kondos G. Platelet aggregation in patients with atrial fibrillation taking aspirin or warfarin. Stroke 1993;24:1458–1461.
136. Grotemeyer K, Scharafinski H, Husstedt I. Two-year follow-up of aspirin responder and aspirin non-responder. A pilot study including 18 post-stroke patients. Thromb Res 1993;71:397–403.
137. Helgason C, Tortorice K, Winkler S. Aspirin response and failure in cerebral infarction. Stroke 1993;24: 345–350.
138. Cipollone F, Patrignani P, Greco A. Differential suppression of thromboxane biosynthesis by indobufen and aspirin in patients with unstable angine. Circulation 1997;96:1109–1116.
139. Mueller M, Salat A, Stangl P. Variable platelet response to low-dose ASA and the risk of limb deter-ioration in patients submitted to peripheral arterial angioplasty. Thromb Haemost 1997;78:1003–1007.
140. Ryan W, Hakenkamp K. Variable response to aspirin measured by platelet aggregation and bleeding time. Lab Med 1991;22:197–202.
141. Akopov S, Grigorian G, Gabrielian E. Dose-dependent aspirin hydrolysis and platelet aggregation in patients with atherosclerosis. J Clin Pharmacol 1992;32:133–135.
142. Tohgi H, Konno S, Tamura B. Effects of low to high doses of aspirin on platelet aggregability and metabolites of thromboxane-A_2 and prostacyclin. Stroke 1992;23:1400–1404.
143. Taylor D, Barnett H, Haynes R. Low-dose and high-dose acetylsalicylic acid for patients undergoing carotid endarterectomy: a randomised controlled trial. Lancet 1999;353:2179–2184.
144. The Canadian Cooperative Study Group. A randomised trial of aspirin and sulfinpyrazone in threat-ened stroke. N Engl J Med 1978;297:1246–1249.
145. De La Cruz J, Bellido I, Camara F. Effect of acetylsalicyclic acid on platelet aggregation in male and female whole blood: an in vitro study. Scand J Haematol 1986;36:394–397.
146. Cooke G, Bray P, Hamlington J. Pl^{A2} polymorphism and efficacy of aspirin. Lancet 1998;351:1253.
147. Santos MT, Valles J, Aznar J, et al. Prothrombotic effects of erythrocytes on platelet reactivity. Reduc-tion by aspirin. Circulation 1997;95:63–68.
148. Valles J, Santos M, Aznar J. Erythrocyte promotion of platelet reactivity dcereases the effectiveness of aspirin as an antithrombotic therapeutic modality. Circulation 1998;97:350–355.
149. Sorli P, Garcia-Palmieri M, Costas R. Hematocrit and risk of coronary artery disease: the Puerto Rico Health Program. Am Heart J 1981;101:456–61.

150. Meade E, Smith W, DeWitt D. Differential inhibition of prostaglandin endoperoxide synthase (cyclo-oxygenase) isozymes by aspirin and other non-steroidal anti-inflammatory drugs. J Biol Chem 1993; 268:6610–6614.
151. Vane J. Inhibition of prostaglandin synthesis as a mechanism of action for aspirin-like drugs. Nature 1971;231:232–235.
152. Smith W, DeWitt D. Biochemistry of prostaglandin endoperoxide H synthase-1 and synthase-2 and their differential susceptibility to nonsteroidal anti-inflammatory drugs. Semin Nephrol 1995;15:179–194.
153. Karim S, Habib A, Levy-Toledano S. Cyclooxygenases-1 and -2 of endothelial cells utilize exogenous or endogenous arachidonic acid for transcellular production of thromboxane. J Biol Chem 1996;271: 12,042–12,048.
154. Weber A, Zimmermann K, Meyer-Kirchrath J, Schror K. Cyclooxygenase-2 in human platelets as a possible factor in aspirin resistance. Lancet 1999;353:900.
155. Vane J, Bakhe YS, Botting R. Cyclooxygenase 1 and 2. Ann Rev Pharmacol Toxicol 1998;38:97–120.
156. Vejar M, Fragasso G, Hackett D. Dissociation of platelet activation and spontaneous myocardial ischemia in unstable angina. Thromb Haemost 1990;63:163–168.
157. Chesebro JH, Fuster V, McGoon DC, et al. Trial of combined warfarin and dipyridamole or aspirin therapy in prosthetic heart valve replacement: danger of aspirin compared with dipyridamole. Am J Cardiol 1983;51:1537–1541.
158. Coumadin Aspirin Reinfarction Study (CARS) Investigators. Randomised double-blind trial of fixed low-dose warfarin with aspirin after myocardial infarction. Lancet 1997;350:389–396.
159. Cohen M, Adams PC, Parry G, et al. Combination antithrombotic therapy in unstable rest angina and non-Q-wave infarction in nonprior aspirin users. Primary end points analysis from the ATACS trial. Circulation 1994;89:81–88.
160. Oler A, Whooley MA, Oler J, Grady D. Adding heparin to aspirin reduces the incidence of myocardial infarction and death in patients with unstable angina. JAMA 1996;276:811–815.
161. Anand S, Yusuf S, Pogue J, Weitz J, Flather M, for the OASIS Pilot Study investigators. Long-term oral anticoagulant therapy in patients with unstable angina or suspected non-Q-wave myocardial infarction: organization to assess strategies for ischemic syndromes (OASIS) pilot study results. Circulation 1998;98:1064–1070.
162. Altman R, Rouvier J, Gurfinkel E. Oral anticoagulant treatment with and without aspirin. Thromb Haemost 1995;74(1):506–510.
163. The Post Coronary Artery Bypass Graft Trial Investigators. The effect of aggressive lowering of low-density lipoprotein cholesterol levels and low-dose anticoagulation on obstructive changes in saphenous vein coronary artery bypass grafts. N Engl J Med 1997;336:153–162.
164. Hurlen M, Seljeflot I, Arnesen H. Platelet aggregability after myocardial infarction. Evidence of aspirin non-responsiveness in a subpopulation [abstr]? Eur Heart J 1996;17:262.
165. Poggio ED, Kottke-Marchant K, Welsh PA, Brooks LM, Dela Rosa LR, Topol EJ. The prevalence of aspirin resistance in cardiac patients as measured by platelet aggregation and PFA-100 [abstr]. J Am Coll Cardiol 1999;33(Suppl A):254A.

15

Exercise Testing and Risk Assessment

Christopher R. Cole, MD
and Michael S. Lauer, MD

INTRODUCTON

With the development of advanced imaging modalities, the regular exercise electro-cardiographic (ECG) test has come to be regarded by some as passé. This has been due in large part to the low sensitivity and specificity for the diagnosis of coronary artery disease (CAD). With newer methods of interpretation, however, exercise testing remains a powerful and inexpensive prognostic tool. The use of the exercise test has important implications for risk stratification as a part of prevention strategies and for post-myocardial infarction (MI) management. This chapter focuses primarily on the prognostic implications of exercise testing using cardiovascular events and mortality as endpoints. It examines all aspects of the exercise test including functional capacity, heart rate changes during exercise, blood pressure (BP) response, and more recent methods of computerized interpretation of the exercise ECG.

STANDARD METHODS OF INTERPRETATION

Exercise ECGs are interpreted visually at most centers, with a study being considered abnormal if there is at least 1 mm of horizontal or downsloping ST-segment depression at 60–80 ms after the J-point *(1)*. This approach has been used for decades. Numerous studies

From: *Contemporary Cardiology: Preventive Cardiology:*
Strategies for the Prevention and Treatment of Coronary Artery Disease
Edited by: J. Foody © Humana Press Inc., Totowa, NJ

in which patients have undergone both exercise ECG and coronary angiography have demonstrated poor test accuracy with low sensitivity and specificity (2–6). Most of these studies suffer from inherent sequential workup bias, as patients with negative exercise ECGs are less likely to be referred for coronary angiography; this bias results in inflated sensitivity and deflated specificity (7–11). A recent prospective study of 814 male veterans who agreed to undergo both exercise and coronary angiography demonstrated poor sensitivity (about 45%), but reasonably good specificity (about 85%) for the diagnosis of coronary disease, defined as the presence of at least one 50% coronary stenosis (12).

The poor diagnostic performance of exercise ECG has led many clinicians to routinely request more costly imaging studies, although some groups have argued against this (13). Reasons why the exercise ECG may perform poorly include the following: trying to find the wrong lesion, trying to answer the wrong question, and using the wrong methods.

Trying to find the wrong lesion: exercise ECG relies on the presence of hemodynamically obstructive lesions; a 50% lesion would not be expected to produce stress induced ischemia.

Trying to answer the wrong question: many, if not most patients referred for exercise ECG have some degree of coronary disease; the main question for the clinician is whether their disease is severe enough that either myocardial revascularization or aggressive medical therapy are indicated. This requires knowledge of prognosis, rather than diagnosis. Thus, research on exercise testing should focus much more on prediction of events rather than prediction of angiographic findings.

Using the wrong methods: exercise ECG potentially involves much more than looking at visually assessed ECG changes with exercise. Important non-ECG variables to consider include functional capacity (14), heart rate (15–18) and BP (19,20) responses, and arrhythmias (21); some of these variables have been tightly linked with prognosis. Some researchers have proposed using computerized measures of ST-segment changes adjusted for heart rate (HR) (22).

FUNCTIONAL CAPACITY

A direct relationship between functional capacity and survival has been well established in a number of prospective, population-based studies (23–34). In the clinical setting, exercise capacity has also proven to be a powerful and independent predictor of cardiac morbidity and mortality and all-cause mortality (14,35–46).

Exercise capacity is usually estimated in the stress lab based on published tables (1). The standard unit is the MET, or metabolic equivalent, which is the amount of oxygen consumed at rest. In a typical adult, 1 MET equals 3.5 mL/kg/min of oxygen uptake. Direct measurement of exercise capacity is possible using sophisticated gas exchange analysis, which in clinical practice is primarily used among patients with severe heart failure (47–50). Concern has been raised that estimated exercise capacity is inherently inaccurate, particularly when standard treadmill protocols are used, in which case it tends to be systematically overestimated (51).

A functional classification for an individual may be determined based on the workload achieved. Exercise capacity is strongly correlated with age and gender; therefore, any classification scheme must take these important confounders into account. The classification system in use at the Cleveland Clinic is shown in Table 1. A classification using directly measured oxygen uptake is presented in Table 2 (51a).

Table 1
Exercise Capacity Classifications by Age and Sex

Women					
Age	Poor	Fair	Average	Good	High
20–29	<7.5	8–10.3	10.3–12.5	12.5–16	>16
30–39	<7	7–9	9–11	11–15	>15
40–49	<6	6–8	8–10	10–14	>14
50–59	<5	5–7	7–9	9–13	>13
60–69	<4.5	4.5–6	6–8	8–11.5	>11.5
70–79	<3.5	3.5–4.5	4.5–6.5	6.5–8	> 8
≥80	<2.5	2.5–4	4–5.5	5.5–7	> 7
Men					
Age	Poor	Fair	Average	Good	High
20–29	<8	8–11	11–14	14–17	>17
30–39	<7.5	7.5–10	10–12.5	12.5–16	>16
40–49	<7	7–8.5	8.5–11.5	11.5–15	>15
50–59	<6	6–8	8–11	11–14	>14
60–69	<5.5	5.5–7	7–9.5	9.5–13	>13
70–79	<4.5	4.5–5.5	5.5–8	8–9.5	>9.5
≥80	<3.5	3.5–4.5	4.5–6.5	6.5–7.5	>7.5

For any given age (in years) and workload (in METs) the exercise capacity can be classified into one of five categories.

Table 2
Functional Classification of Patients Based on Measured Gas Exchange

Severity of impairment	Functional class	VO_{2max} (mL/kg/min)
None to mild	A	>20
Mild to moderate	B	16–20
Moderate to severe	C	10–15
Severe	D	<10

Modified from ref. 51a.

There have been a number of clinical studies that have used exercise capacity as a predictor of mortality. The Seattle Heart Watch Study (36) was a prospective study of 1852 men with a known history of CAD. After treadmill testing they were followed for 3 yr, during which time there were 195 deaths. One of the most powerful predictors of death was poor exercise capacity (as measured by a short duration of exercise). This remained true in both univariate and multivariate analysis of clinical and exercise data.

Subsequently, Bruce and associates (39) prospectively followed 3611 men and 547 women with no known CAD for 10 yr. In asymptomatic men they found that any clinical risk factor (age >55, hypertension, tobacco use) when combined with two or more exercise variables (angina on the treadmill, HR <90% age-predicted maximum, double product <80% predicted, >20% difference between observed $VO_{2\,max}$ and that expected for a healthy person of similar age) predicted a 33-fold increase in the combined endpoint of worsened angina, MI, coronary artery bypass surgery, or death.

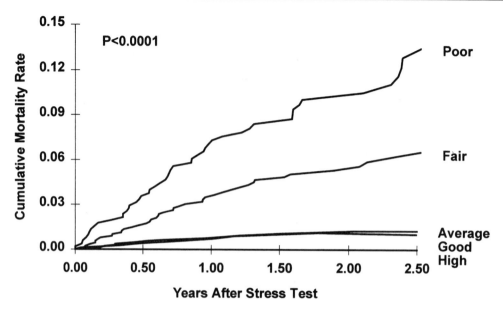

Fig. 1. Kaplan-Meier plot relating age- and gender-specific estimated functional capacity to total all-cause mortality. Taken from ref. *14.*

In a study by Podrid and colleagues *(38),* 142 men with a history of CAD and a strongly positive exercise test (>2 mm ST-segment depression) were divided into three groups by duration of exercise during a Bruce protocol treadmill test. Men who exercised 1–6 min ($\cong$6 METs) had a significant increase in mortality when compared to those exercising 6–9 min ($\cong$8 METs) or >9 min ($\cong$11 METs). There were no survival differences between the two groups of higher functional capacity. A low workload is also predictive of cardiac events as demonstrated by Swada and co-workers *(52),* who showed an increased cardiac event rate in patients achieving less than 6 METs workload.

Weiner and associates have looked extensively at the Coronary Artery Surgery Study (CASS) registry in regard to exercise capacity *(41–44).* Most recently, they reported the 16-yr follow- up on 3086 men and 747 women who underwent maximal treadmill testing and coronary angiography *(44).* The subjects were divided into high-, intermediate-, and low-risk groups on the basis of exercise testing. Men in the high- or intermediate-risk groups had 16-yr survival rates of 61% and 56%, respectively, whereas men in the low-risk group had only a 38% survival rate ($p < 0.0001$). The results for women were similar (79, 73, and 44%, respectively $p < 0.0001$). Among men, 12-yr survival was improved by coronary artery bypass surgery vs. medical therapy in the high-risk subgroup (69% vs. 55%, respectively, $p = 0.0025$), but the two therapies were similar in the other two subgroups. Among women, neither medical nor surgical therapy improved 12-yr survival rates in any of the three subgroups.

In the only study to take into account evidence of myocardial perfusion defects, Snader and colleagues *(14)* found, in 3400 patients with no history of diagnosed CAD undergoing exercise single photon emission computed tomography (SPECT) thallium testing, that patients with average or better functional capacity classifications (Table 1) had a 2.5-yr mortality of <2% compared with 6 and 14%, respectively, in individuals who were in the fair and poor groups (Fig. 1). Of note, more than 81% of the 108 deaths during

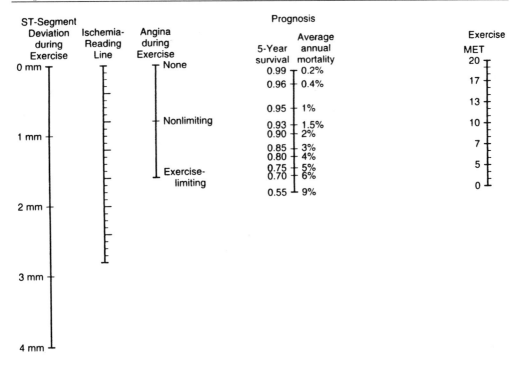

Fig. 2. Duke treadmill exercise score nomogram. See text for details. Taken from ref. *54*.

follow-up occurred in the fair- and poor-capacity groups. The thallium scan was also predictive of mortality in this study. In multivariable analyses including clinical, exercise, and thallium variables, estimated exercise capacity was the strongest predictor of death ($\chi^2 = 34, p < 0.0001$), with the only other predictors being age ($\chi^2 = 28, p < 0.0001$), male gender ($\chi^2 = 17, p < 0.0001$), and abnormal thallium perfusion ($\chi^2 = 5, p = 0.03$). Estimated functional capacity and thallium sum score were roughly equivalent predictors of cardiac mortality.

The Duke nomogram (Fig. 2) is a risk stratification tool that incorporates exercise capacity with ST-segment deviation and symptoms on the treadmill to predict 5-yr mortality. The nomogram was derived by regression analysis *(53)* and has been validated prospectively *(54)*, although some researchers have not found a correlation with mortality *(55)*.

To estimate prognosis for an individual patient using the nomogram, a line is first drawn from the maximum amount of ST-segment depression during exercise to the observed degree of angina. A mark is made on the ischemia-reading line where these lines intersect. From this mark, a line is drawn to the workload achieved on the exercise line. The intersection of this line and the prognosis line provides a risk assessment for survival.

ECG DATA

Visual ST-Segment Interpretation

The classic method of interpretation of the exercise ECG test focuses solely on ST-segment depression. An abnormal response is typically defined as ST-segment depression ≥ 1 mm that is horizontal or downsloping or upsloping ST-segment depression ≥ 1.5–2.0 mm.

The pathophysiology of the ST-segment change is thought to be due to a current of ischemia from the affected myocardial cells resulting in a net depression.

Ellestad and Wan *(35)* retrospectively examined the predictive capability of ST-segment depression in 2700 patients who had undergone exercise treadmill testing for cardiovascular morbidity or mortality. There was no association between a positive test and mortality, but there was an association between an early onset of ST-segment depression and mortality in univariate analysis.

In more than 3600 white men enrolled in the Lipid Research Clinic Prevalence Study, a positive exercise test was predictive of cardiac and all-cause mortality in univariate analysis *(116)*. When stratified for age and cardiac risk factors, the test was also predictive. In both this study and the previous study, no adjustments were made for functional capacity. Other investigations have not been able to demonstrate an association between standard visual ST-segment analysis and mortality *(56–59)*.

Heart Rate Adjustment of the ST-Segment

Because standard visual ST-segment analysis is imprecise and fails to take workload into account, it has been argued that heart-rate adjusted, computerized ST-segment measurements may improve the diagnostic and prognostic capabilities of exercise ECG *(22)*. Two specific measures have been described, the ST-segment/heart rate (ST/HR) index and the ST/HR slope.

The ST/HR index is the simplest approach, in which the change in ST-segment depression during exercise is divided by the difference between peak and resting heart rates. This index is easy to calculate and can be applied to patients undergoing staggered protocols, like the Bruce or modified Bruce.

The ST/HR slope is derived by seeking the maximal change in ST-segment depression as a function of HR change during exercise. To be valid, this measure requires a gradual graded protocol, like the Cornell protocol.

There is considerable controversy as to whether computerized ST-segment measurements adjusted for HR changes represent a viable alternative to visually read ST segments. Although some researchers have found that computerized and/or HR-adjusted ST-segment analyses can significantly improve the diagnostic properties of the exercise-ECG *(58–62)*, others have been unable to confirm this *(12,63,64)*. There have been two major studies relating computerized ST-HR measures to prognosis, one from the Framingham Offspring Study *(56)* and the other from the Multiple Risk Factor Intervention Trial (MRFIT) study *(57,58)*: both showed that standard visual ST-segment analyses failed to predict events, whereas computerized ST-HR measures did.

Okin and associates *(56)* followed 3168 asymptomatic men and women enrolled in the Framingham Offspring Study for 4 yr. All participants underwent maximum exercise testing at baseline with comparison made between the ST/HR index and standard visual ST-segment analysis. Although visual ST-segment analysis was not effective in predicting coronary events (sudden death, MI, or new-onset angina) the ST/HR index was highly predictive.

The association of the ST/HR index and death was further examined in 6000 men enrolled in the usual care arm of the MRFIT trial *(57,58)*. All participants underwent maximum exercise testing at enrollment. After 7 yr of follow-up there were 109 deaths. Visual ST-segment analysis was not predictive of death in this population, whereas the ST/HR index was predictive.

Q-Waves

Although there is an association between Q-waves on the resting ECG and mortality *(65)*, the presence or absence of Q-waves on the resting ECG does not alter the diagnostic accuracy of exercise induced ST-segment depression *(66)*.

QT Dispersion

QT dispersion (QTD) is defined as the time difference between the shortest QT interval in any lead and the longest QT interval in any other lead. The presence of QDT > 60 ms in addition to standard criteria has been proposed as a method of increasing the specificity of the exercise test for diagnosis of CAD *(67)*.

R-Wave Changes

R-waves may change in amplitude during exercise. Leroy *(68)* investigated the prognostic value of these changes in 303 post-MI patients over 4 yr of follow-up. Although there was a significant correlation of increased R-wave amplitude during exercise and three-vessel CAD and with the extent of ST-segment depression during exercise there was no relation to mortality. There was also an association with angina at follow-up but not with recurrent infarction. Several studies have been published on the diagnostic value of R-wave amplitude changes with mixed results *(69–74)*.

T-Wave Changes

The T-wave will normally decrease gradually in early exercise and begin to increase in amplitude at maximal exercise. At 1 min into recovery they should be back to baseline. A T-wave increase of 2.5 mm or greater in lead V2 may increase the sensitivity of the exercise test *(75)*. Although not a common finding, deep T-wave inversion (≥8 mm depression) associated with downsloping ST-segment depression of ≥1 mm is associated with an increased incidence of three-vessel and left-main disease *(76)*. T-wave inversion <8 mm is a less-specific finding and may be a normal variant.

T-Wave Alternans

T-wave alternans (TWA) is characterized by microvolt beat-to-beat changes in the T-wave amplitude *(77,78)*. It has been demonstrated to have prognostic significance for ventricular tachycardia for patients with the long-QT syndrome *(79–81)* and in patients with ischemic cardiac disease *(82)*.

Recent studies have focused on T-wave alternans during exercise testing. Individuals who are at increased risk of ventricular arrhythmias will have the sudden onset of sustained TWA at a heart rate lower than that of controls (<110 beats per minute [bpm] or <70% maximum predicted HR) *(83)*. Among patients referred for electrophysiology testing (EPS), TWA has been demonstrated to be a better predictor than EPS of ventricular tachycardia (VT) or death *(84)*. Other studies of the prognostic capability of TWA in other populations are ongoing *(85)*.

U-Wave Inversion

If they are upright at baseline, U-wave inversion during exercise may be a marker of ischemia, left ventricular (LV) hypertrophy, or diastolic dysfunction *(86–90)*. There are no prognostic studies to date of U-wave inversion.

Left Bundle-Branch Block

Approximately 0.5% of patients undergoing exercise testing will develop transient left bundle-branch block (LBBB). Grady and associates *(91)* examined the prognostic significance of this finding using a control cohort study. They selected 70 patients who developed exercise-induced LBBB and matched them to 70 control subjects based on age, sex, prior history of CAD, and standard risk factors. In 4 yr of follow-up, there were seven deaths, five of which occurred in the exercise-induced LBBB group. There were also higher rates of need for revascularization and implantation of pacemaker or defibrillator in the group that had transient LBBB. The adjusted relative risk (RR) of developing one of these endpoints was 2.78 (95% confidence interval 1.16–6.65).

Arrhythmias

The occurrence of exercise-induced arrhythmia is generally a marker of worse outcome. Supraventricular arrhythmias have been associated with increased mortality *(68)* as have VT, and fibrillation *(92,93)*. However, not all investigators have found an association between VT and mortality *(94,95)*.

Various groups have reported conflicting results regarding the diagnostic and prognostic significance of exercise-induced ventricular ectopy (e.g., premature ventricular complexes [PVCs] or bigeminy) *(21,96–98)*. Califf and colleagues *(96)* found that the 236 patients out of 1293 consecutive treadmill patients with simple ventricular arrhythmias (at least one PVC, but without paired complexes or VT) had a higher incidence of significant CAD (57 vs. 44%), three vessel disease (31 vs. 17%) and abnormal LV function (43 vs. 24%) than did patients without ventricular arrhythmias. In the 620 patients with significant CAD, patients with paired complexes or VT had a higher 3-yr mortality (25%) than did patients with simple ventricular arrhythmias (17%) and patients with no ventricular arrhythmias (10%). In patients with nonsignificant CAD, ventricular ectopy had no prognostic significance.

Schweikert and co-workers *(21)* demonstrated an association between ventricular ectopy and thallium defects but not severe CAD or 2-yr mortality. Two cohorts consisting of adults without heart failure or known severe resting ventricular ectopic activity were studied. The first cohort consisted of adults ($n = 2743$) who underwent maximal exercise thallium stress testing. The second cohort consisted of adults ($n = 423$) who underwent coronary angiography within 90 ds of treadmill testing. In the thallium cohort, exercise-induced ventricular ectopic activity was associated with a greater frequency of thallium defects (35.2% vs. 18.7%, odds ratio 2.35, 95% confidence interval [CI] 1.62–3.42, $p < 0.001$); after adjusting for possible confounders, this association persisted (for any defect adjusted odds ratio 1.66, 95% CI 1.09–2.53, $p = 0.02$). There was no association between exercise-induced ventricular ectopic activity and mortality during 2-yr of follow-up. In the angiographic cohort, there was no association of exercise-induced ventricular ectopy with severe CAD (19% vs. 20%, odds ratio 0.93, 95% CI 0.41-2.09, p = not significant).

In 1486 patients from the CASS study *(97)*, there was no association between mortality and ventricular ectopy after stratification by severity of CAD. In the 80 patients of 1160 consecutive patients *(98)* who developed frequent (greater than or equal to 10% of beats in any 1 min) or repetitive (greater than or equal to three beats in a row) ventricular ectopic beats there was no difference in mortality when followed over 5 yr.

HEART RATE

HR Rise During Exercise

Maximal exercise HR is related to peak workload in a linear fashion and has been demonstrated to have similar prognostic capabilities to workload achieved *(68)*. Researchers have argued that peak HR is a better prognostic marker than METs because it is a measured value, whereas the workload achieved is usually estimated.

Chronotropic Incompetence

The term chronotropic incompetence refers to an attenuated HR response to exercise. Over 20 yr ago, Ellestad performed an exercise test on a 51-yr-old athletic man who had a normal exercise tolerance for age and no symptoms or ST-segment depression during exercise *(99)*. A short time after the exercise test, the man suffered sudden cardiac death; an autopsy revealed severe two-vessel coronary disease with an 80% left anterior descending (LAD) artery stenosis. Of note, the patient had only reached a maximum HR of 110 beats/min during exercise. Later, analyzing follow-up of 2700 patients undergoing exercise testing, Ellestad and his colleagues noted that patients with a slow HR during exercise were more likely to suffer an acute coronary event than patients with ischemic ST-segment depression and a normal HR response *(35)*. Other groups also reported worse prognosis among patients with attenuated exercise heart responses *(100)*, as well as larger burdens of myocardial scar as noted by radionuclide imaging *(101)*.

As imaging modalities like thallium scintigraphy and stress echocardiography became more popular, interest on the HR response to exercise focused away from prognosis and more toward its impact on test accuracy for the diagnosis of CAD. A number of groups have found that an impaired HR response to exercise is associated with reduced test sensitivity *(102–104)*. Indeed, many exercise laboratories will report out tests in which patients fail to reach 85% of their age-predicted maximum HR as being "nondiagnostic." Although such a term does at least indirectly imply the need for further testing, it does not carry the ominous connotation as the phrase "evidence of myocardial ischemia."

The physiology behind the HR response to exercise is a complex one which relates to perturbations in resting and exercise sympathetic and parasympathetic tone and neurohormonal milieu. A detailed discussion of the mechanisms underlying normal and abnormal HR responses to exercise is beyond the scope of this review, but can be found elsewhere *(105)*.

The most important determinant of exercise HR response to exercise is age, with decreasing maximal HRs achievable as people get older. The relationship between peak HR and age in a healthy individual has been found to be an inverse linear one; a number of groups have reported on linear equations for estimating peak heart, with 220 minus age in years being one of the more popularly used in clinical exercise laboratories. A commonly used definition of chronotropic incompetence is failure to reach 85% of the age-predicted peak HR.

A major limitation of this approach is that the estimated peak HR has a high standard deviation and therefore may be difficult to apply to individuals, as opposed to populations *(106)*. There are other problems with using ability to reach 85% of the age-predicted maximum HR as a measure of chronotropic incompetence. In addition to age, other important predictors of the HR response to exercise is resting HR and physical fitness, both factors that themselves are predictive of coronary heart disease risk (CHD) *(31,106–109)*.

Data from the Framingham Heart Study have shown that ability to reach a target HR is influenced by these two variables and even by age itself *(16)*. Therefore, any effort to relate chronotropic incompetence to prognosis or diagnosis suffers an inherent risk of serious confounding.

To help account for these potential confounding factors Wilkoff and Miller developed a marker called the chronotropic index *(110)*. The index takes advantage of the linear relation between exercise HR increase and metabolic work. Before exercise, a person has a certain metabolic reserve (MR), which is the difference between his or her peak oxygen consumption (or exercise capacity) and rest oxygen consumption, which is typically 3.5 mL/kg/min, or 1 MET. As exercise progresses, that MR is used up. Analogously, at rest there is a potential HR reserve, which is the difference between the peak attainable HR (as estimated, e.g., by 220 minus age) and the resting HR. As exercise progresses, HR reserve, like the MR, is used up as well.

During any given stage of exercise, the percent MR used can be expressed as:

$$\%MR \text{ used} = [(METs_{stage} - METs_{rest})/(METs_{peak} - METs_{rest})] \times 100$$

In an analogous fashion, for the percent HR reserve (HRR) used at any given stage of exercise can be expressed as

$$\%HRR \text{ used} = [(HR_{stage} - HR_{rest})/(220 - age - HR_{rest})] \times 100$$

Wilkoff and Miller have shown that in a group of healthy, nonhospitalized adults a plot of HRR used to MR used during different stages of exercise reveals a tight linear relationship with a slope of approximately one with a 95% CI of 0.8–1.3 *(110)*. The calculated value of this slope, which has been termed as the chronotropic index *(16,111)*, is independent of stage of exercise considered. Thus, chronotropic incompetence can be defined as a percent HRR used to percent MR used ratio of <0.8; this is referred to as a low chronotropic index. The advantage of using this approach to assess chronotropic response is that it accounts for age, functional capacity, and resting HR; *it is not merely a reflection of physical fitness or exercise time.*

One possible problem with this method is that except for patients undergoing sophisticated gas-exchange analyses, exercise capacity in METs is estimated, and not directly measured. Among patients who undergo symptom-limited testing, one can consider the ratio of HRR used to MR used at peak exercise, when by definition the proportion of MR used has a value of 1. Using this approach the chronotropic index is based entirely on directly measured variables, i.e., resting HR, peak HR, and age *(112)*. Because the value of the chronotropic index is independent of stage of exercise considered, this measure at least indirectly takes into account effects of functional capacity as well *(110)*.

A study by Brener and colleagues examined the association of chronotropic response to exercise and angiographic severity of coronary disease *(18)*. Among 475 patients who underwent exercise testing and coronary angiography within 180 days, peak heart, percent target HR achieved, and the chronotropic index were all closely related to the number of diseased coronary arteries. Also of note, despite the anatomic relationship between the right coronary artery and the sinus node, there was no association between isolated disease of the proximal right coronary artery and chronotropic response. In contrast, after adjusting for age and gender, stenosis in the proximal LAD artery was strongly associated with peak HR (for each 10 beats/min decrement, odds ratio [OR] 1.23, 95% CI 1.07–1.41, $p = 0.03$), percent target HR achieved (for each 10% decrement, OR 1.44, 95% CI 1.15–1.81,

$p = 0.02$), and chronotropic index (for each 0.2 decrement, OR 1.6, 95% CI 1.03–1.54, $p = 0.02$).

Lauer studied 1575 healthy male participants of the Framingham Heart Study who underwent graded exercise testing according to the Bruce protocol and were followed for nearly 8 yr. *(16)*. There were 327 who failed to reach 85% of their age-predicted maximum HR; of these 21 (6%) died and 44 (14%) experienced an incident CHD event. In contrast, of the 1248 subjects who reached their target HR, only 34 (3%) died and only 51 (4%) experienced CHD events. The chronotropic index also stratified subjects well for prediction of death and coronary heart disease events. After adjusting for ST-segment changes and standard cardiovascular risk factors, all-cause mortality was predicted by the change in HR with exercise ($p = 0.04$) and by the chronotropic index as measured during stage 2 of exercise ($p = 0.05$).

Although these studies showed that chronotropic incompetence was predictive of mortality among healthy adults, the possibility that this was merely a manifestation of MI could not be excluded. Therefore, Lauer and associates studied 231 consecutive adults (mean age 57, 146 men) who underwent stress echocardiography at the Cleveland Clinic Foundation and who were not taking beta blockers *(113)*. After 41 mo of follow-up, 41 patients died, had a nonfatal MI, or underwent myocardial revascularization at least 3 mo after the stress test. Failure to reach 85% of the age-predicted maximum HR was predictive of events (RR 2.47, 95% CI 1.28–4.79, $p = 0.007$) as was a chronotropic index <0.8 (RR 2.44, 95% CI 1.31–4.55, $p = 0.005$). Even after adjusting for myocardial ischemia by echocardiography and other possible confounders, failure to reach 85% of the target HR remained predictive (adjusted RR 2.20, 95% CI 1.11–4.37, $p = 0.02$) as was a low chronotropic index (adjusted RR 1.85, 95% CI 0.98–3.47, $p = 0.06$).

These findings were conformed in a population of 1877 men and 1076 women who underwent SPECT thallium exercise testing *(17)*. No one was taking beta blockers and no one had undergone prior cardiac invasive procedures or had a history of congestive heart failure (CHF). Failure to reach 85% of the age-predicted maximum HR was noted in 316 (11%) patients, whereas a low chronotropic index was noted in 762 (26%); thallium perfusion defects were found in 612 (21%). Death during 2 yr of follow-up occurred in 91 patients. Even after adjusting for thallium evidence of ischemia and other possible confounders, failure to reach 85% of the age-predicted maximum HR was predictive of death (adjusted RR 1.84, 95% CI 1.13–3.00, $p = 0.01$) as was a low chronotropic index (adjusted RR 2.19, 95% CI 1.43–3.44, $p = 0.0003$). Of note, a low chronotropic index by itself was as ominous a sign as thallium perfusion defects; the presence of both was associated with a particularly poor prognosis (Fig. 3).

It is unclear why chronotropic incompetence is associated with an adverse outcome. Previous investigators had argued that slower HRs during exercise represents a compensatory mechanism for hearts beset by a heavy ischemic burden, but the ability to predict events many years after testing argues that the mechanism must be more complex *(99)*. Nonetheless, there must be some relation to ischemia, given the association of chronotropic incompetence with angiographic severity of coronary disease *(18)* and with thallium perfusion defects *(101)* and the improvement of chronotropic response with myocardial revascularization *(114)*. Another possible mechanism might be that subtle alterations of autonomic tone are themselves markers, if not outright contributors, to the severity and activity of atherosclerosis. Investigations in this area have included consideration of the Bezold-Jarish reflex *(115)*, decreased vagal activity at rest *(116)*, and the relation

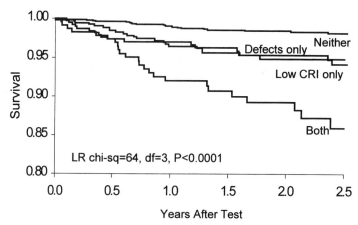

Fig. 3. Kaplan-Meier plot relating chronotropic incompetence (CRI), thallium defects, or both to all-cause mortality. Taken from ref. *17*.

between resting HR and coronary disease risk *(106)*. Investigators have argued that the relationship between chronotropic incompetence and outcome may parallel the associations between exercise HR responses and severity of neurohormonal alterations in patients with CHF *(117,118)*.

Heart Rate Recovery

Not only is the HR increase during exercise important but the HR fall after exercise has important prognostic implications as well. A recent study examined this association between HR recovery immediately following exercise and mortality *(15)*. Cole and associates followed 2428 consecutive adults who underwent symptom-limited exercise thallium testing for 6 yr. HR recovery was defined as the change in HR from peak exercise to 1 min of recovery. An abnormal HR recovery was defined as ≤12 beats/min. The endpoint of the study was all-cause mortality.

In 6 yr of follow-up there were 213 deaths. In univariate analysis a low HR recovery strongly predicted mortality (Fig. 4; mortality at 6 yr 19% vs. 5%; RR 3.96; 95% CI 3.02–5.19; $p < 0.0001$). Even after adjusting for age, gender, medications, thallium perfusion defects, hypertension, diabetes, smoking, resting HR, chronotropic response during exercise, and workload achieved a low HR recovery remained highly predictive of death (adjusted relative risk 2.00; 95% CI 1.49–2.68; $p < 0.001$).

These findings held true if HR recovery was considered as a continuous variable or log-transformed value and also when stratified by age, gender, history of CAD, thallium perfusion defects, use of beta blockers, or vasodilating drugs. Even in patients with completely normal thallium scans an abnormal HR recovery was significantly predictive of mortality. Although a minority of patients (26%) had an abnormal HR recovery, the majority of deaths (56%) were among those who had an abnormally low value. This is in marked contrast to most risk factors, which although they identify high-risk groups, predict only a minority of events.

The prognostic potential of HR recovery also held true in a larger population of healthy young adults undergoing submaximal exercise testing *(119)*. There were 5234 healthy adults with no known heart disease, who were followed for 12 yr following submaximal exercise testing. An abnormal HR recovery was defined as a less than 42 beat fall in HR

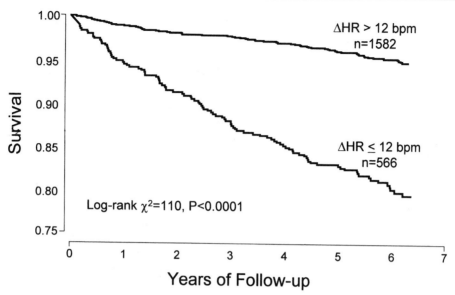

Fig. 4. Kaplan-Meier plot relating HR recovery to all-cause mortality. Based on data from ref. *15*.

2 min into recovery. Those with abnormal HR recovery had a 2.5-fold increase in mortality over the study period (10% vs. 4%). These findings remained true even after adjustment for multiple confounding risk factors.

The potential mechanisms for why HR recovery predicts mortality relate to vagal activity. Imai and colleagues studied the HR recovery after maximal and submaximal exercise in both normal individuals, athletes, and patients with heart failure *(120)*. In all groups the fall in HR immediately after exercise was markedly prolonged following atropine administration but not with beta blockade, suggesting that HR recovery is primarily a function of the parasympathetic nervous system. This effect was independent of age and exercise intensity but was more pronounced in athletes and attenuated in those with heart failure. These studies would seem to suggest that increased HR recovery is a marker of increased parasympathetic activity that has been associated with a reduction in the risk of death *(121)*.

BLOOD PRESSURE (BP)

An exaggerated BP response to exercise (or "exercise hypertension") has been associated with a higher risk of developing hypertension at rest *(122,123)*. Based on exercise test data recording in healthy adults in the Framingham Offspring Study, we have defined exercise hypertension as a peak systolic BP of at least 210 mmHg in men and 190 mmHg in women *(124)*. Previous reports regarding its prognostic significance have shown conflicting results *(125–131)*.

A report from a Veteran Administration clinic in which exercise testing had been performed in normotensive subjects found that exercise hypertension was associated with a greater likelihood of echocardiographic LV hypertrophy *(132)*. This potential association was analyzed in detail among the Framingham Offspring cohort and found to be largely, although not entirely, confounded by age, gender, and resting BP *(124)*.

Snader and associates studied 594 adults who underwent exercise testing and coronary angiography within 90 d of one another at the Cleveland Clinic Foundation *(14)*; all increased systolic BP during exercise by at least 10 mmHg. Exercise hypertension was present in 196 patients (33%). Severe coronary disease was less common in patients with exercise hypertension (14% vs. 25%, odds ratio 0.51, 95% CI 0.32–0.81, $p = 0.004$). When resting and exercise types of hypertension were considered together, resting hypertension was associated with a greater likelihood of severe CAD, whereas exercise hypertension was independently associated with a lower likelihood. After adjusting for resting BP, age, gender, other coronary risk factors, and exercise capacity, exercise hypertension remained predictive of a lower likelihood of severe coronary disease (adjusted OR 0.58, 95% CI 0.34–0.97, $p = 0.04$).

Among 3445 adults evaluated for known or suspected CAD, exercise hypertension was associated with a lower likelihood of myocardial perfusion abnormalities as assessed by thallium scanning and was not associated with an increased mortality rate *(19)*. Exercise hypertension was defined as a peak systolic BP of $\geq$210 mmHg in men and $\geq$190 mmHg in women and was present in 39% of the population. Patients with exercise induced hypertension were less likely to have either fixed or reversible thallium perfusion defects (16% vs. 25%; odds ratio [OR] 0.58; 95% confidence interval [CI] 0.49–0.69; $p < 0.001$) as well as reversible defects only (OR 0.71; 95% CI 0.57–0.90; $p < 0.001$). There was no association between exercise-induced hypertension and mortality during 6 yr of follow-up. These findings suggest that among clinical populations exercise hypertension is not an ominous finding and may even be a benign one.

CONCLUSION

There is a wealth of often-overlooked information contained in the exercise test. The focus of exercise test interpretation should turn away from the ST-segment and toward exercise capacity, HR, and other autonomic markers. Using these parameters, the exercise test can be an important tool for risk stratification and prevention. Future research is needed into how to use more expensive imaging tests more judiciously.

REFERENCES

1. Fletcher GF, Balady G, Froelicher VF, et al. Exercise standards. A statement for healthcare professionals from the American Heart Association. Writing Group. Circulation 1995;91:580–615.
2. Detrano R, Froelicher VF. Exercise testing: uses and limitations considering recent studies. Prog Cardiovasc Dis 1988;31:173–204.
3. Detrano R, Gianrossi R, Mulvihill D, et al. Exercise-induced ST segment depression in the diagnosis of multivessel coronary disease: a meta analysis. J Am Coll Cardiol 1989;14:1501–1508.
4. Detrano R, Gianrossi R, Froelicher V. The diagnostic accuracy of the exercise electrocardiogram: a meta-analysis of 22 years of research. Prog Cardiovasc Dis 1989;32:173–206.
5. Detrano R. Variability in the accuracy of the exercise ST-segment in predicting the coronary angiogram: how good can we be? J Electrocardiol 1992;24:54–61.
6. Gianrossi R, Detrano R, Mulvihill D, et al. Exercise-induced ST depression in the diagnosis of coronary artery disease. A meta-analysis. Circulation 1989;80:87–98.
7. Philbrick JT, Horwitz RI, Feinstein AR. Methodologic problems of exercise testing for coronary artery disease: groups, analysis and bias. Am J Cardiol 1980;46:807–812.
8. Philbrick JT, Horwitz RI, Feinstein AR, et al. The limited spectrum of patients studied in exercise test research. Analyzing the tip of the iceberg. JAMA 1982;248:2467–2470.
9. Choi BC. Sensitivity and specificity of a single diagnostic test in the presence of work-up bias [see comments]. J Clin Epidemiol 1992;45:581–586.
10. Diamond GA. Reverend Bayes' silent majority. An alternative factor affecting sensitivity and specificity of exercise electrocardiography. Am J Cardiol 1986;57:1175–1180.

11. Ransohoff DF, Feinstein AR. Problems of spectrum and bias in evaluating the efficacy of diagnostic tests. N Engl J Med 1978;299:926–930.
12. Froelicher VF, Lehmann KG, Thomas R, et al. The electrocardiographic exercise test in a population with reduced work-up bias: diagnostic performance, computerized interpretation, and multivariable freedom. Ann Intern Med 1998;128:965–974.
13. Christian TF, Miller TD, Bailey KR, Gibbons RJ. Exercise tomographic thallium-201 imaging in patients with severe coronary artery disease and normal electrocardiograms [see comments]. Ann Intern Med 1994;121:825–832.
14. Snader CE, Marwick TH, Pashkow FJ, et al. Importance of estimated functional capacity as a predictor of all-cause mortality among patients referred for exercise thallium single-photon emission computed tomography: report of 3,400 patients from a single center. J Am Coll Cardiol 1997;30:641–648.
15. Cole CR, Blackstone EH, Pashkow FJ, et al. Heart rate recovery immediately after exercise as a predictor of mortality. N Engl J Med 1999;341:1351–1357.
16. Lauer MS, Okin PM, Larson MG, et al. Impaired heart rate response to graded exercise. Prognostic implications of chronotropic incompetence in the Framingham Heart Study. Circulation 1996;93:1520–1526.
17. Lauer MS, Francis GS, Okin PM, et al. Impaired chronotropic response to exercise stress testing as a predictor of mortality. JAMA 1999;281:524–529.
18. Brener SJ, Pashkow FJ, Harvey SA, et al. Chronotropic response to exercise predicts angiographic severity in patients with suspected or stable coronary artery disease. Am J Cardiol 1995;76:1228–1232.
19. Campbell L, Marwick TH, Pashkow FJ, et al. Usefulness of an exaggerated systolic blood pressure response to exercise in predicting myocardial perfusion defects in known or suspected coronary artery disease. Am J Cardiol 1999;84:1304–1310.
20. Lauer MS, Pashkow FJ, Harvey SA, et al. Angiographic and prognostic implications of an exaggerated exercise systolic blood pressure response and rest systolic blood pressure in adults undergoing evaluation for suspected coronary artery disease. J Am Coll Cardiol 1995;26:1630–1636.
21. Schweikert RA, Pashkow FJ, Snader CE, et al. Association of exercise-induced ventricular ectopic activity with thallium myocardial perfusion and angiographic coronary artery disease in stable, low-risk populations. Am J Cardiol 1999;83:530–534.
22. Okin PM, Kligfield P. Heart rate adjustment of ST segment depression and performance of the exercise electrocardiogram: a critical evaluation. J Am Coll Cardiol 1995;25:1726–1735.
23. Peters RK, Cady LD, Jr., Bischoff DP, et al. Physical fitness and subsequent myocardial infarction in healthy workers. JAMA 1983;249:3052–3056.
24. Paffenbarger RS Jr, Hyde RT, Wing AL, Hsieh CC. Physical activity, all-cause mortality, and longevity of college alumni. N Engl J Med 1986;314:605–613.
25. Leon AS, Connett J, Jacobs DR Jr, Rauramaa R. Leisure-time physical activity levels and risk of coronary heart disease and death. The Multiple Risk Factor Intervention Trial. JAMA 1987;258:2388–2395.
26. Ekelund LG, Haskell WL, Johnson JL, et al. Physical fitness as a predictor of cardiovascular mortality in asymptomatic North American men. The Lipid Research Clinics Mortality Follow-up Study. N Engl J Med 1988;319:1379–1384.
27. Blair SN, Kohl HWD, Paffenbarger RS Jr, et al. Physical fitness and all-cause mortality. A prospective study of healthy men and women. JAMA 1989;262:2395–2401.
28. van Saase JL, Noteboom WM, Vandenbroucke JP. Longevity of men capable of prolonged vigorous physical exercise: a 32 year follow up of 2259 participants in the Dutch eleven cities ice skating tour. Br Med J 1990;301:1409–1411.
29. Arraiz GA, Wigle DT, Mao Y. Risk assessment of physical activity and physical fitness in the Canada Health Survey mortality follow-up study. J Clin Epidemiol 1992;45:419–428.
30. Paffenbarger RS Jr, Hyde RT, Wing AL, et al. The association of changes in physical-activity level and other lifestyle characteristics with mortality among men. N Engl J Med 1993;328:538–545.
31. Lakka TA, Venalainen JM, Rauramaa R, et al. Relation of leisure-time physical activity and cardiorespiratory fitness to the risk of acute myocardial infarction. N Engl J Med 1994;330:1549–1554.
32. Lee IM, Hsieh CC, Paffenbarger RS Jr. Exercise intensity and longevity in men. The Harvard Alumni Health Study. JAMA 1995;273:1179–1184.
33. Blair SN, Kohl HW 3rd, Barlow CE, et al. Changes in physical fitness and all-cause mortality. A prospective study of healthy and unhealthy men. JAMA 1995;273:1093–1098.
34. Lissner L, Bengtsson C, Bjorkelund C, Wedel H. Physical activity levels and changes in relation to longevity. A prospective study of Swedish women. Am J Epidemiol 1996;143:54–62.
35. Ellestad MH, Wan MK. Predictive implications of stress testing. Follow-up of 2700 subjects after maximum treadmill stress testing. Circulation 1975;51:363–369.

36. Bruce RA, DeRouen T, Peterson DR, et al. Noninvasive predictors of sudden cardiac death in men with coronary heart disease. Predictive value of maximal stress testing. Am J Cardiol 1977;39:833–840.

37. McNeer JF, Margolis JR, Lee KL, et al. The role of the exercise test in the evaluation of patients for ischemic heart disease. Circulation 1978;57:64–70.

38. Podrid PJ, Graboys TB, Lown B. Prognosis of medically treated patients with coronary-artery disease with profound ST-segment depression during exercise testing. N Engl J Med 1981;305:1111–1116.

39. Bruce RA, Hossack KF, DeRouen TA, Hofer V. Enhanced risk assessment for primary coronary heart disease events by maximal exercise testing: 10 years' experience of Seattle Heart Watch. J Am Coll Cardiol 1983;2:565–753.

40. McKirnan MD, Sullivan M, Jensen D, Froelicher VF. Treadmill performance and cardiac function in selected patients with coronary heart disease. J Am Coll Cardiol 1984;3:253–261.

41. Weiner DA, Ryan TJ, McCabe CH, et al. Prognostic importance of a clinical profile and exercise test in medically treated patients with coronary artery disease. J Am Coll Cardiol 1984;3:772–779.

42. Weiner DA, Ryan TJ, McCabe CH, et al. The role of exercise testing in identifying patients with improved survival after coronary artery bypass surgery. J Am Coll Cardiol 1986;8:741–748.

43. Weiner DA, Ryan TJ, McCabe CH, et al. Value of exercise testing in determining the risk classification and the response to coronary artery bypass grafting in three-vessel coronary artery disease: a report from the Coronary Artery Surgery Study (CASS) registry. Am J Cardiol 1987;60:262–266.

44. Weiner DA, Ryan TJ, Parsons L, et al. Long-term prognostic value of exercise testing in men and women from the Coronary Artery Surgery Study (CASS) registry. Am J Cardiol 1995;75:865–870.

45. Bogaty P, Dagenais GR, Cantin B, et al. Prognosis in patients with a strongly positive exercise electrocardiogram. Am J Cardiol 1989;64:1284–1288.

46. Morris CK, Ueshima K, Kawaguchi T, et al. The prognostic value of exercise capacity: a review of the literature. Am Heart J 1991;122:1423–1431.

47. Mancini DM, Eisen H, Kussmaul W, et al. Value of peak exercise oxygen consumption for optimal timing of cardiac transplantation in ambulatory patients with heart failure. Circulation 1991;83:778–786.

48. Aaronson KD, Mancini DM. Is percentage of predicted maximal exercise oxygen consumption a better predictor of survival than peak exercise oxygen consumption for patients with severe heart failure? J Heart Lung Transplant 1995;14:981–989.

49. Mancini D, Katz S, Donchez L, Aaronson K. Coupling of hemodynamic measurements with oxygen consumption during exercise does not improve risk stratification in patients with heart failure. Circulation 1996;94:2492–2496.

50. Myers J, Gullestad L, Vagelos R, et al. Clinical, hemodynamic, and cardiopulmonary exercise test determinants of survival in patients referred for evaluation of heart failure. Ann Intern Med 1998;129:286–293.

51. Myers J, Buchanan N, Walsh D, et al. Comparison of the ramp versus standard exercise protocols. J Am Coll Cardiol 1991;17:1334–1342.

51a. Weber KT, Janicki JS, McElroy PA. Determination of aerobic capacity and the severity of chronic cardiac and circulatory failure. Circulation 1987;76(Suppl VI):40–46.

52. Sawada SG, Ryan T, Conley MJ, et al. Prognostic value of a normal exercise echocardiogram. Am Heart J 1990;120:49–55.

53. Mark DB, Hlatky MA, Harrell FE Jr, et al. Exercise treadmill score for predicting prognosis in coronary artery disease. Ann Intern Med 1987;106:793–800.

54. Mark DB, Shaw L, Harrell FE Jr, et al. Prognostic value of a treadmill exercise score in outpatients with suspected coronary artery disease. N Engl J Med 1991;325:849–853.

55. Nallamothu N, Pancholy SB, Lee KR, et al. Impact on exercise single-photon emission computed tomographic thallium imaging on patient management and outcome. J Nucl Cardiol 1995;2:334–338.

56. Okin PM, Anderson KM, Levy D, Kligfield P. Heart rate adjustment of exercise-induced ST segment depression. Improved risk stratification in the Framingham Offspring Study. Circulation 1991;83:866–874.

57. Okin PM, Prineas RJ, Grandits G, et al. Heart rate adjustment of exercise-induced ST-segment depression identifies men who benefit from a risk factor reduction program. Circulation 1997;96:2899–2904.

58. Okin PM, Grandits G, Rautaharju PM, et al. Prognostic value of heart rate adjustment of exercise-induced ST segment depression in the multiple risk factor intervention trial. J Am Coll Cardiol 1996;27:1437–1443.

59. Cole CR, Pashkow FJ, Snader CE, et al. Computerized ST/HR index is a better predictor of mortality than standard ST or thallium (Abstract). J Am Coll Cardiol 1999;33:542A.

60. Okin PM, Kligfield P. Identifying coronary artery disease in women by heart rate adjustment of ST-segment depression and improved performance of linear regression over simple averaging method with comparison to standard criteria. Am J Cardiol 1992;69:297–302.
61. Okin PM, Kligfield P. Effect of precision of ST-segment measurement on identification and quantification of coronary artery disease by the ST/HR index. J Electrocardiol 1992;24:62–67.
62. Ribisl PM, Liu J, Mousa I, et al. Comparison of computer ST criteria for diagnosis of severe coronary artery disease. Am J Cardiol 1993;71:546–551.
63. Lachterman B, Lehmann KG, Detrano R, et al. Comparison of ST segment/heart rate index to standard ST criteria for analysis of exercise electrocardiogram. Circulation 1990;82:44–50.
64. Herbert WG, Dubach P, Lehmann KG, Froelicher VF. Effect of beta-blockade on the interpretation of the exercise ECG: ST level versus delta ST/HR index. Am Heart J 1991;122:993–1000.
65. Cullen K, Stenhouse NS, Wearne KL, Cumpston GN. Electrocardiograms and 13 year cardiovascular mortality in Busselton study. Br Heart J 1982;47:209–212.
66. Miranda CP, Herbert WG, Dubach P, et al. Post-myocardial infarction exercise testing. Non-Q wave versus Q wave correlation with coronary angiography and long-term prognosis. Circulation 1991;84: 2357–2365.
67. Stoletniy LN, Pai RG. Value of QT dispersion in the interpretation of exercise stress test in women. Circulation 1997;96:904–910.
68. Leroy F, Lablanche JM, Bauters C, et al. Prognostic value of changes in R-wave amplitude during exercise testing after a first acute myocardial infarction. Am J Cardiol 1992;70:152–155.
69. Bonoris PE, Greenberg PS, Christison GW, et al. Evaluation of R wave amplitude changes versus ST-segment depression in stress testing. Circulation 1978;57:904–910.
70. Bonoris PE, Greenberg PS, Castellanet MJ, Ellestad MH. Significance of changes in R wave amplitude during treadmill stress testing: angiographic correlation. Am J Cardiol 1978;41:846–851.
71. Battler A, Froelicher V, Slutsky R, Ashburn W. Relationship of QRS amplitude changes during exercise to left ventricular function and volumes and the diagnosis of coronary artery disease. Circulation 1979;60:1004–1013.
72. Cheng SL, Ellestad MH, Selvester RH. Significance of ST-segment depression with R-wave amplitude decrease on exercise testing. Am J Cardiol 1999;83:955–969.
73. Hollenberg M, Zoltick JM, Go M, et al. Comparison of a quantitative treadmill exercise score with standard electrocardiographic criteria in screening asymptomatic young men for coronary artery disease. N Engl J Med 1985;313:600–606.
74. Wagner S, Cohn K, Selzer A. Unreliability of exercise-induced R wave changes as indexes of coronary artery disease. Am J Cardiol 1979;44:1241–1246.
75. Lee JH, Crump R, Ellestad MH. Significance of precordial T-wave increase during treadmill stress testing. Am J Cardiol 1995;76:1297–1299.
76. Chikamori T, Doi YL, Furuno T, et al. Diagnostic significance of deep T-wave inversion induced by exercise testing in patients with suspected coronary artery disease. Am J Cardiol 1992;70:403–406.
77. Verrier RL, Stone PH. Exercise stress testing for T wave alternans to expose latent electrical instability [editorial]. J Cardiovasc Electrophysiol 1997;8:994–997.
78. Hohnloser SH, Klingenheben T, Zabel M, et al. T wave alternans during exercise and atrial pacing in humans. J Cardiovasc Electrophysiol 1997;8:987–993.
79. Schwartz PJ, Malliani A. Electrical alternation of the T-wave: clinical and experimental evidence of its relationship with the sympathetic nervous system and with the long Q-T syndrome. Am Heart J 1975;89:45–50.
80. Surawicz B, Fisch C. Cardiac alternans: diverse mechanisms and clinical manifestations. J Am Coll Cardiol 1992;20:483–499.
81. Zareba W, Moss AJ, le Cessie S, Hall WJ. T wave alternans in idiopathic long QT syndrome. J Am Coll Cardiol 1994;23:1541–1546.
82. Salerno JA, Previtali M, Panciroli C, et al. Ventricular arrhythmias during acute myocardial ischaemia in man. The role and significance of R-ST-T alternans and the prevention of ischaemic sudden death by medical treatment. Eur Heart J 1986;7:63–75.
83. Rosenbaum DS, Albrecht P, Cohen RJ. Predicting sudden cardiac death from T wave alternans of the surface electrocardiogram: promise and pitfalls. J Cardiovasc Electrophysiol 1996;7:1095–1111.
84. Gold MR, Bloomfield DM, Anderson KP, et al. T wave alternans predicts arrhythmia vulnerability in patients undergoin electrophysiology study [abstract]. Circulation 1998;98(Suppl):I-647–I-648.

85. Klingenheben T, Cohen RJ, Peetermans J, Hohnloser SH. Predictive value of T-wave alternans in patients with congestive heart failure. Circulation 1998;98(Suppl):I–864.

86. Chikamori T, Kitaoka H, Matsumura Y, et al. Clinical and electrocardiographic profiles producing exercise-induced U-wave inversion in patients with severe narrowing of the left anterior descending coronary artery. Am J Cardiol 1997;80:628–632.

87. Choo MH, Gibson DG. U waves in ventricular hypertrophy: possible demonstration of mechano-electrical feedback. Br Heart J 1986;55:428–433.

88. Gerson MC, Phillips JF, Morris SN, McHenry PL. Exercise-induced U-wave inversion as a marker of stenosis of the left anterior descending coronary artery. Circulation 1979;60:1014–1020.

89. Gerson MC, McHenry PL. Resting U wave inversion as a marker of stenosis of the left anterior descending coronary artery. Am J Med 1980;69:545–550.

90. Salmasi AM, Salmasi SN, Nicolaides AN, et al. The value of exercise-induced U-wave inversion on ECG chest wall mapping in the identification of individual coronary arterial lesions. Eur Heart J 1985; 6:437–443.

91. Grady TA, Chiu AC, Snader CE, et al. Prognostic significance of exercise-induced left bundle-branch block. JAMA 1998;279:153–156.

92. Berntsen RF, Gunnes P, Rasmussen K. Pattern of coronary artery disease in patients with ventricular tachycardia and fibrillation exposed by exercise-induced ischemia. Am Heart J 1995;129:733–738.

93. de Paola AA, Gomes JA, Terzian AB, et al. Ventricular tachycardia during exercise testing as a predictor of sudden death in patients with chronic chagasic cardiomyopathy and ventricular arrhythmias. Br Heart J 1995;74:293–295.

94. Casella G, Pavesi PC, Sangiorgio P, et al. Exercise-induced ventricular arrhythmias in patients with healed myocardial infarction. Int J Cardiol 1993;40:229–235.

95. Yang JC, Wesley RC Jr, Froelicher VF. Ventricular tachycardia during routine treadmill testing. Risk and prognosis. Arch Intern Med 1991;151:349–353.

96. Califf RM, McKinnis RA, McNeer JF, et al. Prognostic value of ventricular arrhythmias associated with treadmill exercise testing in patients studied with cardiac catheterization for suspected ischemic heart disease. J Am Coll Cardiol 1983;2:1060–1067.

97. Sami M, Chaitman B, Fisher L, et al. Significance of exercise-induced ventricular arrhythmia in stable coronary artery disease: a coronary artery surgery study project. Am J Cardiol 1984;54:1182–1188.

98. Busby MJ, Shefrin EA, Fleg JL. Prevalence and long-term significance of exercise-induced frequent or repetitive ventricular ectopic beats in apparently healthy volunteers. J Am Coll Cardiol 1989;14: 1659–1665.

99. Ellestad MH. Chronotropic incompetence. The implications of heart rate response to exercise (compensatory parasympathetic hyperactivity?) [editorial]. Circulation 1996;93:1485–1487.

100. Hinkle LE Jr, Carver ST, Plakun A. Slow heart rates and increased risk of cardiac death in middle-aged men. Arch Intern Med 1972;129:732–748.

101. Hammond HK, Kelly TL, Froelicher V. Radionuclide imaging correlatives of heart rate impairment during maximal exercise testing. J Am Coll Cardiol 1983;2:826–833.

102. Heller GV, Ahmed I, Tilkemeier PL, et al. Influence of exercise intensity on the presence, distribution, and size of thallium-201 defects. Am Heart J 1992;123:909–916.

103. Beleslin BD, Ostojic M, Stepanovic J, et al. Stress echocardiography in the detection of myocardial ischemia. Head- to-head comparison of exercise, dobutamine, and dipyridamole tests. Circulation 1994;90:1168–1176.

104. Marwick TH, Nemec JJ, Pashkow FJ, et al. Accuracy and limitations of exercise echocardiography in a routine clinical setting. J Am Coll Cardiol 1992;19:74–81.

105. Hammond HK, Froelicher VF. Normal and abnormal heart rate responses to exercise. Prog Cardiovasc Dis 1985;27:271–296.

106. Dyer AR, Persky V, Stamler J, et al. Heart rate as a prognostic factor for coronary heart disease and mortality: findings in three Chicago epidemiologic studies. Am J Epidemiol 1980;112:736–749.

107. Paffenbarger RS, Hale WE. Work activity and coronary heart mortality. N Engl J Med 1975;292: 545–550.

108. Willich SN, Lewis M, Lowel H, et al. Physical exertion as a trigger of acute myocardial infarction. Triggers and Mechanisms of Myocardial Infarction Study Group. N Engl J Med 1993;329:1684–1690.

109. Mittleman MA, Maclure M, Tofler GH, et al. Triggering of acute myocardial infarction by heavy physical exertion. Protection against triggering by regular exertion. Determinants of Myocardial Infarction Onset Study Investigators. N Engl J Med 1993;329:1677–1683.

110. Wilkoff BL, Miller RE. Exercise testing for chronotropic assessment. Cardiol Clin 1992;10:705–717.
111. Lauer MS, Pashkow FJ, Larson MG, Levy D. Association of cigarette smoking with chronotropic incompetence and prognosis in the Framingham Heart Study. Circulation 1997;96:897–903.
112. Okin PM, Lauer MS, Kligfield P. Chronotropic response to exercise. Improved performance of ST-segment depression criteria after adjustment for heart rate reserve. Circulation 1996;94:3226–3231.
113. Lauer MS, Mehta R, Pashkow FJ, et al. Association of chronotropic incompetence with echocardiographic ischemia and prognosis [In Process Citation]. J Am Coll Cardiol 1998;32:1280–1286.
114. Chin CF, Messenger JC, Greenberg PS, Ellestad MH. Chronotropic incompetence in exercise testing. Clin Cardiol 1979;2:12–18.
115. Mark AL. The Bezold-Jarisch reflex revisited: clinical implications of inhibitory reflexes originating in the heart. J Am Coll Cardiol 1983;1:90–102.
116. Hayano J, Yamada A, Mukai S, et al. Severity of coronary atherosclerosis correlates with the respiratory component of heart rate variability. Am Heart J 1991;121:1070–1079.
117. Francis GS, Goldsmith SR, Ziesche S, et al. Relative attenuation of sympathetic drive during exercise in patients with congestive heart failure. J Am Coll Cardiol 1985;5:832–839.
118. Colucci WS, Ribeiro JP, Rocco MB, et al. Impaired chronotropic response to exercise in patients with congestive heart failure. Role of postsynaptic beta-adrenergic desensitization. Circulation 1989;80:314–323.
119. Cole C, Foody J, Blackstone E, Lauer M. Heart rate recovery after submaximal exercise testing as a predictor of mortality in a cardiovascularly healthy cohort. Ann Intern Med 2000;132:552–555.
120. Imai K, Sato H, Hori M, et al. Vagally mediated heart rate recovery after exercise is accelerated in athletes but blunted in patients with chronic heart failure. J Am Coll Cardiol 1994;24:1529–1535.
121. Schwartz PJ, La Rovere MT, Vanoli E. Autonomic nervous system and sudden cardiac death. Experimental basis and clinical observations for post-myocardial infarction risk stratification. Circulation 1992;85:I77–I91.
122. Dlin RA, Hanne N, Silverberg DS, Bar-Or O. Follow-up of normotensive men with exaggerated blood pressure response to exercise. Am Heart J 1983;106:316–320.
123. Wilson MF, Sung BH, Pincomb GA, Lovallo WR. Exaggerated pressure response to exercise in men at risk for systemic hypertension. Am J Cardiol 1990;66:731–736.
124. Lauer MS, Levy D, Anderson KM, Plehn JF. Is there a relationship between exercise systolic blood pressure response and left ventricular mass? The Framingham Heart Study. Ann Intern Med 1992;116:203–210.
125. Irving JB, Bruce RA, DeRouen TA. Variations in and significance of systolic pressure during maximal exercise (treadmill) testing. Am J Cardiol 1977;39:841–848.
126. Filipovsky J, Ducimetiere P, Safar ME. Prognostic significance of exercise blood pressure and heart rate in middle-aged men. Hypertension 1992;20:333–339.
127. Fagard RH, Pardaens K, Staessen JA, Thijs L. Prognostic value of invasive hemodynamic measurements at rest and during exercise in hypertensive men. Hypertension 1996;28:31–36.
128. Fagard R, Staessen J, Thijs L, Amery A. Relation of left ventricular mass and filling to exercise blood pressure and rest blood pressure. Am J Cardiol 1995;75:53–57.
129. Morrow K, Morris CK, Froelicher VF, et al. Prediction of cardiovascular death in men undergoing noninvasive evaluation for coronary artery disease. Ann Intern Med 1993;118:689–695.
130. Mundal R, Kjeldsen SE, Sandvik L, et al. Exercise blood pressure predicts cardiovascular mortality in middle- aged men. Hypertension 1994;24:56–62.
131. Mundal R, Kjeldsen SE, Sandvik L, et al. Exercise blood pressure predicts mortality from myocardial infarction. Hypertension 1996;27:324–329.
132. Gottdiener JS, Brown J, Zoltick J, Fletcher RD. Left ventricular hypertrophy in men with normal blood pressure: relation to exaggerated blood pressure response to exercise. Ann Intern Med 1990;112:161–166.

16

Electron Beam Tomography in the Prevention of Coronary Artery Disease

Arthur Agatston, MD

INTRODUCTION

As technology advances, the noninvasive imaging of preclinical and subclinical disease holds great promise for the early detection of the atherosclerotic process and for monitoring its progression after prevention strategies are instituted (*1*). Electron beam computed tomography (EBT) acquires images in 50–100 ms compared with 500 ms plus for conventional computed tomography (CT) scanners. Just as a camera with a fast shutter speed can stop action, the EBT acquires images of the beating heart without motion artifact. This allows detection and precise quantification of small deposits of coronary calcium.

From: *Contemporary Cardiology: Preventive Cardiology:*
Strategies for the Prevention and Treatment of Coronary Artery Disease
Edited by: J. Foody © Humana Press Inc., Totowa, NJ

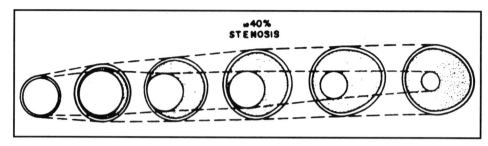

Fig. 1. This series of diagrams illustrates coronary remodeling as coronary atherosclerotic plaque grows *(10)*. The lumen is not compromised until there is 40% or more cross-sectional stenosis. A "lumengram" will not reflect much of the mural atherosclerotic process.

We review the role of EBT in the detection of coronary atherosclerosis and in the prevention of coronary events.

PATHOPHYSIOLOGIC CONCEPTS

Because coronary disease has a long incubation period, there is a significant window of opportunity for the detection of the atherosclerotic process and for monitoring its progress before coronary events occur. Vietnam and Korean casualty studies *(2,3)* and the Bogalusa heart study *(4)* have shown that raised coronary atherosclerotic lesions are commonly found in arterial walls in early adulthood. The necropsy studies of Bill Roberts *(5)* have documented that by the time clinical events occur whether the presentation is sudden death, acute myocardial infarction (MI), or angina pectoris, there is diffuse coronary atherosclerosis involving all three major coronary arteries. Dr. Roberts and colleagues dissected the coronaries into 5 mm segments. They invariably found diffuse obstructive disease in those dying with clinical coronary disease *(6,7)*. Initially, these data appeared to be in conflict with the angiographer's experience of often finding one- or two-vessel disease at angiography in those presenting with clinical coronary artery disease (CAD) *(8,9)*. This apparent conflict has been resolved by the work of Glagov and associates *(10)*. Unlike earlier postmortem coronary studies, Dr. Glagov fixed the coronary arteries at systemic perfusion pressures, thus examining them in a more physiologic state. He demonstrated that early atherosclerotic lesions grow outward rather than into the coronary lumen. He found that as a result of this coronary remodeling, the lumen is typically not compromised until there is greater than 40% cross-sectional obstruction (Fig. 1). This pathophysiology has been confirmed with in vivo studies using intravascular ultrasound *(11)*. These studies have demonstrated the presence of complicated plaques in areas that appear angiographically normal due to the process of coronary remodeling demonstrated by Glagov. Thus, the "lumenogram" misses a good deal of the atherosclerotic process that takes place in the vessel wall. It may appear normal in the face of extensive coronary atherosclerosis.

THE IDEAL CORONARY SCREENING TEST

An ideal coronary screening test would be one that could noninvasively image and quantify coronary atherosclerosis early in its natural history and allow monitoring of its progression or lack thereof in response to risk factor interventions over a relatively short time interval. In addition, such a test should be safe, inexpensive, and reproducible. Does the presence and quantity of coronary calcium reflect the coronary plaque burden and if so, can it be accurately imaged and quantified and tracked noninvasively?

THE PATHOLOGY OF CORONARY CALCIUM

Postmortem studies have shown that the sole cause of coronary calcification is intimal atherosclerosis and that the quantity of coronary calcium reflects the total atherosclerotic plaque burden (12). In 1961, Blankenhorn (13) reported results from a study of 3500 coronary segments from 89 hearts in which he found that coronary calcium was invariably associated with intimal atherosclerosis that caused some degree of lumenal narrowing. His review of the literature found no reports of Monckeberg's medial sclerosis associated with the coronaries. Subsequent studies have confirmed his findings with rare exception.

Because of the potential to identify coronary calcium noninvasively using fluoroscopy, many necropsy studies were performed that studied the relationship between coronary calcification and coronary atherosclerosis in the 1960s and 1970s. These studies demonstrated that the extent of coronary calcium reflected total atherosclerotic plaque burden and were related to coronary events (14–17). Eggen and co-workers (18) measured the mean percentage area of raised atherosclerotic plaques and the mean surface area of coronary calcium in those dying of cardiovascular and noncardiovascular causes. The surface area of coronary calcium was measured from postmortem radiographs. They found that the percentage of surface area covered by atherosclerotic plaque and by coronary calcium was much larger in those dying of cardiovascular diseases as compared to noncardiovascular causes. The relative percentage of coronary surface area covered by plaque in those dying coronary vs. noncoronary deaths was actually higher for calcified plaque than for raised atherosclerotic lesions. The relative percentages between cases and controls for coronary calcium were greatest in those dying young (9:1 in the fourth and fifth decades) and decreased in those dying later but was still 2:1 for those dying in their seventh decade. This study suggests that as a marker for clinical coronary disease, calcium is just as good or even better than raised noncalcified atherosclerotic plaques.

Which plaques tend to be calcified? In the 1990s it has become clear that there are two families of plaques (19). Those that are soft due to a large cholesterol ester pool—called fibrous plaques—and those that have ruptured and remodeled after intra- and/or extra-plaque hemorrhage, which are called complicated plaques. The latter plaques are larger and are more likely to be calcified. Kragel and colleagues (20), in a quantitative pathology study found that larger, more obstructive plaques have greater percentages of calcium. Calcium was absent or minimal in plaques that were 0–20% obstructive and increased exponentially in more obstructive plaques. McCarthy and associates (17) found that calcifications were present in 16 of 19 total occlusions found at autopsy. The three cases without calcification had recent infarcts (less than 6 mo) and it was felt these fresh plaques had not had time to calcify. Warburton (15) found coronary calcium in 23 of 24 complete occlusions. These reports are consistent with recent intravascular ultrasound (IVUS) studies (21,22) showing that the hemorrhagic plaques associated with acute coronary events tend not to be calcified. There are no studies yet of the time duration between plaque rupture and the appearance of calcium.

A limitation of conventional pathology studies of coronary calcium is that early calcium deposits are washed out by routine histologic preparations that decalcify the specimens. The quantity of calcium and its association with atherosclerosis is therefore underestimated (23). Performing EBT on the postmortem coronary before it undergoes histological preparation circumvents this limitation. Mautner and associates *(24)* have shown that the EBT calcium score used to quantify coronary calcium (*see* below) has a close correlation with the quantity of calcium found histologically.

Recently, EBT postmortem studies have been performed to examine the quantitative relationship between coronary calcium and plaque burden. Simons and colleagues *(25)* quantified the area of coronary calcium from 38 coronary segments taken from thirteen hearts by counting the number of pixels with Hounsfield units (the standard measure of density on CT scans) greater than 130. Total atherosclerotic plaque burden was quantified by planimetering the total area of plaque under light microscopy after sectioning the coronaries into 3 mm segments. They found a good correlation between the whole heart, coronary artery, and segmental coronary atherosclerotic plaque area and coronary calcium area by EBT.

Sangiorgi and colleagues *(26)* used a nondecalcifying methodology to fix and study 723 3-mm coronary artery segments from 37 coronary arteries. A significant relationship was found between calcium plaque area measured histologically and atherosclerotic plaque area on a per heart basis ($r = .87, p < 0.0001$), per artery basis (left anterior descending [LAD]: $r = .89, p < 0.0001$; left circumflex: $r = .7, p < 0.001$; and RCA: $r = .89$, $p < 0.0001$) and per-segment basis ($r = .52, p < 0.0001$).

Thus, postmortem studies indicate that (1) the presence of coronary calcium is invariably associated with intimal atherosclerosis, (2) calcium tends to be associated with larger, complicated plaques (post plaque rupture), (3) coronary calcification is dramatically more extensive in those dying cardiovascular deaths compared to those dying from noncardiovascular causes, and (4) the total area of coronary calcium correlates well with total plaque burden.

FLUOROSCOPY STUDIES OF CORONARY CALCIUM

Fluoroscopy studies of coronary calcium were predominantly oriented toward the prediction of obstructive disease rather than quantifying the extent of preclinical disease in primary prevention. The sensitivity for obstructive disease was poor in young subjects but specificity was good while in older subjects sensitivity improved while specificity was poor *(27)*. In these studies, calcium was reported as being present or absent and not quantified. The decreasing specificity in older subjects is due to their high prevalence of coronary atherosclerosis *(12)*. Detrano and colleagues *(28)* studied the ability of digital subtraction fluoroscopy to detect nonobstructive and obstructive disease. They found a sensitivity of 83% and a specificity of 79%.

One large study of the prognostic value of fluoroscopy was performed using the Duke data bank. Margolis and associates *(29)* reviewed the records of 800 consecutive patients who underwent both fluoroscopy and coronary angiography and were followed for an average of 5 yr. Calcium was scored as either present or absent. Margolis found that the prevalence of coronary calcium increased in relation to the number of vessels involved with obstructive lesions. The presence of coronary calcium was a predictor of future cardiac events. Its predictive value was found to be independent of the number of angiographically involved vessels as well as independent of age, gender, left ventricular function, and the results of exercise testing.

The detection of calcification of the aortic arch on chest X-ray *(30)* and of the abdominal aorta on abdominal X-ray *(31)* in patients in their fourth and fifth decade has also been found to be associated with future cardiovascular events.

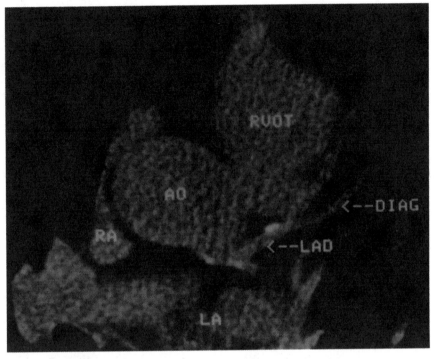

Fig. 2. EBT scans demonstrating calcific deposits (arrowheads) in the left main and LAD. AO = aorta, RVOT = right ventricular outflow tract, LA = left atrium, RA = right atrium, LAD = left anterior descending artery, DIAG = diagonal.

EBT TECHNIQUE

Conventional CT scanners acquire images by rotating an X-ray tube mechanically around the patient. Images are acquired in 1–2 s for conventional scanners and down to 600 ms for "spiral scanners" using partial scanning techniques. When these instruments are used to scan a moving target such as the heart, the resulting image is blurred due to motion artifacts. In contrast, EBT technology eliminates moving parts by rotating an "electron beam" to produce X-rays. The rotating electron beam is swept across a series of one to four semicircular tungsten targets located beneath the patient. Images are acquired in 100 ms using consecutive 3 mm or 1.5 mm thick slices. This speed freezes the motion of the heart and the coronary arteries, thus eliminating motion artifacts *(32)*.

EBT CORONARY CALCIUM PROTOCOL

In 1988, a scanning protocol was developed specifically for imaging of the coronary arteries without the use of contrast media *(33)*. Each slice is acquired in 100 ms and is electrocardiogram gated to diastole. From 20–40 contiguous 3 mm slices are acquired using one or two breath holds. Sequential slices are obtained by table incrementation. The heart is scanned beginning at the base of the aorta and down 12 cm toward the cardiac apex. The unopacified coronary arteries are thus imaged due to the relatively high CT number of flowing blood compared to the periarterial fat. The high density of calcium results in the detection of even very small (1 mm^2) calcified plaques (Fig. 2). The conventional density scale used in all CT imaging is the Hounsfield unit. The threshold for

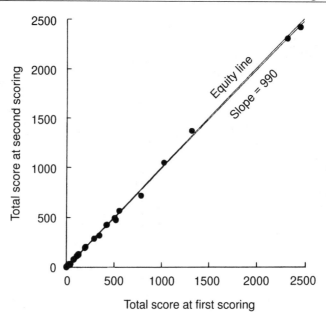

Fig. 3. Intraoberver agreement of two blinded EBT readings of calcium score *(34)*.

a coronary calcium lesion is usually set at a density of 130 Hounsfield units having an area $\geq$1 mm^2. Based on this, a calcium score has been used to quantify the total mass of coronary calcium in the following manner. A "region of interest" is placed around all lesions within the coronary artery. Automated measurements of the lesion area in square millimeters and the maximal computed tomography density in Hounsfield units are determined and recorded. Each lesion is then assigned a density score based on the Hounsfield units as follows: Hounsfield unit 130–199 = 1, 200–299 = 2, 300–399 = 3, and $\geq$400 = 4. A score for each lesion is then calculated by multiplying the density number by the area. The total coronary artery calcium score is the sum of all the individual lesion scores.

In contrast to coronary angiography, stress thallium, stress echo, and carotid intima-medial thickness, the continuous coronary calcium score facilitates automated, fast, easy, and precise quantification. The learning curve for observers is short and inter- and intra-observer agreement is excellent *(34)* (Fig. 3). It is important to appreciate the fact that EBT calcium scores will not differ significantly between tests performed at major medical centers and nonacademic centers.

Reproducibility of EBT has been evaluated by performing sequential studies on the same patient after they have gotten off and then back on the scanning console *(35–37)*. These studies show some problems with reproducibility at low calcium scores—those less than 10. At scores above 10, however, reproducibility is excellent. When determining an initial risk profile, reproducibility is not a problem because small differences in scores do not significantly change the population percentile into which an individual falls. For tracking the progression of disease in individuals, however, other quantification methods in addition to the calcium score such as numbers of lesions, their location, and lesion volumes may be necessary to add precision.

A close correlation between the total coronary calcium score and the quantity of coronary calcium found at postmortem has been documented by Mautner and associates *(24)*.

CORONARY CALCIUM AND EARLY ATHEROSCLEROSIS

Although the orientation of cardiologists has been to detect only obstructive CAD, for the primary prevention of coronary events it is necessary to detect the atherosclerosis at an earlier stage. It would clearly be ideal to detect, quantify, and monitor the progression of coronary artery atherosclerosis before it becomes obstructive. Possibly because coronary atherosclerosis is underestimated by angiography (8), it has been demonstrated that compared with completely normal coronary arteries, even near-normal and mildly diseased vessels predict coronary events (38).

There is also evidence that the prognostic power of obstructive coronary disease as seen on angiographyis due not to the progression of obstructive lesions but because obstructive lesions are surrogate markers for the total extent of coronary atherosclerosis, which include nonobstructive plaques (39). This concept is consistent with the work of Little and co-workers (40) and of Ambrose (41) that demonstrates that it is most often the smaller, nonobstructive plaques that lead to acute coronary events. Nakagomi and colleagues in a study of 350 consecutive patients sent for elective coronary angiography demonstrated a strong positive correlation between the number of vessels with obstructive disease and an atherosclerosis extent score (39). The latter score was based on the percentage of the coronary artery length involved by atheroma defined as any luminal irregularity. This work indicates that when multiple obstructive lesions are present then there are likely to be many nonobstructive and potentially obstructive or occlusive plaques as well.

Can EBT coronary calcium detect and quantify early atherosclerosis? Fallavollita and co-workers (42) performed EBT coronary scans in 98 patients (age 53 ± 12) in whom coronary angiography revealed luminal irregularities less than or equal to 50% diameter stenosis (59 patients), or completely normal coronary arteries (39 patients). Patients with early disease had a mean calcium score of 135 ± 330 (range 0–1719) compared to a mean score of 2.5 ± 4.8 (range 0–19.5) in those with no luminal irregularities. Schmermund and associates (43) studied 49 patients (age 47 ± 12) from the Mayo Clinic EBT database who, on angiography, had normal or near normal coronary arteries (no stenosis ≥20% diameter stenosis, and/or luminal dilatation). Seventy-three percent of patients with near-normal coronaries had coronary calcium by EBT compared with 39% with normal coronaries ($p = 0.02$). We looked at the association of the number of calcified lesions and the calcified plaque volume with the number of coronary segments with luminal irregularities defined as >5% diameter stenosis (44). Good correlations were found for both the number of calcified lesions ($r = .68$, $p < 0.0001$) and the calcified plaque volume ($r = .65$, $p < 0.0001$). These studies showing that coronary calcium scanning can detect early disease are consistent with population studies looking for preclinical markers of atherosclerosis in the young. In the Muscatine Young Adult Follow-up Survey, Mahoney and colleagues (45) found coronary calcium to be present in 31% of young men and 10% of young women (mean age 33). These researchers found that increased body mass index measured during childhood (mean age 15), and increased body mass index, increased blood pressure, and low high-density lipoprotein (HDL) measured in young adult life (mean age 27) predicted the presence of coronary calcium. Coronary artery calcium was also found in very young patients with homozygous familial hypercholesterolemia. Schmidt and associates (46) correlated the level of cholesterol and the age of patients with the severity of coronary calcium by EBT in 17 patients with homozygous familial hypercholesterolemia (age 28 ± 13). They found a good correlation between the coronary calcium

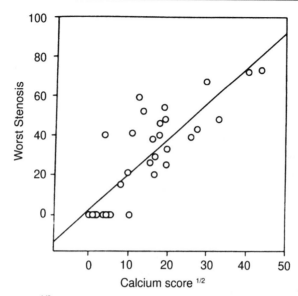

Fig. 4. Calcium score$^{1/2}$ and worst stenosis in 36 asymptomatic subjects, $r = 0.85$ *(49)*.

score and the cholesterol-year score ($r = .77; p < .0001$). In 29 youths (age 14 ± 3) with familial heterozygous hypercholesterolemia (mean cholesterol = 5.95 mmol/L) Gidding and co-workers *(47)* found the presence of coronary calcium in 24% of the subjects. These studies in the young and very young indicate that EBT coronary scanning can detect coronary atherosclerosis at an early stage, years before it is likely to cause a coronary event.

EBT AND OBSTRUCTIVE DISEASE

Does EBT coronary calcification detection predict obstructive disease? Many studies comparing EBT and coronary angiography have been reported. Kaufman and associates *(48)* studied 163 patients with a spectrum of coronary disease on coronary angiography. They found that sensitivity, specificity, and overall accuracy for obstructive disease were 86, 81, and 83%, respectively. For discriminating between those with either nonobstructive and/or obstructive disease, the respective percentages were 81, 86, and 83. Arguably the best indication of the ability of a diagnostic test using a continuous variable to discriminate between the presence or absence of disease is the area under the receiver operating characteristic (ROC) curve. A perfect test would have an area of 1.0. The areas under receiver operating characteristic curves for EBT coronary calcium score were 0.90 for both any disease and for obstructive disease in the foregoing study. These results indicate excellent discrimination of the EBT coronary calcium score for both nonobstructive and obstructive disease.

Guerci and colleagues *(49)* looked at the relationship of EBT coronary calcium score to angiographic findings in both asymptomatic and symptomatic adults. They studied 36 asymptomatic subjects who consented to cardiac catheterization and 54 age- and sex-matched symptomatic control patients. A significant relationship was found between the calcium score and the worst angiographic stenosis for both asymptomatic subjects ($r = .85, p < 0.0001$) and for symptomatic controls ($r = .51, p = 0.0001$, Fig. 4) . An algorithm for the identification of three vessel angiographic disease using a combination of EBT calcium score and risk factor analysis was developed by Schmermund and col-

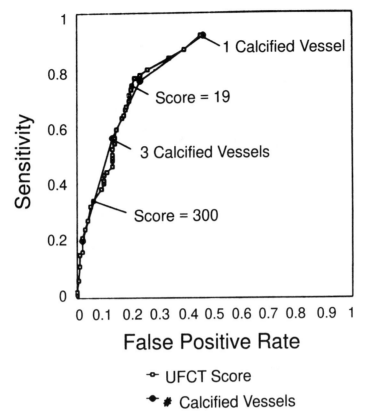

Fig. 5. Receiver-operating characteristic curves for ultrafast computed tomography (UFCT) calcium score of calcified vessels. The false-positive rate represents one specificity. Area under the curve, representing the ability to detect patients with obstructive disease, is 0.82 *(51)*.

leagues *(50)*. Two hundred and ninety-one patients with suspected, but not previously known, CAD were studied. Sixty-eight (23%) of the cohort had three-vessel disease. Receiver operating characteristic curves showed EBT to be superior to clinical risk factors at predicting three-vessel disease (area under curve 0.86 vs. 0.77, $p = 0.002$). A "noninvasive index" incorporating the risk factors of diabetes and male sex showed a small increment in predictive value (area under curve 0.88).

The largest study of the relationship of the EBT coronary calcium score to coronary arteriographic findings was a multicenter study *(51)* of 710 patients from seven medical centers. The findings were concordant with both earlier and subsequent angiographic EBT studies. Of the patients studied, 427 had significant angiographic disease and 404 (95%) of these had coronary calcium on EBT. As the log of the calcium score increased, the probability of multivessel obstructive disease increased ($p < 0.0001$, Fig. 5). The area under the ROC curve for prediction of obstructive disease was 0.82, again indicating excellent discrimination. As in other studies, those with obstructive CAD without coronary calcium on EBT tended to have one vessel disease.

EBT VS. CONVENTIONAL RISK FACTORS

Guerci and associates *(52)* also studied the relative value of the conventional risk factors and the EBT calcium score for predicting angiographic disease. Two hundred and

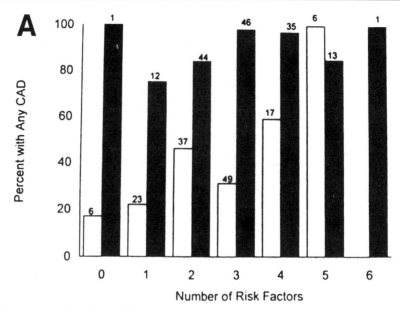

Fig. 6A. Percentage of patients with any coronary disease as a function of the number of risk factors and the coronary calcium score. Solid bars refer to patients with calcium scores below 80%. Open bars refer to patients with calcium scores <80. Numbers at the top of each bar refer to the number of patients in each group. The likelihood of any coronary disease was independent of the number of risk factors for patients with calcium scores below 80, whereas the likelihood of any coronary disease was related to the number of risk factors for those with calcium scores <80. The value of p refers to the difference between the likelihood of disease among those with calcium scores above and below 80%, after adjustment for the number of risk factors. $p < 0.001$ (52).

ninety patients with suspected, but not known, CAD undergoing coronary angiography and EBT were included. Age, the ratio of total cholesterol to high-density lipoprotein, and coronary calcium score were significantly and independently associated with the presence of any CAD and of obstructive CAD. Cigarette smoking was significantly associated with any CAD and diabetes was significantly associated with obstructive CAD. A coronary calcium score of ≥ 80 was associated with an increased likelihood of any coronary disease regardless of the number of risk factors and a calcium score of ≥ 170 was associated with an increased likelihood of obstructive disease regardless of the number of risk factors ($p < 0.001$, Figs. 6A and 6B).

Kennedy and co-workers (53) also compared the coronary calcium score with traditional risk factors to determine their independent predictive power for the diagnosis of obstructive angiographic CAD in symptomatic patients. In 158 patients, 43% of whom had obstructive disease, they found that coronary calcification was a stronger predictor of angiographic CAD than were the standard risk factors. The area under the ROC curves were 0.74 for coronary calcium vs. 0.68 for the risk factors ($p = 0.008$).

FALSE NEGATIVE STUDIES

The false negative rate tends to be higher in younger age groups, running around 10%, whereas in older age groups it is less than 5%. Smokers are commonly found in the group of patients with coronary events but without coronary calcium (22). This may be because

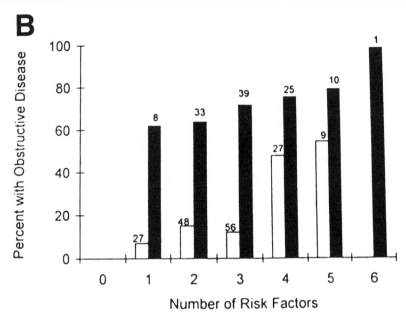

Fig. 6B. Percentage of patients with obstructive coronarv disease as a function of the number of risk factors and the coronary calcium score. Solid bars refer to patients with calcium scores ≥170; open bars refer to patients with calcium scores <170. Numbers at the top of each bar refer to the number of patients in each group. No patient with obstructive disease had no risk factors. Interpretation as in Fig. 6A *(52)*.

smoking is associated with only marginally more coronary atherosclerosis than is present in nonsmokers. This is in contrast to aortic atherosclerosis, which is much more extensive in smokers than nonsmokers *(54)*. It appears that smoking is important as a coronary risk factor more because of its thrombogenic risk than because of its atherosclerotic risk *(55,56)*. This explains why the risk of coronary events in smokers returns to baseline within 1–2 yr of stopping smoking *(57)*. This also explains why smoking shows up as a cause of MI in patients who are then found to have normal coronary arteries. This phenomenon is particularly common in younger patients. Other thrombogenic risk factors should be looked for in patients who experience coronary events without significant coronary risk factors and without extensive coronary artery atherosclerosis by either EBT or coronary angiography. We have identified a 26-yr-old and a 62-yr-old (both nonsmokers) who sustained acute myocardial infarctions with minimal atherosclerosis but with the presence of anticardiolipin antibody and with elevated protein C respectively. Ozner and colleagues studied platelet function in 13 middle-aged patients who had coronary events without established coronary risk factors *(58)*. They found that abnormal platelet function was present in a high percentage of these patients who tended to have minimal or no atherosclerosis on coronary arteriography and unremarkable conventional coronary risk factors. Schmermund and associates *(22)* looked at the relationship between coronary atherosclerosis and coronary calcium in patients with acute coronary syndromes using intravascular ultrasound and EBT. They found that the vast majority of those with acute coronary syndromes had coronary calcium by EBT, but that those with negative EBTs tended to have minimal or no atherosclerotic plaque formation. This line of evidence indicates that EBT as well as coronary angiography quantifies the atherogenic risk for coronary events but cannot quantify the thrombogenic risk. Other methods will be required to identify those groups in addition to smokers who are at risk for coronary events despite only mild coronary atherosclerosis. EBT may be the ideal technique for addressing this problem by identifying patients who have survived into later adulthood with extensive coronary atherosclerosis who have not had coronary events. Comparing the thrombogenic risk profile in these patients with others who have had events with mild atherosclerosis may shed important light on nonatherogenic causes of MI.

Thus, angiographic studies are concordant with pathology studies, showing that EBT coronary calcium quantification indicates the total atherosclerotic burden. Although it does not predict luminal stenosis on a site-by-site basis, it is a good predictor of significant stenosis within the coronary tree. Its major limitation is the identification of those patients destined for events in whom thrombogenic mechanisms predominate over atherogenic mechanisms.

STRESS TESTING AND EBT

Kajinami and associates *(59)* performed EBT on 251 consecutive patients who underwent elective coronary angiography and stress thallium for suspected CAD. As in previous studies they found that as significant CAD increased from zero- to three-vessel disease, the total calcium score increased significantly. By ROC analysis, quantification of coronary artery calcification with EBT predicted angiographically confirmed coronary stenosis as well as thallium in those greater than 70 and better than thallium in those between 40 and 60 yr old.

Zuo-Xiang He and colleagues *(60)* prospectively studied 411 patients who underwent EBT and stress myocardial perfusion tomography (SPECT). None of the patients with calcium scores less than 10 had positive SPECT imaging. For patients with scores of 11–100, 101–399, and greater than or equal to 400 the percentages with abnormal SPECTs were 2.6%, 11.3%, and 46% ($p < 0.0001$), respectively. They concluded that the coronary calcium score identifies a high risk group of asymptomatic subjects who have clinically important silent ischemia.

POPULATION STUDIES

If EBT coronary calcium quantification reflects total atherosclerotic burden, how is this reflected in studying asymptomatic and symptomatic populations? We studied *(33)* 584 patients, 109 with and 475 without CAD. In all age groups, there was a significantly and dramatically higher calcium score in those with vs. those without clinical coronary disease (Table 1). We also compared the prevalence of coronary calcium in asymptomatic men and women *(61)*. We scanned 1396 males and 502 females (age range 14–88 yr). The prevalence of calcium, and the distribution of total calcium scores were compared for men and women at 5- and 10-yr intervals. The prevalence of calcium in women was half that of men, until the age of 60 yr when the difference diminished. The mean total calcium score distributions of men between the ages of 40 and 69 yr were virtually identical to those of women between the ages of 50 and 79. The quantitative data obtained by EBT showed very close agreement with autopsy studies of coronary calcium. The differences in prevalence and extent of coronary calcium appear to be parallel to those observed in the clinical incidence of CAD in men and women.

Table 1
Calcification in Coronary Disease Versus No Coronary Disease by Age in 584 Subjects

| | Age group (yr) | | | |
	30–39	40–49	50–59	60–69
No of patients				
No CAD	110	181	116	68
CAD	3	17	54	35
Prevalence				
No CAD	25%	39%	73%	74%
CAD	100%	88%	96%	100%
Total calcium score (raw)				
No CAD	5 ± 2	27 ± 9	83 ± 14	187 ± 38
CAD	132 ± 91	291 ± 93	462 ± 95	786 ± 115
Total calcium score (LN)[a]				
No CAD	0.24 ± 0.05	0.42 ± 0.05	1.14 ± 0.09	1.43 ± 0.13
CAD	1.80 ± 0.42	1.87 ± 0.24	2.04 ± 0.13	2.66 ± 0.09
Lesion number (raw)				
No CAD	0.6 ± 0.15	1.6 ± 0.33	4.6 ± 0.55	7.1 ± 1.07
CAD	6.7 ± 1.2	11.4 ± 2.5	14.4 ± 2.0	25.3 ± 2.7
Lesion number (SQRT)				
No CAD	0.8 ± 0.05	1.1 ± 0.07	1.0 ± 0.11	2.3 ± 0.19
CAD	2.6 ± 0.22	3.0 ± 0.40	3.4 ± 0.25	4.8 ± 0.27
	$p < 0.01$	$p < 0.0001$	$p < 0.0001$	$p < 0.0001$

[a]$p < 0.0001$ over all ages. Values are expressed as mean values ± standard error of the mean; CAD = clinical coronary artery disease; lesion number = number of coronary calcific densities reported; LN = logarithmic transformed data; prevalence = prevalence of reported coronary calcium by computed tomography; raw = raw data; SQRT = square root transformed data (33).

PROSPECTIVE STUDIES

The fluoroscopy study of Margolis and associates (29) mentioned earlier indicated the potential for the detection of the presence of coronary calcium to independently predict future cardiovascular events. Detrano and co-workers (62) performed digital subtraction cinefluoroscopy on 1461 high-risk asymptomatic adults and followed them prospectively for 8 yr. The presence of coronary artery calcium was an independent predictor of coronary endpoints. Neither Margolis nor Detrano quantified coronary calcium, which is difficult to do using fluoroscopy.

EBT has the advantage of precise and reproducible quantification of coronary calcium. Detrano and co-workers (63) studied 491 symptomatic patients who had undergone coronary angiography with EBT. Thirteen CHD-related deaths and 8 nonfatal acute infarctions occurred over 30 ± 13 mo. The EBT coronary calcium score correlated well with the presence of obstructive disease on angiography ($p = 0.0001$). The EBT calcium score predicted coronary events as well as did the number of angiographically affected arteries.

We followed 367 asymptomatic subjects for 5.9 ± 1.4 yr (64). The mean age was 52 ± 13. Nineteen sustained coronary events including MI, angina with a positive angiogram, coronary bypass surgery, and PTCA. The mean calcium scores in those with compared to those without events were 509 ± 435 and 76 ± 206, respectively ($p < 0.0001$). The odds ratios for those having events with total calcium score cutoffs of 0, 50, and 100 was 14.9 ($p < 0.0005$), 11.1 ($p < 0.0001$) and 9.8 ($p < 0.0001$), respectively. The Kaplan-

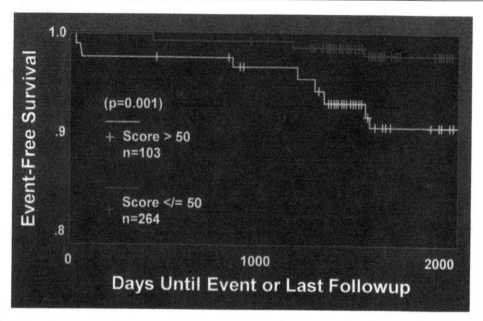

Fig. 7. Event free survival in those with calcium scores greater than 50 (*top line*) compared to those with calcium scores less than 50 (*lower line*).

Meier curve for a calcium score cutoff of 50 is shown in Fig. 7. It can be appreciated that most of the separation between groups occurred after several years.

Arad and colleagues *(65)* performed EBTs on 1173 asymptomatic subjects, free from a history of clinical CAD, with a mean age of 52. They were followed for 19 mo and 18 patients sustained 26 cardiac events during this period. The sensitivities and specificities for an event for calcium scores of 100, 160, and 680 were 89%, 89%, and 50% and 77%, 82%, and 95%, respectively. Odds ratios ranged from 20.0–35.4 for a coronary event ($p < 0.0001$ for all). Detrano and associates *(66)* also followed a cohort of 1196 asymptomatic, older high-risk asymptomatic patients (mean age 66). There were 46 coronary events recorded over 41 mo. The relative risk for an event for a calcium score greater than 44 was 2.4. An ROC curve constructed with a combination of calcium score and risk factors was 0.71 ± 0.04. This did not differ significantly from a score derived from risk factors alone, a finding that is discordant from other studies. Subjects were recruited knowing they were at high risk for events and were told of the results of coronary fluoroscopy and EBT. The number of subjects who acted on this information by taking aspirin, statins, and other preventive measures was not reported.

EBT AND PROGRESSION OF CAD

The progression of CAD by angiography has been used as a surrogate for coronary events in clinical trials. Waters and colleagues *(67)* looked at the relationship between the angiographic progression of coronary atherosclerosis and clinical endpoints in 335 patients after a mean follow-up of 44 ± 10 mo. They found coronary progression to be a strong and independent predictor of future coronary events and concluded that it is indeed justified as a surrogate marker in clinical trials. Janowitz and co-workers *(68)* studied the potential of EBT to track the progression of coronary calcium. They followed 10 asymptomatic patients with coronary calcium and 10 patients with clinical CAD with sequential

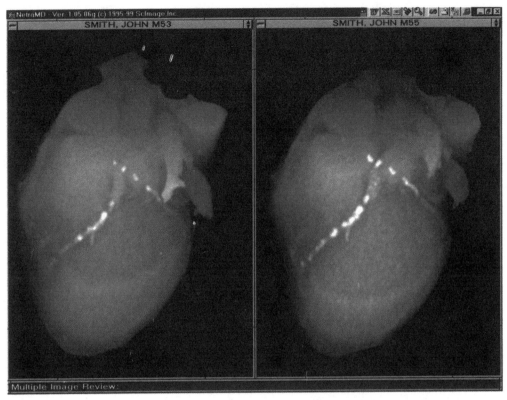

Fig. 8. Serial studies performed one and one half years apart. Left anterior descending artery, diagonally at left of heart; right coronary artery at right. (Reproduced with permission from Tracey Callister.)

scans 1 yr apart. It was found that the progression of calcified plaques could be easily tracked on a one-to-one basis. Overall, patients with clinical CAD had an increase in total calcium score of 44% at 1 yr and those with coronary calcium but without clinical disease progressed at a mean rate of 22%. With current work stations that can perform rapid three-dimensional reconstructions, the progression of coronary calcium can be monitored easily and accurately (Fig. 8). Callister and associates *(69)* used a volume score to assess coronary artery calcium on EBT scans separated by at least 12 mo and correlated its progression with treatment using HMG-CoA reductase inhibitors. Forty-four patients who were untreated increased their calcium volume by $52 \pm 36\%$ ($p < 0.001$). Patients who were treated with statins but with LDLs of greater than 120 mg/dL after treatment progressed at a rate of $25 \pm 22\%$ ($p < 0.001$) . Those who were treated and achieved LDLs of less than 120 mg/dL had a net regression with a decrease in mean calcium volume of $-7 \pm 23\%$ ($p = 0.01$). Figure 9 shows the relationship of the degree of LDL lowering vs. change in calcium volume score.

THE TOTALITY OF EVIDENCE

The evaluation of a risk factor for predicting cardiovascular events should be based on the totality of evidence. The parameters used to assess a new risk factor include (1) biologic credibility, (2) dose response relationship, (3) strength of association, (4) concordance of studies, and (5) quality of studies *(70)*.

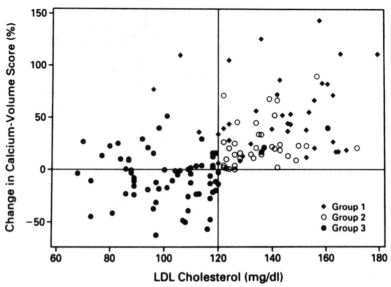

Fig. 9. Scatter plot of the percent change in the calcium–volume score at 1 yr in relation to the average LDL-C level for all patients. All untreated patients (group 1) and treated patients with average LDL-C levels of at least 120 mg/dL (group 2) had increased scores, whereas 63% of treated patients with average LDL-C levels below 120 mg/dL (group 3) had decreased scores *(1)*.

Because coronary calcification is actually part of the atherosclerotic process and correlates well with total plaque burden in pathology studies, its biologic credibility is well established. The dose-response relationship between coronary calcium and the quantity of atherosclerosis seen pathologically, angiographically, and by the clinical measures of positive stress testing and clinical events has also been clearly and repeatedly demonstrated. The strength of association between coronary calcium score and both anatomic and clinical measures of atherosclerosis is in the same order of magnitude as that of smoking and lung cancer. There is excellent concordance within and between the pathologic, angiographic and clinical EBT literature.

The overall quality of studies is also excellent. The ideal study of the prognostic significance of coronary calcium, however, has not been performed. This study would take a randomly selected population, scan them, and not let the subjects or the physicians know the calcium score. The population could then be followed to find the precise relationship between coronary calcium score and future events. Such a study, however, can no longer be justified on ethical grounds because of the volume of evidence indicating the clinical significance of coronary calcium.

Most of the correlational descriptive studies and case control studies of coronary calcium do not suffer from the limitations of such studies when they are used to examine risk factors such as cholesterol level or interventions such as hormone replacement therapy (HRT) or taking antioxidant vitamins. Biases are present in the later studies because subjects are self-selected or selected by their physicians for various treatments and/or lifestyle changes. Measurements of many of the risk factors have substantial variability. Cholesterol and other lipid levels may vary over short periods of time and may not reflect the subject's long-term levels, which may change acutely at the time of illness. Recall bias for certain exposures may also introduce error. For these reasons, large and expen-

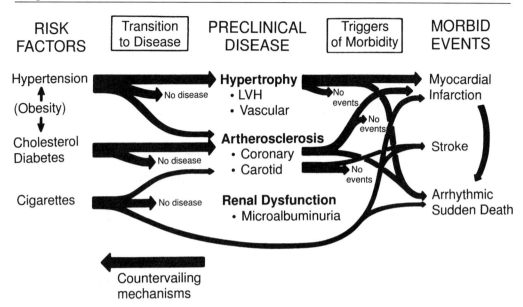

Fig. 10. Concept of the relationship of preclinical disease to risk factors and morbid events. The presence of preclinical disease is invariably a better predictor of morbid events than are the conventional risk factors.

sive clinical trials are necessary to determine if there are significant associations between exposures and events.

For the presence of coronary calcium in case-control studies or angiographic correlational studies, the subjects and physicians were unaware of their calcium scores. They therefore could not change potentially confounding variables in response to such knowledge. In addition, these scores do not change significantly from week to week, month to month, or test to test on the same day. In contrast, for prospective studies of the significance of coronary calcium, knowledge of the score may lead to lifestyle changes and therapeutic interventions (such as aspirin administration) by the patient and/or physician, thus introducing confounding variables.

Although there are legitimate differences of opinion concerning what calcium score thresholds require what treatments (71), the totality of evidence clearly shows that high scores are indications for aggressive risk-factor interventions. For this reason, it has been proposed that the EBT coronary calcium score should be incorporated into the National Cholesterol Education Program guidelines (72,73).

THE FUTURE—THE NEW PREVENTION STRATEGY

Currently, a "new prevention strategy" is emerging based on the noninvasive imaging of preclinical disease and advanced blood testing of new lipid and nonlipid risk factors. The concept that the detection of preclinical disease should play an important role in prevention screening was reviewed by Devereux and Alderman (1) (see Fig. 10). It makes pathophysiological sense that the presence of actual pathologic changes in target organs should be better predictors of clinical events than are risk factors. This has been borne out by the medical literature. In the Framingham Study (74), left ventricular mass was a better predictor of morbidity and mortality than blood pressure and was independent of other risk factors as well. In a similar manner, the presence of preclinical disease in

The New Prevention Strategy

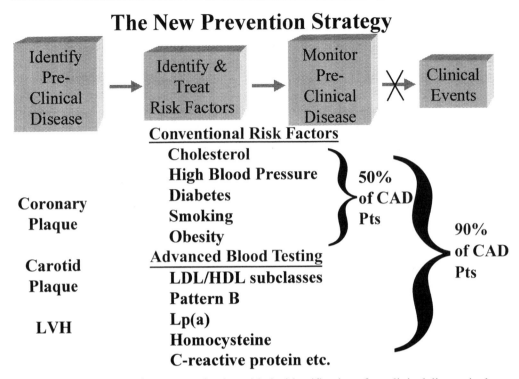

Fig. 11. The new prevention strategy begins with the identification of preclinical disease in those at a minimal threshold of risk based on the conventional risk factors. If disease is present, risk factors will be treated and the effect on progression of preclinical disease monitored. If preclinical disease progresses (as seen in Fig. 8), more aggressive treatment of the conventional and/or the new risk factors is indicated. If preclinical disease is controlled, clinical disease is unlikely.

the carotid artery as indicated by increased intima-medial thickness has been shown to be a better predictor of MI and stroke in older asymptomatic individuals than are the conventional risk factors *(75)*. The relative risk between the highest vs. lowest quintile of intima-medial thickness was 3.87 ($p < 0.001$). The strong predictive value of EBT for future coronary events was discussed previously.

The ability of EBT, using 3-dimensional reconstructions, to track atherosclerosis progression with serial studies allows physicians to tailor therapy to each individual. As impressive as the statin trials have been, it should be appreciated that they decrease coronary events by only 20–40% *(76)*. This means that the majority of patients who take statins and are destined for coronary events still have them. Current evidence from low-fat diet trials is not convincing that such diets can decrease the risk of coronary events beyond that attained by the statins *(77)*.

Strategies that include new blood tests for the atherogenic lipid profile (gradient gel electrophoresis for LDL size), as well as tests for lipoprotein(a), homocysteine, c-reactive protein, and other potential risk factors show promise for adding therapies to the statins that will decrease coronary events well beyond the levels attained by statin treatment alone *(78)*. It is often difficult to set goals of lipid and blood pressure lowering as well as goals of diet and exercise for individual patients. By monitoring coronary atherosclerosis with serial EBT examinations, both the patient and the physician can get the feedback required to optimize treatment (Fig. 11). Wong and associates *(79)* demonstrated that this feedback can help motivate beneficial lifestyle behaviors including aspirin usage, weight loss, and decreasing dietary fat intake. If there is progression in calcified plaque on serial studies (Fig. 9), then either more aggressive therapy of known risk factors or the search for additional modifiable risk factors is indicated. If there is no progression, then the patient and physician can feel confident that the risk of a coronary event has been minimized.

In conclusion, a combination of better noninvasive imaging of the presence and progression of preclinical atherosclerosis and the identification and treatment of the traditional and the new risk factors, will facilitate the prevention of the great majority of cardiovascular events.

REFERENCES

1. Devereux RB, Alderman MH. Role of preclinical cardiovascular disease in the evolution from risk factor exposure to development of morbid events. Circulation 1993;88:1444–1455.
2. McNamara JJ, Molot MA, Stremple IF, Cutting RT. Coronary artery disease in combat casualties in Vietnam. JAMA 1971;216:1185–1187. 21. Strong JP. Coronary atherosclerosis in soldiers: a clue to the natural history of atherosclerosis in the young. JAMA 1986;256:2863–2866.
3. Enos WF, Holmes RH, Beyer J. Coronary disease among United States soldiers killed in action in Korea: preliminary report. JAMA 1953;152:1090–1093.
4. Berenson GS, Srinivasan SR, Bao W, et al. Association between multiple cardiovascular risk factors and atherosclerosis in children and young adults. The Bogalusa Heart Study. N Engl J Med 1998;338:1690–1692.
5. Roberts WC, Jones AA. Quantitation of coronary artery narrowing at necropsy in sudden coronary death: analysis of 31 patients and comparison with 25 control subjects. Am J Cardiol 1979;44:39–45.
6. Wames CA, Roberts WC. Comparison at necropsy by age group, of amount and distribution of narrowing by atherosclerotic plaque in 2995 5 mm long segments of 240 major coronary arteries in 60 men aged 31 to 70 years with sudden coronary death. Am Heart J 1994;108:431–435.
7. Cabin HS, Roberts WC. Quantitative comparison of extent of coronary narrowing and size of healed myocardial infarct in 33 necropsy patients with clinically recognized and in 28 with clinically unrecognized (silent) previous acute myocardial infarction. Am J Cardiol 1982;50:677–680.
8. Arnett EN, Isner JM, Redwood DR, et al. Coronary artery narrowing in coronary heart disease: comparison of cineangiographic and necropsy findings. Ann Intern Med 1979;91:350–356.
9. Waller BF, The eccentric coronary atherosclerotic plaque: morphologic observations and clinical relevance. Clin Cardiol 1989;12:14–20.
10. Glagov S, Weisenberg E, Zarins CK, et al. Compensatory enlargement of human atherosclerotic coronary arteries. N Engl J Med 1987;316:1371–1375.
11. Tobis JM, Mallery J, Mahon D, et al. Intravascular ultrasound imaging of human coronary arteries in vivo. Circulation 1991;83:913–926.
12. Rifkin RD, Parisi AF, Folland E. Coronary calcification in the diagnosis of coronary artery disease. Am J Cardiol 1979;44:141–146.
13. Blankenhorn DH. Coronary calcification: a review. Am J Med Sci 1961;242:1–9.
14. Beakenkopf WG, Daoud AS, Love BM. Calcification in the coronary arteries and its relation to arteriosclerosis and myocardial infarction. Am J Radiol 1964;92:865–871.
15. Warburton RK, Tampas JP, Soule AB, et al. Coronary artery calcification: its relationship to coronary artery stenosis and myocardial infarction. Radiology 1968;91:109–115.
16. Frink RJ, Achor RWP, Brown AL, et al. Significance of calcification of the coronary arteries. Am J Cardiol 1970;26:241–247.
17. McCarthy JH, Palmer FJ. Incidence and significance of coronary artery calcification. Br Heart J 1974;36:499–506.
18. Eggen DA, Strong JP, McGill KC. Coronary calcification: relationship to clinically significant coronary lesions and race, sex and topographical distribution. Circulation 1965;32:948–955.
19. Fuster V, Badimon L, Badimon JJ, Chesebro JH. The pathogenesis of coronary artery disease and the acute coronary syndromes (first of two parts). N Engl J Med 1992;326:242–250.

20. Kragel AH, Reddy SG, Wittes JT, et al. Morphomeuic analysis of the composition of atherosclerotic plaques in the four major epicardial coronary arteries in acute myocardial infarction and in sudden coronary death. Circulation 1989;80:1747–1756.

21. Mintz GS, Pichard AD, Popma JJ, et al. Determinants and correlates of target lesion calcium in coronary artery disease: a clinical, angiographic and intravascular ultrasound study. J Am Coll Cardiol 1997;29: 268–274.

22. Schmermund A, Baumgart G, Görge G, et al. Coronary artery calcium in acute coronary syndromes: a comparative study of electron beam CT, coronary angiography, and intracoronary ultrasound in survivors of acute myocardial infarction and unstable angina. Circulation 1997;96:1461–1469.

23. Fitzpatrick LA, Severson A, Edwards WD, Ingram RT. Diffuse calcification in human coronary arteries: association of osteopontin with atherosclerosis. J Clin Invest 1994;1597–1604.

24. Mautner SL, Mautner GC, Froehlich J, et al. Coronary artery disease: prediction with in vitro electron beam CT. Radiology 1994;192:625–630.

25. Simons DB, Schwartz RS, Edwards WD, et al. Noninvasive definition of anatomic coronary artery disease by ultrafast computed tomographic scanning: a quantitative pathologic comparison study. J Am Coll Cardiol 1992;20:1118–1126.

26. Sangiorgi G, Rumberger JA, Severson A, et al. Arterial calcification and not lumen stenosis is highly correlated with atherosclerotic plaque burden in humans: a histologic study of 723 coronary artery segments using non-decalcifying methodology. J Am Cardiol 1998;31:126–133.

27. Uretsky BF, Rifkin RD, Sharma SC, et al. Value of fluoroscopy in the detection of coronary stenosis: influence of age, sex and number of vessels calcified on diagnostic efficacy. Am Heart J 1988;115:323–333.

28. Detrano R, Markovic D, Simpfendorfer C, et al. Digital subtraction fluoroscopy: a new method of detecting coronary calcifications with improved sensitivity for the prediction of coronary disease. Circulation 1985;71:725–732.

29. Margolis JR, Chen M, Kong Y, et al. The diagnostic and prognostic significance of coronary artery calcification. A report of 800 cases. Radiology 1980;137:609–616.

30. Witteman JCM, Kannel WB, Wolf PA, et al. Aortic calcified plaques and cardiovascular disease: The Framingham Study. Am J Cardiol 1990;66:1060–1064.

31. Witteman JCM, Kok FJ, Saase Van JLCM, et al. Aortic calcification as a predictor of cardiovascular mortality. Lancet 1986;2:1120–1122.

32. Gould RG. Principles of ultrafast computed tomography: historical aspects, mechanism of action and scanner characteristics. In: Stanford W, Rumberger JA, eds. Ultrafast Computed Tomography in Cardiac Imaging: Principles and Practice. Futura Publishing, Mount Kisco, NY, 1992, pp. 1–16.

33. Agatston AS, Janowitz WR, Hildner FJ, et al. Quantification of coronary artery calcium using ultrafast computed tomography. J Am Coll Cardiol 1990;15:827–832.

34. Kaufmann RB, Sheedy PF II, Breen JF, et al. Detection of heart calcification with electron beam CT: interobserver and intraobserver reliability for scoring quantification. Radiology 1994;190:347–352.

35. Bielak LF, Kaufmann RB, Moll PP, et al. Small lesions in the heart identified at electron beam CT: calcification or nose? Radiology 1994;192:631–636.

36. Devries S, Wolfkiel C, Shah V, et al. Reproducibility of the measurement of coronary calcium with ultrafast computed tomography. Am J Cardiol 1995;75:973–977.

37. McCollough CH, Kaufmann RB, Cameron BM, et al. Electron beam CT: use of a calibration phantom to reduce variability in calcium quantification. Radiology 1995;196:159–165.

38. Kemp HG, Kronmal RA, Vlietstra RE, Frye RL. Seven year survival of patients with normal or near normal coronary arteriograms: a CASS registry study. J Am Coll Cardiol 1986;7:479–483.

39. Nakagomi A, Celermajer DS, Lumley T, Freedman SB. Angiographic severity of coronary narrowing is a surrogate marker for the extent of coronary arthrosclerosis. Am J Cardiol 1996;78:516–519.

40. Little WC, Constantiescu M, Applegate RI, et al. Can coronary angiography predict the site of a subsequent myocardial infarction in patients with mild-to-moderate coronary artery disease? Circulation 1988;78:1157–1166.

41. Ambrose JA, Tannenbaum MA, Alexopoulos D, et al. Angiographic progression of coronary artery disease and the development of myocardial infarction. J Am Coll Cardiol 1988;12:56–62.

42. Fallavollita JA, Kumar K, Brody AS, et al. Detection of coronary artery calcium to differentiate patient with early coronary atherosclerosis from luminally normal arteries. Am J Cardiol 1996;78:1281–1283.

43. Schmermund A, Rumberger JA, Colter JF, et al. Angiographic correlates of "spotty" coronary artery calcium detected by electron-beam computed tomography in patients with normal or near-normal coronary angiograms. Am J Cardiol 1998;82:508–511.

44. Agatston AS, Janowitz WR, Kaplan G, et al. Ultrafast computed tomography-detected coronary calcium reflects the angiographic extent of coronary arterial atherosclerosis. Am J Cardiol 1994;74:1272–1274.
45. Mahoney LT, Burns TL, Stanford W, et al. Coronary risk factors measured in childhood and young adult life are associated with coronary artery calcification in young adults: the Muscatine Study. Am Coll Cardiol 1996;27:277–284.
46. Schmidt HH, Hill S, Makariou EV, et al. Relation of cholesterol-year score to severity of calcific atherosclerosis and tissue deposition in homozygous familial hypercholesterolemia. Am J Cardiol 1996; 77:575–580.
47. Gidding SS, Bookstein LC, Chomka EV. Usefulness of electron beam tomography in adolescents and young adults with heterozygous familial hypercholesteromia. Circulation 1998;98:2580–2583.
48. Kaufmann RB, Peyser PA, Sheedy PF, et al. Quantification of coronary artery calcium by electron beam computed tomography for determination of severity of angiographic coronary artery disease in younger patients. J Am Coll Cardiol 1995;25:626–632.
49. Guerci AD, Spadaro LA, Popma JJ, et al. Relation of coronary calcium score by electron beam computed tomography to arteriographic findings in asymptomatic and Budoff symptomatic adults. Am J Cardiol 1997;79:128–133.
50. Schmermund A, Bailey KR, Rumberger JA, et al. An algorithm for noninvasive identification of angiographic three-vessel and/or left main coronary artery disease in symptomatic patients on the basis of cardiac risk and electron-beam computed tomograpic calcium scores. J Am Coll Cardiol 1999;33:444–452.
51. Budoff MJ, Georgiou D, Brody A, Agatston AS, et al. Ultrafast computed tomography as a diagnostic modality in the detection of coronary artery disease. Circultation 1996;93:898–904.
52. Guerci AD, Spadaro LA, Goodman KJ, et al. Comparison of electron beam computed tomography scanning and conventional risk factor assessment for the prediction of angiographic coronary artery disease. J Am Coll Cardiol 1998;32:673–679.
53. Kennedy J, Shavelle R, Wang S, et al. Coronary calcium and standard risk factors in symptomatic patient referred for coronary angiography. Am Heart J 1998;135:696–702.
54. Strong JP, Richard ML. Cigarette smoking and atherosclerosis in autopsied men. Atherosclerosis 1976; 23:451–476.
55. Fuster V, Chesebro JH, Frye RL, Elveback LR. Platelet survival and the development of coronary artery disease in the young adult: effects of cigarette smoking, strong family history and medical therapy. Circulation 1981;63:546–550.
56. Hung J, Lam JYT, Lacoste L, Letchacovski G. Cigarette smoking acutely increases platelet thrombus formation in patients with coronary artery disease taking aspirin. Circulation 1995;92:2432–2436.
57. Kennedy J, Shavelle R, Wang S, et al. Coronary calcium and standard risk factors in symptomatic patient referred for coronary angiography. Am Heart J 1998;135:696–702.
58. Ozner M, Ahn YS, Meyerberg RJ. Chronic platelet activation and acute coronary syndromes in 13 middle aged patients. J Clin Appl Thromb 1997;3:46–53.
59. Kajinami K, Seki H, Takekoshi N, Mabuchi H. Noninvasive prediction of coronary atherosclerosis by quantification of coronary artery calcification using electron beam computed tomography: comparison with electrocardiographic and thallium exercise stress test results. J Am Coll Cardiol 1995;26:1209–1221.
60. He ZX, Hedrick TD, Pratt CM, et al. Severity of coronary artery calcification by eltectron beam tomography predicts silent myocardial ischemia. Circulation 2000;101:244–251.
61. Janowitz WR, Agatston AS, Kaplan G, Viamonte M Jr. Differences in prevalence and extent of coronary artery calcium detected by ultrafast computed tomography in asymptomatic men and women. Am J Cardiol 1993;72(3):247–254.
62. Detrano RC, Wong ND, Tang W, et al. Prognostic significance of cardiac cinefluoroscopy for coronary calcific deposits in asymptomatic high risk subjects. J Am Coll Cardiol 1994;24:354–358.
63. Detrano R, Hsiai T, Wang S, et al. Prognostic value of coronary calcification and angiographic stenoses in patients undergoing coronary angiography. J Am Coll Cardiol 1996;27:285–290.
64. Agatston AS, Janowitz WR, Kaplan G, et al. Electron beam CT coronary calcium predicts future coronary events. Circulation 1996;94:I–360A.
65. Arad Y, Spadaro LA, Goodman K, et al. Predictive value of electron beam computed tomography of the coronary arteries. 19 month follow-up of 1173 asymptomatic subjects. Circulation 1996;93(11): 1951–1953.
66. Detrano RC, Wong ND, Doherty TM, et al. Coronary calcium does not accurately predict near-term future coronary events in high-risk adults. Circulation 1999;99:2633–2638.
67. Waters D, Craven CE, Lesperance J. Prognostic significance of progression of coronary atherosclerosis. Circulation 1993;87:1067–1075.

68. Janowitz WR, Agatston AS, Viamonte M. Comparison of serial quantitative evaluation of calcified coronary artery plaque by ultrafast computed tomography in persons with and without obstructive coronary artery disease. Am J Cardiol 1991;681:1–6.

69. Callister TQ, Raggi P, Cooil B, et al. Effect of HMG-CoA reductase inhibitors on coronary artery disease as assessed by electron-beam computed tomography. N Engl J Med 1998;339(27):1972–1978.

70. Hennekens CH, Buring JE. Statistical association and cause-effect relationships. In: Mayrent SL, ed. Epidemiology in Medicine. Little, Brown and Co., Boston/Toronto, 1987, pp. 30–53.

71. Rumberger JA, Brundage BH, Rader DJ, Kondos G. Electron beam computed tomographic coronary calcium scanning: a review and guidelines for use in asymptomatic persons. Mayo Clin Proc 1999;74: 243–252.

72. Grundy SM. Age as a risk factor: you are as old as your arteries. Am J Cardiol 1999;83(10):1455–1457.

73. Grundy SM. Primary prevention of heart disease-integrating risk assessment with intervention. Circulation 1999;100:988–998.

74. Koren MJ, Devereux RB, Casale PN, et al. Relation of left ventricular mass and geometry to morbidity and mortality in men and women with essential hypertension. Ann Intern Med. 1991;114:345–352.

75. O'Leary DH, Polak JF, Kronmal RA, et al. Carotid atherosclerosis as quantified by measuring the intimal-medial thickness is a superior predictor of myocardial infarction and stroke compared to the conventional risk factors. Cardiovascular Health Study Collaborative Research Group. N Engl J Med 1999;340(1):14–22.

76. Superko HR. Beyond LDL-C reduction. Circulation 1996;94:2351–2354.

77. Corr LA, Oliver MF. The low fat/low cholesterol diet is ineffective. Eur Heart J 1997;18:18–22.

78. Superko HR. The new thinking on lipids and coronary artery disease. Curr Opin Cardiol 1997;12: 180–187.

79. Wong ND, Detrano RC, Diamond G, et al. Does coronary artery screening by electron beam computed tomography motivate potentially beneficial lifestyle behaviors? Am J Cardiol 1996;78:1220–1223.

17

A Multidisciplinary Model for Aggressive Risk Factor Control in Cardiovascular Disease

Joseph P. Frolkis, MD, PHD

CONTENTS

INTRODUCTION
BACKGROUND
RATIONALE
CONCLUSION
REFERENCES

INTRODUCTION

Critical recent insights into the epidemiology, pathophysiology, and treatment of cardiovascular disease (CVD) have served to underscore the value of primary and secondary prevention efforts. At the same time, there is growing awareness that a troubling gap exists between accepted standards for risk factor assessment and control and actual clinical practice. This is particularly so for traditional care settings in which the physician is the source of preventive services. The resulting context creates an opportunity to develop innovative and effective models for the detection and modification of CVD risk factors. This chapter reviews the background and rationale for the creation of a Preventive Cardiology Program, summarizes the design of the program developed at The Cleveland Clinic Foundation, and describes representative clinical outcomes from our initial cohort.

BACKGROUND

CVD Epidemiology

Approximately 1 million deaths yearly are attributable to CVD, making it the leading cause of mortality in the United States *(1)*. Coronary heart disease (CHD) causes more than half of all CVD deaths, making it alone the overall national leader in mortality *(2)*. In addition to mortality, of course, CVD imposes a terrible of burden of suffering on those who survive, including the loss of normal ventricular function in half of those with a

From: *Contemporary Cardiology: Preventive Cardiology:
Insights into the Prevention and Treatment of Coronary Artery Disease*
Edited by: J. Foody © Humana Press Inc., Totowa, NJ

history of myocardial infarction *(3)*, and significant functional impairment in many of the 4 million stroke survivors *(4)*. This sobering human cost is accompanied by a staggering financial one, with current estimates of combined direct and indirect annual CVD expenses approaching $300 billion *(5)*.

Recent epidemiological trends in CVD have important implications for the future of preventive cardiology. There has been a marked decrease in age-adjusted mortality rates for both CHD and stroke in the United States over the last 30 yr *(2)*, probably as a result of decreased levels of serum cholesterol *(6)*, blood pressure *(7)*, and cigarette smoking *(8)*. Improved survival rates for initial myocardial infarction (MI), and more effective secondary prevention in those who have experienced an initial event also contribute to this trend *(9)*. These improved survival rates, however, combined with the increasing prevalence of CVD with age and the concurrent rise in the percentage of the population that is elderly, have produced a paradoxical *increase* in the overall prevalence of CVD which is projected to continue into the next century *(10)*. Thus, the population at risk for both initial and recurrent CVD events, and therefore likely to benefit from aggressive risk factor control, will increase in the future.

These population trends have been accompanied by a growing understanding of the epidemiological behavior of the risk factors for CVD. It is now appreciated, for instance, that CVD is unlikely to occur when a patient has only a single risk factor. Much more commonly, two or more such factors co-occur in a given patient *(1,11,12)*. The presence of multiple CVD risk factors significantly increases the relative and absolute risks of CVD and CHD in both men and women *(13)*, and it has become apparent that risk factors are at least additive, and probably synergistic, in their effects *(14,15)*. Such findings clarify the multifactorial nature of CVD, and underscore the importance of simultaneously assessing all risk factors in a given patient in the process of estimating future risk *(13,16)*.

Effectiveness of Risk Factor Control

In addition to the scientific data on the potent and interactive nature of CVD risk factors and the increasing population burden of CVD, there is consistent and encouraging evidence about the reduction of CVD incidence that can be produced through control of the modifiable risk factors for the disease. Although a complete review of the supporting literature is beyond the scope of this chapter, it may be helpful to briefly summarize the current consensus on several of the major traditional CVD risk factors that are amenable to modification in the preventive cardiology setting.

The five major clinical studies published to date examining the effects of lipid lowering with the 3-hydroxy-3-methylglutaryl coenzyme A (HMG-CoA) reductase inhibitors (the "statin trials") for both primary and secondary prevention have demonstrated striking reductions in relative risks for morbid and mortal CVD events for men and women across a wide range of ages and lipid levels *(17–21)*. Each of these trials also documented a statistically significant decrease in the need for revascularization procedures. In addition, the three secondary prevention trials *(18,20,21)* found a significant decrease in cerebrovascular events in patients treated with statins, an effect supported by studies documenting regression of carotid atherosclerosis as a result of aggressive lipid lowering *(22,23)*, and by a recent meta-analysis showing that cholesterol lowering with the statins reduces the risk of stroke *(24)*.

The reduction in risk for CVD events that accompanies cigarette cessation *(25,26)*, control of elevated blood pressure *(27–31)*, and the use of antithrombotic agents *(32,33)* is similarly well documented and unequivocal. Each of these risk factors confers a two- to threefold increase in risk for CVD when it is present and untreated.

Dietary therapy remains a cornerstone of treatment for those at risk for CVD and for patients with documented disease, as proposed in the guidelines of the National Cholesterol Education Program (NCEP) *(34)*. The potential impact of altered patterns of nutrient intake was confirmed by the results of a recent follow-up report of a trial involving a so-called "Mediterranean" diet. Patients randomized to such treatment enjoyed 50–70% reductions in risk for morbid and mortal CVD events when compared with patients who ate a prudent Western diet *(35)*.

It has long been recognized that diabetes is a potent risk factor for CHD, stroke, and peripheral arterial disease (PAD), which occur twice as often in diabetic men and up to four times as often in diabetic women as in their nondiabetic counterparts *(1,36)*. CVD is the leading cause of mortality in diabetes, causing 80% of all deaths; CHD is responsible for 75% of all CVD—related mortality in diabetics *(37)*. It is now recognized that even diabetics without documented CHD have a risk for MI comparable to nondiabetics who have already suffered an MI *(38)*. Such evidence has fueled calls to lower cholesterol in diabetics to the same level as in patients with diagnosed CHD (<100 mg/dL) *(38,39)*. In fact, there is agreement that strict control of all the traditional risk factors is critical in modifying CVD occurrence in diabetics. One recent study showed that although the prevalence of CVD was constant across increasing quartiles of glycohemoglobin in a diabetic population, it was strongly associated with age, hypertension, cigarette use, and the ratio of total:high-density lipoprotein cholesterol (TC:HDL-C) *(40)*.

Physical inactivity doubles risk for both CVD mortality and CHD morbidity *(41)*. Increased physical activity, in turn, decreases all-cause mortality, CVD mortality, and CVD morbidity *(42–45)*. The beneficial effects of exercise have been documented in both genders, the elderly, and smokers, even when performed at moderate levels *(42,45, 46)*. In addition to enhancing fibrinolytic activity, improving carbohydrate metabolism, and lowering weight, blood pressure, and serum triglyceride (TG) levels *(47)*, a recent study showed that exercise was an independent predictor of decreased angiographic progression of CHD *(48)*.

Obesity increases CVD risk both directly and indirectly. It has been known for some time that obesity is indirectly causal via its effect on hypertension, diabetes, elevated TGs, and low levels of HDL-C, and its association with physical inactivity and diets high in cholesterol and saturated fats *(49–51)*. More recently, it has been noted that much of the excess CVD risk associated with obesity is accounted for by the pattern of central adiposity, probably through the mechanism of insulin resistance *(50,51)*. Although most patients cannot maintain successful weight loss *(52,53)*, it is now recognized that CVD risk factors like hypertension, hypercholesterolemia, and glucose intolerance can be favorably altered by even modest reductions in excess weight *(49,53)*.

There is an extensive literature demonstrating a causal linkage between various psychosocial factors and CVD. Hostility *(54)*, depression *(55–57)*, hopelessness *(58)*, worry *(59)*, and social isolation *(60,61)* have all been shown to be associated with total and CVD mortality and to nonfatal and total CHD incidence. Psychosocial factors are thought to affect CVD risk both directly and indirectly. Direct effects are hypothesized to be mediated by the process of cardiovascular reactivity, whereby exaggerated responses to stress by the sympathetic and pituitary-adrenal axis produce ischemic and arrhythmogenic events *(62)*. Indirect effects include facilitating poor lifestyle choices concerning cigarette use, physical inactivity, and overweight *(63)*. Psychosocial factors have an impact on CVD risk comparable to other major risk factors, increasing incidence from two- to four-fold *(62,63)*. Although major clinical trials are lacking in this area, behavior modification and stress management interventions have demonstrated favorable effects in secondary prevention studies *(56,64)*. Because psychological issues can negatively affect compliance with efforts to modify other CVD risk factors, systems to assess and address these issues must be built into preventive cardiological care.

The Limits of Intervention

Several lines of scientific inquiry have shed new light on the pathophysiology of CVD, with important implications for preventive cardiology. It is now known that most acute coronary events are caused by the rupture of "vulnerable" atherosclerotic plaques with subsequent superimposed thrombosis *(65)*. Such plaques are characterized by a large lipid core, a thinned fibrous cap heavily infiltrated by matrix-degrading macrophages, and a paucity of smooth muscle cells *(66)*. Perhaps most strikingly, it appears that the majority of the lesions responsible for such events are not the severely stenotic targets of interventional procedures such as coronary artery bypass grafting (CABG) and balloon angioplasty, but lesions of mild to moderate severity producing stenosis of 70% or less *(67)*. Furthermore, results of the so-called "regression trials" *(68)* and the growing recognition of the role of endothelial dysfunction *(69,70)* and plaque stabilization *(71)* have helped explain the marked reductions in clinical events that accompany aggressive lipid lowering even in the absence of dramatic angiographic change. Combined with the striking relative risk reductions for morbid and mortal CVD events demonstrated in the statin trials described earlier, these recent insights have validated the critical role of preventive practices and even fueled calls for comparative trials of lipid lowering versus revascularization *(72)*.

RATIONALE

The Treatment Gap

It has been demonstrated previously that CVD is prevalent and costly, that it is associated with risk factors that are easily measured and amenable to modification, and that such modification is both effective and based on plausible pathophysiological hypotheses. These facts alone would provide substantial justification for coordinated preventive cardiology programs that focus on risk factor control. Current patterns of clinical practice, however, offer additional proof of the need for such programs.

Based on scientific data like that presented earlier, major professional organizations and expert panels have issued guidelines for the assessment and treatment of CVD risk factors *(73–77)*. Unfortunately, there is consistent data demonstrating that patients are not deriving the benefit of these clinical guidelines *(78,79)*. For hypercholesterolemia, it has been shown that fewer than one-third of those who need treatment are receiving it, even if one includes rudimentary dietary advice *(80)*. Even in patients documented to be at high risk, physicians are not inquiring about the presence of risk factors *(81–84)* or initiating appropriate therapy when they are found to be present *(82,84,85)*. This is true for patients on the coronary care unit (CCU) *(84)*, awaiting bypass *(81)*, prior to discharge from a CHD-related hospitalization *(78)*, or treated in the community *(86,87)*. When hyperlipidemia is treated, even in patients with known CHD, NCEP targets for LDL cholesterol are being met less than 20% of the time *(88–90)*. Similar data exist for the other risk factors *(87)*. It is estimated, for instance, that fewer than 30% of smokers receive documented counseling about cigarette cessation prior to leaving the hospital after myocardial infarction *(91)*, while one study *(84)* found that fewer than 5% of smokers admitted to a CCU had been counseled. The rates of use of beta blockers (45%), angiotensin-converting enzyme (ACE) inhibitors (59%), and aspirin (77%) post-MI are similarly disappointing *(91)*. National data from the National Health and Nutrition Examination Survey (NHANES) suggest that from 1991 to 1994 substantial decreases occurred in awareness (from 73–68%), rates of treatment (from 55–54%), and control (from 29–27%) of blood pressure *(76)*. A recent study of the ambulatory treatment of hypertension found that only 25% of patients were adequately controlled, even using older cutpoints of 140/90 mmHg *(92)*.

Awareness of and concern about this "treatment gap" between recommended guidelines and actual practice is growing *(93,94)*. There is, in addition, increasing recognition that the results of carefully controlled clinical trials are not always applicable to the reality of everyday patient care. In response, efforts have been initiated to analyze barriers to the implementation of risk factor management *(93)*. Such barriers include the structural and reimbursement realities of attempting to provide preventive services in the setting of a busy practice or acute care facility. Physicians, the traditional source of preventive services, have limited time, little confidence in their knowledge concerning prevention, and no financial incentive to provide such services. Physicians also overestimate their own compliance with screening guidelines. While physicians can be quite knowledgeable about the content of specific guidelines and believe generally in the importance of prevention, they comply with recommendations only 20–60% of the time *(95–98)*. Accordingly, it has been found that traditional continuing medical education (CME) is often ineffective in changing physician behavior *(94,99,100)*. The weight of the evidence suggests that making physicians the focus of improved risk factor management may be problematic.

Nontraditional Models of Care

One model that has emerged as an effective solution to the inadequate implementation of aggressive risk factor control is the multidisciplinary team in which the nurse acts as the case manager, with physician supervision *(101)*. Although the structure of such teams varies across institutions and practice settings, they often include dieticians, pharmacists, and psychologists *(102–106)*. Such programs have had success in the management of hypertension *(107,108)*, diabetes *(109)*, smoking cessation *(110–112)*, congestive heart failure (CHF) *(113)*, and hyperlipidemia *(102–106,114–117)*. Simultaneous modification of all risk factors present in a given patient has also proven effective *(104,117)*.

In addition to this documented clinical effectiveness, nurse-managed programs have shown promise in terms of cost effectiveness *(93,106,118–120)*, probably due to a combination of lower salaries for nonphysician professionals, use of standardized clinical algorithms, and improved patient compliance. These characteristics make such programs potentially attractive to managed care providers, although to date preventive services remain undervalued and poorly reimbursed for both physicians and nurses. Because clinical trial results have demonstrated that risk factor modification reduces future CVD events and the need for costly, interventional, hospital-based care, it may be that preventive services can gain more acceptance when viewed as a cost-saving component of an overall health care system.

Organization of a Preventive Cardiology Program

DESIGN AND FUNCTION

The Cleveland Clinic Foundation is one of the largest clinical group practices in the United States and a leading heart treatment center. In 1997, the Cleveland Clinic had over 1.3 million hospital and clinic visits, more than 44,000 hospital admissions, and over 38,000 surgical cases. Over 4000 cardiac procedures are performed annually, with referral from Northeast Ohio accounting for 70% of patients. The Preventive Cardiology Program at The Cleveland Clinic Foundation is organized as a section within the Department of Cardiology. The majority of referrals to the program come from Cleveland Clinic cardiologists, with the remainder coming from cardiothoracic surgeons, vascular medicine physicians, and primary care physicians.

The Preventive Cardiology Program is built around a multidisciplinary team that focuses on the nurse as the case manager. Team members include physicians, nurses, physician's assistants, dietitians, exercise physiologists, and psychologists. Specialists in lipidology, hypertension, diabetes, exercise, and smoking cessation developed detailed clinical algorithms for the treatment of each of the major modifiable risk factors, including lipids, blood pressure, diabetes, and exercise. These algorithms are logical, straightforward, and clearly outlined on pocket-sized laminated cards that can be carried for reference. The algorithms are based on national standards of care, but are intended as guidelines, not requirements. In this way, the algorithms provide a framework for treatment, but permit physicians and nonphysician professionals practice latitude based on their own clinical judgment. This combination of structure and flexibility also allows physicians from different specialties (cardiology, nephrology, endocrinology, and general medicine) to rotate through the clinic while maintaining essentially standardized care. In addition, all staff members undergo training prior to beginning work in the program so that the rationale for the aggressive assessment and treatment of CVD risk factors embodied in the algorithms can be fully explicated.

Prior to their initial visit, patients are mailed a detailed questionnaire assessing demographics, socioeconomic status, cardiovascular history, general medical and surgical history, family history, medication use, and information on diet, exercise, and use of nicotine and alcohol. Patients also complete three psychosocial questionnaires designed to assess levels of anxiety, depression, and hostility. At the initial visit, all forms are reviewed and a more detailed history obtained in a nurse-run interview. A directed physical examination is performed by the nurse and confirmed by the attending physician. A comprehensive laboratory profile is obtained on all patients at the time of the initial visit. Once the data from the home forms and nurse-directed history are entered into the computer and the physical examination performed, a comprehensive assessment and preventive treatment plan is formulated by the nurse and reviewed by the physician. Referral to on-site colleagues in nutrition services, cardiac rehabilitation, and psychology are initiated when appropriate for treatment programs targeting cigarette cessation, exercise, lipid lowering, blood pressure control, diabetes management, and stress reduction. Most patients are referred to a registered dietitian at their initial visit for instruction in reducing saturated fat and cholesterol intake. Additional nutritional recommendations are provided as indicated for the management of hypertension, diabetes, or excess weight.

Follow-up visits are scheduled at 90-day intervals until the targets established at the initial visit are met, and appropriate laboratory studies are obtained 1 wk prior to such visits to permit review at the time of the visit and concurrent incorporation into the treatment plan. Follow-up visits are shorter, but conform to the same general format. The nurse takes an interval history, verifies current medications, reviews the laboratory studies obtained the previous week, and performs a focused physical examination (weight, blood pressure [BP], body-mass index [BMI], waist-to-hip ratio [WHR]). These data are displayed with comparable results from prior visits on a trend sheet, generated by the computer, so that interval progress (or lack thereof) can be easily reviewed by both the patient and the nurse. Following the clinical algorithms, the nurse can then institute any necessary changes in the treatment plan. Physicians are available for consultation or to see the patient at the discretion of the nurse.

It was recognized early in the program's development that efficient data management would be a key to its success. An innovative graphical interface was created that could seamlessly support the clinical, regulatory, research, and communicative functions of data retrieval and application. By organizing information into nine Oracle® database tables, and entering all data online at the time of the clinical visit, the computer is able to generate contemporaneous reports that both meet regulatory reimbursement guidelines and the goal of providing prompt feedback to patients and referring physicians. Such summary reports are produced separately for patients and physicians after the initial visit. After follow up visits, physicians receive copies of the letter sent to patients. Because information can be exported from the database directly into commercially available statistical software packages, the computer interface also provides an ongoing opportunity to pose and answer questions that can then inform clinical research or modification of the practice based on valid outcome data.

INITIAL RESULTS

In an effort to document the impact of the program on risk factor modification, we have begun to analyze data from the initial cohort of almost 1500 patients seen in the Preventive Cardiology unit. Patients were middle aged (mean age 56), overweight (mean BMI 29), and hyperlipidemic (mean TC 240; mean low-density lipoprotein cholesterol [LDL-C] 147). Approximately half (51%) had documented CHD, and a similar number had hypertension (48%). Reflecting the national data reported earlier, rates of risk factor control at entry were low. Fifty-five percent of patients known to be hypertensive had baseline blood pressures above 140 mmHg systolic or 90 mmHg diastolic. Fifty-three percent of diabetic patients had entry fasting blood glucose values above 140 mg/dL. Seventy-nine percent of patients with documented CHD had entry LDL-C levels above 100 mg/dL.

Analysis of change in risk factor values from entry to 12 mo revealed significant decreases in BMI, total cholesterol, LDL-C, TGs, systolic BP, and diastolic BP, and an increase in HDL-C (all $p = 0.0001$). Actual risk factor change included a mean drop in LDL-C of 30 mg/dL, and a fall in mean systolic BP of 5.5 mmHg. The impact of the program on attainment of risk factor targets was examined for cholesterol and BP in those patients who had both initial and 1-yr values available. For patients with CHD who entered the program with LDL-C values above 100 mg/dL, 37% had reached the NCEP target of less than 100 mg/dL. For hypertensive patients who entered the program out of control, 35% had normalized their blood pressure.

CURRENT CHALLENGES

Our initial experience corroborates earlier reports in demonstrating that a multidisciplinary model of providing preventive cardiology care can be practical and effective. It extends those findings, which resulted from clinical trials, by applying this model to a "real world" clinical practice. Despite these results, we have identified several barriers to full implementation of the preventive cardiology concept. Because we believe these developmental challenges are generalizable across practice settings, they are outlined as follows as an aid to researchers planning a similar undertaking.

Attrition. Results from our initial cohort reveal a persistent decline in the rate of follow-up visits across the first year, so that only 20–30% of patients eventually returned at the 12-mo mark. This is of potential concern for both clinical care and research. We have examined the groups who did and did not return for all visits and found that the latter group was older and had a higher rate of CHD. While this does not eliminate the issue of selection bias, it at least demonstrates that—if anything—sicker patients are more likely to return for follow-up care. We have also found that there was no difference in terms of LDL-C lowering between the two groups, supporting the contention that risk factor modification was effective independent of visit compliance. The decline in visit compliance is perhaps to be expected in a referral practice, where the initial assessment and treatment plan may be the only intervention requested or necessary. We hypothesize that many patients prefer to return to their referring or primary care physicians for ongoing care and implementation of the treatment plan. Clearly, in order to document the long-term effectiveness of the program in maintaining lower risk factor levels and, ultimately, decreased rates of clinical events, more thorough follow-up is necessary. As mentioned previously, because this is a medical practice and not a clinical trial, the structure and funding that both mandate and permit close tracking of patients in the latter setting is not available for efforts such as ours. Interventions are being designed to allow further investigation of this issue.

Referral, Territoriality, and Missed Opportunities. As discussed earlier, risk factors are inadequately assessed whether patients are followed by primary care physicians *(80)* or cardiovascular specialists *(85)*. When treatment is initiated, patients frequently fail to reach goals *(88,90)*, a finding confirmed by our initial cohort data as reported above. Nonetheless, inadequate numbers of such patients are referred to specialized programs such as the one just described. A crucial challenge for these programs, therefore, is to understand and overcome the barriers to referral. One obvious barrier is economic threat. Primary care physicians, under an increasing regulatory burden and with falling incomes, may be loathe to relinquish even temporary control of such common medical problems as hyperlipidemia, hypertension, and diabetes. Specialists in cardiology and cardiovascular surgery may be fearful of alienating their primary care referral base by referring patients to preventive cardiology.

Another barrier may be simple miscommunication. It has been suggested *(78)* that cardiovascular specialists assume that primary care physicians will manage risk factors after a CVD event or intervention, and do not want to risk offending them (see earlier) by initiating such treatment themselves. At the same time, primary care physicians conclude that if the cardiovascular specialist has not initiated therapy for risk factors, such treatment must not be of significance. We have begun to explore possible solutions to this set of barriers. First, as mentioned earlier, we are scrupulous about providing rapid (same day) feedback to referring physicians about our assessment and proposed treatment plans for their patients. Second, we are investigating the possibility of "exporting" our program to the primary care health centers affiliated with the Cleveland Clinic. This would allow patients—even those initially evaluated at our program—to receive their ongoing risk factor management under the supervision of their personal physician in a geographically and psychologically accessible location. At the same time, the use of the standardized algorithms would insure a systemwide high level of care. Finally, by including these affiliated sites in the database, the same capacity to generate reports to physicians and patients would be maintained, and clinical data would be available for research purposes. Third, we are working to incorporate preventive cardiology services into the "usual care" offered to cardiology patients prior to hospital discharge. The interval immediately after a medical event or procedure has been identified as a "window" when patients are more open to lifestyle modification, and providing risk factor assessment and treatment during this period could maximize early compliance. It would also signal primary care physicians that such treatment constitutes a key component of ongoing cardiovascular care, and could thereby increase physician adherence with national guidelines.

CONCLUSION

1. CVD remains the leading cause of death in the United States.
2. The prevalence of CVD is likely to increase into the next century, with a larger and older population requiring secondary preventive services.
3. CVD is usually associated with *multiple* risk factors, which interact to increase the likelihood of an initial or recurrent event.
4. Modification of CVD risk factors has been proven to decrease the incidence of CVD, for both primary and secondary prevention.
5. Most "vulnerable" atherosclerotic lesions, while responsible for clinical CVD, are not severely stenotic. The benefits of plaque stabilization and restoration of normal endothelial function have demonstrated that these lesions are amenable to risk factor modification.
6. Nationally, even patients at high risk for CVD are inadequately screened and insufficiently treated for traditional CVD risk factors.
7. Physicians may not be the best—and certainly should not be the sole–providers of preventive cardiological care.
8. A preventive cardiology program utilizing a multidisciplinary team for the aggressive management of CVD risk factors is effective in decreasing risk factor burden and attaining recommended treatment targets.
9. Important barriers remain that must be overcome before the potential impact of preventive cardiology can be fully realized. Innovative solutions will have to incorporate the fiscal and logistic realities of current medical practice in order to succeed.

REFERENCES

1. Levy D, Wilson P. Atherosclerotic cardiovascular disease: an epidemiologic perspective. In: Topol E, ed. Textbook of Cardiovascular Medicine. Lippincott-Raven, Philadelphia, PA, 1998, pp. 12–30.
2. National Center for Health Statistics. Vital Statistics of the United States. Washington, DC, US Government Printing Office, Public Health Service, 1993.
3. Castelli WP. Lipids, risk factors and ischaemic heart disease. Atherosclerosis 1996;124(9):S1–S9.
4. Wolf P. Cerebrovascular risk. In: Izzo J, Black H, eds. Hypertension Primer: The Essentials of High Blood Pressure. Lippincott Williams & Wilkins, Baltimore, MD, 1999, pp. 203–207.
5. AHA. Statistical Update, American Heart Association. 1999.
6. Johnson CL, Rifkind BM, Sempos CT, et al. Declining serum total cholesterol levels among US adults. The National Health and Nutrition Examination Surveys. JAMA 1993;269(23):3002–3008.
7. Thom T, Roccella E. Trends in blood pressure control and mortality. In: Izzo J, Black H, eds. Hypertension Primer: The Essentials of High Blood Pressure. Lippincott Williams & Wilkins, Baltimore, MD, 1999, pp. 268–270.
8. Goldman L, Cook EF. The decline in ischemic heart disease mortality rates. An analysis of the comparative effects of medical interventions and changes in lifestyle. Ann Intern Med 1984;101(6):825–836.

9. Rosamon WD, Chambless LE, Folson AR, et al. Trends in the incidence of myocardial infarction and in mortality due to coronary heart disease, 1987 to 1994. N Engl J Med 1998;339(13):861–867.

10. Kelly DT. Paul Dudley White International Lecture. Our future society. A global challenge. Circulation 1997;95(11):2459–2464.

11. Kannel W. The Framingham experience. In: Marmot M, Elliott P, eds. Coronary Heart Disease Epidemiology: From Aetiology to Public Health. Oxford University Press, New York, 1992, pp. 67–82.

12. Kannel W, Wilson W. Cardiovascular risk factors and hypertension. In: Izzo J, Black H, eds. Hypertension Primer: The Essentials of High Blood Pressure. Lippincott Williams & Wilkins, Baltimore, MD, 1999, pp. 199–202.

13. Lowe LP, Greenland P, Ruth KJ, et al. Impact of major cardiovascular disease risk factors, particularly in combination, on 22-year mortality in women and men. Arch Intern Med 1998;158(18):2007–2014.

14. Califf RM, Armstrong PW, Carver JR, et al. 27th Bethesda Conference: matching the intensity of risk factor management with the hazard for coronary disease events. Task Force 5. Stratification of patients into high, medium and low risk subgroups for purposes of risk factor management. J Am Coll Cardiol 1996;27(5):1007–1019.

15. Kannel WB, Wilson PW. An update on coronary risk factors. Med Clin North Am 1995;79(5):951–971.

16. Ballantyne CM. Current thinking in lipid lowering. Am J Med 1998;104(6A);33S–41S.

17. Downs JR, Clearfield M, Weis S, et al. Primary prevention of acute coronary events with Lovastatin in men and women with average cholesterol levels. JAMA 1998;279:1615–1622.

18. Sacks FM, Pfeffer MA, Moye LA, et al. The effect of pravastatin on coronary events after myocardial infarction in patients with average cholesterol levels. Cholesterol and Recurrent Events Trial investigators. N Engl J Med 1996;335(14):1106–1110.

19. Shepherd J, Cobbe SM, Ford I, et al. Prevention of coronary heart disease with pravastatin in men with hypercholesterolemia. West of Scotland Coronary Prevention Study Group. N Engl J Med 1995; 333(20):1301–1307.

20. The Long-Term Intervention with Pravastatin in Ischaemic Disease (LIPID) Study Group. Prevention of cardiovascular events and death with pravastatin in patients with coronary heart disease and a broad range of initial cholesterol levels. N Engl J Med 1998;339(19):1349–1357.

21. The Scandinavian Simvastatin Survival Study (4S). Randomized trial of cholesterol lowering in 4444 patients with coronary heart disease. Lancet 1994;344(8934):1383–1389.

22. Furberg CD, Adams HP Jr, Applegate WB, et al. Effect of lovastatin on early carotid atherosclerosis and cardiovascular events. Asymptomatic Carotid Artery Progression Study (ACAPS) Research Group. Circulation 1994;90(4):1679–1687.

23. Furberg CD, Byington RP, Crouse JR, et al. Pravastatin, lipids, and major coronary events. Am J Cardiol 1994;73(15):1133–1134.

24. Herbert PR, Gaziano JM, Chan KS, et al. Cholesterol lowering with statin drugs, risk of stroke, and total mortality. An overview of randomized trials. JAMA 1997;278(4):313–321.

25. Department of Health and Human Services. The Health Benefits of Smoking Cessation: A Report of the Surgeon General, Rockville, MD, 1990.

26. Department of Health and Human Services. Services. The health consequences of smoking: cardiovascular disease. A Report of the Surgeon General. Rockville, MD, 1983.

27. SHEP Cooperative Research Group. Prevention of stroke by antihypertensive drug treatment in older persons with isolated systolic hypertension. Final results of the Systolic Hypertension in the Elderly Program (SHEP). JAMA 1991;265(24):3255–3264.

28. Collins R, Peto R, MacMahon S, et al. Blood pressure, stroke, and coronary heart disease. Part 2, short-term reductions in blood pressure: overview of randomized drug trials in their epidemiological context. Lancet 1990;335(8693):827–838.

29. Cutler J, Psaty B, MacMahon S, et al. Public health issues in hypertension control: what has been learned from clinical trials. In: Laragh J, Brenner B, eds. Hypertension: Pathophysiology, Diagnosis and Management, 2nd ed. Raven Press, New York, 1995, vol. 1, 253–270

30. Hebert PR, Fiebach NH, Eberlein KA, et al. The community-based randomized trials of pharmacologic treatment of mild-to-moderate hypertension. Am J Epidemiol 1988;127(3):581–590.

31. Hebert PR, Moser M, Jayer J, et al. Recent evidence on drug therapy of mild-to-moderate hypertension and decreased risk of coronary heart disease. Arch Intern Med 1993;153(5):578–581.

32. Pasternak RC, Grundy SM, Levy D, et al. 27th Bethesda Conference: matching the intensity of risk factor management with the hazard for coronary disease events. Task Force 3. Spectrum of risk factors for coronary heart disease. J Am Coll Cardiol 1996;27(5):978–990.

33. Hennekens CH, Dyken ML, Fuster V. Aspirin as a therapeutic agent in cardiovascular disease: a statement for healthcare professionals from the American Heart Association. Circulation 1997;96(8): 2751–2753.
34. Summary of the second report of the National Cholesterol Education Program (NCEP) Expert Panel on Detection, Evaluation, and Treatment of High Blood Cholesterol in Adults (Adult Treatment Panel II) [comment]. JAMA 1993;269(23):3015–3023.
35. Lorgeril MD, Salen P, Martin J-L, et al. Mediterranean diet, traditional risk factors and the rate of cardiovascular complications after myocardial infarction: Final Report of the Lyon Diet Heart Study. Circulation 1999;99:779–785.
36. Garber AJ. Vascular disease and lipids in diabetes. Med Clin North Am 1998;82(4):931–948.
37. Aronson D, Rayfield E. Diabetes. In: Topol E, ed. Textbook of Cardiovascular Medicine. Lippincott-Raven, Philadelphia, PA, 1998, pp. 171–194.
38. Haffner SM, Lehto S, Ronnemaa T, et al. Mortality from coronary heart disease in subjects with type 2 diabetes and in nondiabetic subjects with and without prior myocardial infarction. N Engl J Med 1998;339(4):229–234.
39. Sobel B. Complications of diabetes: macrovascular disease. In: Olefsky J, ed. Current Approaches to the Management of Type 2 Diabetes: A Practical Monograph. National Diabetes Education Initiative, Secaucus, NJ, 1997, pp. 27–30.
40. Meig JB, Singer DE, Sullivan LM, et al. Metabolic control and prevalent cardiovascular disease in non-insulin-dependent diabetes mellitus (NIDDM): The NIDDM Patient Outcome Research Team. Am J Med 1997;102(1):38–47.
41. Powell KE, Thompson PD, Caspersen CJ, et al. Physical activity and the incidence of coronary heart disease. Ann Rev Public Health 1987;8:253–287.
42. Blair SN, Kampert JB, Kohl W 3rd, et al. Influences of cardiorespiratory fitness and other precursors on cardiovascular disease and all-cause mortality in men and women. JAMA 1996;276(3):205–210.
43. Blair SN, Kohl HW 3rd, Barlow CE, et al. Changes in physical fitness and all-cause mortality. A prospective study of healthy and unhealthy men. JAMA 1995;273(14):1093–1098.
44. Erikssen G, Liestol K, Bjornholt J, et al. Changes in physical fitness and changes in mortality. Lancet 1998;352(9130):759–762.
45. Wannamethee SG, Shaper AG, Walker M. Changes in physical activity, mortality, and incidence of coronary heart disease in older men. Lancet 1998;351(9116):1603–1608.
46. NIH Consensus Development Panel on Physical Activity and Cardiovascular Health. Physical activity and cardiovascular health. JAMA 1996;276(3):241–246.
47. Pasternak RC, Grundy SM, Levy D, et al. 27th Bethesda Conference: matching the intensity of risk factor management with the hazard for coronary disease events. Task Force 3. Spectrum of risk factors for coronary heart disease. J Am Coll Cardiol 1996;27(5):978–990.
48. Niebauer J, Hambrecht R, Velich T, et al. Attenuated progression of coronary artery disease after 6 yr of multifactorial risk intervention: role of physical exercise. Circulation 1997;96(8):2534–2541.
49. Eckel RH. Obesity and heart disease: a statement for healthcare professionals from the Nutrition Committee, American Heart Association. Circulation 1997;96(9):3248–3250.
50. Kannel WB, D'Agostino RB, Cobb JL. Effect of weight on cardiovascular disease. Am J Clin Nutr 1996;63(3 Suppl):419S–422S.
51. Schwartz MW, Brunzell JD. Regulation of body adiposity and the problem of obesity. Arterioscler Thromb Vasc Biol 1997;17(2):233–238.
52. Rosenbaum M, Leibel RL, Hirsch J. Obesity. N Engl J Med 1997;337(6):396–407.
53. Stone N. Diet, nutritional issues, and obesity. In: Topol E, ed. Textbook of Cardiovascular Medicine. Lippincott-Raven, Philadelphia, PA, 1998, pp. 31–58.
54. Helmer D, Ragland D, Syme S. Hostility and coronary heart disease. Am J Epidemiol 1991;133:112–122.
55. Barefoot JC, Schroll M. Symptoms of depression, acute myocardial infarction, and total mortality in a community sample. Circulation 1996;93(11):1976–1980.
56. Frasure-Smith N, Lesperance F, Talajic, M. Depression following myocardial infarction. Impact on 6-month survival. JAMA 1993;270(15):1819–1825.
57. Frasure-Smith N, Lesperance F, Talajic, M. Depression and 18-month prognosis after myocardial infarction. Circulation 1995;91(4):999–1005.
58. Everson SA, Kaplan GA, Goldberg DE, et al. Hopelessness and 4-year progression of carotid atherosclerosis. The Kuopio Ischemic Heart Disease Risk Factor Study. Arterioscler Thromb Vasc Biol 1997; 17(8):1490–1495.

59. Kubzansky LD, Kawachi I, Spiro A 3rd, et al. Is worrying bad for your heart? A prospective study of worry and coronary heart disease in the Normative Aging Study. Circulation 1997;95(4):818–824.
60. Berkman LF, Leo-Summers L, Horwitz RI. Emotional support and survival after myocardial infarction. A prospective, population-based study of the elderly. Ann Intern Med 1992;117(12):1003–1009.
61. Olsen O. Impact of social network on cardiovascular mortality in middle aged Danish men. J Epidemiol Commun Health 1993;47(3):176–180.
62. Theorell T. The psycho-social environment, stress, and coronary heart disease. In: Marmot M, Elliot P, eds. Coronary Heart Disease Epidemiology: From Aetiology to Public Health. Oxford University Press, New York, 1992, pp. 256–273.
63. Smith T, Leon A, eds. Coronary Heart Disease: A Behavioral Perspective. Research Press, Champaign, IL. 1992.
64. van Dixhoorn J, Duivenvoorden HJ, Staal JA, et al. Cardiac events after myocardial infarction: possible effect of relaxation therapy. Eur Heart J 1987;8(11):1210–1214.
65. Falk E, Shah PK, Fuster V. Coronary plaque disruption. Circulation 1995;92(3):657–671.
66. Lee RT, Libby P. The unstable atheroma. Arterioscler Thromb Vasc Biol 1997;17:1859–1867.
67. Levine GN, Keaney JF, Vita JA. Cholesterol reduction in cardiovascular disease. N Engl J Med 1995;332(8):511–520.
68. Superko HR, Krauss RM. Coronary artery disease regression: Convincing evidence for the benefit of aggressive lipoprotein management. Circulation 1994;90:1056–1069.
69. Treasure CB, Klein JL, Weintraub WS, et al. Beneficial effects of cholesterol-lowering therapy on the coronary endothelium in patients with coronary artery disease. N Engl J Med 1995;332(8):481–493.
70. Anderson TJ, Meredith IT, Yeung AC, et al. The Effect of cholesterol-lowering and antioxidant therapy on endothelium-dependent coronary vasomotion. N Engl J Med 1995;332(8):488–493.
71. Brown BG, Zhao XQ, Sacco DE, Albers J.J. Lipid lowering and plaque regression: new insights into prevention of plaque disruption and clinical events in coronary disease. Circulation 1993;87(6):1781–1791.
72. Forrester JS, Shah PK. Lipid lowering versus revascularization: an idea whose time (for testing) has come. Circulation 1997;96(4):1360–1362.
73. National Cholesterol Education Program (NCEP) Expert Panel on Detection, Evaluation, and Treatment of High Blood Cholesterol in Adults (Adult Treatment Panel II) (comment). Summary of the second report. JAMA 1993;269(23):3015–3023.
74. 27th Bethesda Conference September 14–15, 1995. Matching the intensity of risk factor management with the hazard for coronary disease events. J Am Coll Cardiol 1996;27(5):957–1047.
75. Report of the Expert Committee on the diagnosis and classification of diabetes mellitus. Diabetes Care 1997;20(7):1183–1197.
76. The sixth report of the Joint National Committee on prevention, detection, evaluation, and treatment of high blood pressure. Arch Intern Med 1997;157(21):2413–2446.
77. Recommendations of the Second Joint Task Force of European and Other Societies on Coronary Prevention. Prevention of coronary heart disease in clinical practice. Eur Heart J 1998;339(19):1349–1357.
78. Pearson TA, Peters TD. The treatment gap in coronary artery disease and heart failure: community standards and the post-discharge patient. Am J Cardiol 1997;80(8B):45H–52H.
79. Greenland P, Grundy S, Pasternak RC, Lenfant C. Problems on the pathway from risk assessment to risk reduction. Circulation 1998;97:1761–1762.
80. Giles WH, Anda RF, Jones DH, et al. Recent trends in the identification and treatment of high blood cholesterol by physicians: progress and missed opportunities. JAMA 1993;269:1133–1138.
81. Miller M, Konkel K, Fitzpatrick D, et al. Divergent reporting of coronary risk factors before coronary artery bypass surgery. Am J Cardiol 1995;75:736–737.
82. The Clinical Quality Improvement Network (CQIN) Investigators. Low incidence of assessment and modification of risk factors in acute care patients at high risk for cardiovascular events, particularly among females and the elderly. Am J Cardiol 1995;76:570–573.
83. Frame PS, Kowulich BA, Llewellyn AM. Improving physician compliance with a health maintenance protocol. J Fam Pract 1984;19:341–344.
84. Frolkis J, Zyzanski S, Schwartz J, Suhan P. Physician non-compliance with the 1993 National Cholesterol Education Program (NCEP-ATPII) Guidelines. Circulation 1998;98:851–855.
85. Cohen MV, Byrne MJ, Levine B, et al. Low rate of treatment of hypercholesterolemia by cardiologist in patients with suspected and proven coronary artery disease. Circulation 1991;83:1294–1304.
86. Campbell NC, Thain J, Deans HG, et al. Secondary prevention in coronary heart disease: baseline survey of provision in general practice. Br J Med 1998;316:1430–1434.

87. McCormick D, Gurwitz JH, Lessard D, et al. Use of aspirin, b-blockers, and lipid-lowering medications before recurrent acute myocardial infarction. Arch Intern Med 1999;159:561–567.
88. Schrott HG, Bittner V, Vittinghoff E, et al. Adherence to National Cholesterol Education Program treatment goals in postmenopausal women with heart disease. The Heart and Estrogen/Progestin Replacement Study (HRS). The HERS Research Group. JAMA 1997;277:1281–1286.
89. Marcelino JJ, Feingold KR. Inadequate treatment with HMG-CoA reductase inhibitors by health care providers. Am J Med 1996;100:605–610.
90. Hoerger TJ, Bala MV, Bray JW, et al. Treatment patterns and distribution of low-density lipoprotein cholesterol levels in treatment-eligible United States adults. Am J Cardiol 1998;82:61–65.
91. Ellerbeck EF, Jencks SF, Radford MJ, et al. Quality of care for Medicare patients with acute myocardial infarction. A four-state pilot study from the Cooperative Cardiovacular Project. JAMA 1995;273: 1509–1514.
92. Berlowitz DR, Ash AS, Hickey EC, et al. Inadequate management of blood pressure in a hypertensive population. N Engl J Med 1998;339(27):1957–1963.
93. Pearson T, McBride P, Houston-Miller N, Smith S. Task Force 8. Organization of Preventive Cardiology Service. J Am Coll Cardiol 1996;27:1039–1047.
94. Hill MN, Levine DM, Whelton PK. Awareness, use, and impact of the 1984 Joint National Committee consensus report on high blood pressure. Am J Public Health 1988;78:1190–1194.
95. Pommerenke FA, Weed DL. Physician compliance: improving skills in preventive medicine practices. Am Fam Physician 1991;43:560–568.
96. Lomas J, Anderson GM, Domnick-Pierr, K, et al. Do practice guidelines guide practice? The effect of a consensus statement on the practice of physicians. N Engl J Med 1989;321:1306–1311.
97. Fix KN, Oberman A. Barriers to following National Cholesterol Educational Program Guidelines: An appraisal of poor physician compliance. Arch Intern Med 1992;152:2385–2387.
98. McBride PE, Pacala JT, Dean J, Plane MB. Primary care residents and the management of hypercholesterolemia. Am J Prev Med 1990;6:71–76.
99. Davis A, Thompson M, Oxman A, Haynes R. Changing physician performance. A systematic review of the effect of continuing medical education strategies. JAMA 1995;274:700–705.
100. Browner WS, Baron RB, Solkowitz S, et al. Physician management of hypercholesterolemia. A randomized trial of continuing medical education. West J Med 1994;161:572–578.
101. Hill MN, Miller NH. Compliance enhancement. A call for multidisciplinary team approaches (editorial). Circulation 1996;93:4–6.
102. Sikand G, Kashyap ML, Yang I. Medical nutrition therapy lowers serum cholesterol and saves medication costs in men with hypercholesterolemia. J Am Diet Assoc 1998;98:889–894.
103. Shaffer J, Wexler LF. Reducing low-density lipoprotein cholesterol levels in an ambulatory care system. Arch Intern Med 1995;155:2330–2335.
104. Haskell WL, Alderman EL, Fair JM, et al. Effects of intensive multiple risk factor reduction on coronary atherosclerosis and clinical cardiac events in men and women with coronary artery disease: The Stanford Coronary Risk Intervention Project (SCRIP). Circulation 1994;89:975–990.
105. Harris DE, Record NB, Gipson GW, Pearson TA. Lipid lowering in a multidisciplinary clinic compared with primary physician management. Am J Cardiol 1998;81:929–933.
106. Schectman G, Wolff N, Byrd JC, et al. Physician extenders for cost-effective management of hypercholesterolemia. J Gen Intern Med 1996;11:277–286.
107. Schultz JF, Sheps SG. Management of patients with hypertension: A hypertension clinic model. Mayo Clin Proc 1994;69:997–999.
108. Reichgott MJ, Pearson S, Hill MN. The nurse practitioner's role in complex patient management: hypertension. J Natl Med Assoc 1983;75:1197–1204.
109. Weinberger M, Kirkman MS, Samsa GP, et al. A nurse-coordinated intervention for primary care patients with non-insulin-dependent diabetes mellitus: impact on glycemic control and health-related quality of life. J Gen Intern Med 1995;10:59–66.
110. Taylor CB, Houston-Miller N, Killen JD, DeBusk RF. Smoking cessation after acute myocardial infarction: effects of a nurse-managed intervention. Ann Intern Med 1990;113:118–123.
111. Taylor CB, Miller NH, Herman S, et al. A nurse-managed smoking cessation program for hospitalized smokers. Am J Public Health 1996;86:1557–1560.
112. Miller NH, Smith PM, DeBusk RF, et al. Smoking cessation in hospitalized patients. Results of a randomized trial. Arch Intern Med 1997;157:409–415.
113. Lasater M. The effect of a nurse-managed CHF clinic on patient readmission and length of stay. Home Healthc Nurse 1996;14:351–356.

114. Blair TP, Bryant FJ, Bocuzzi S. Treating hyperlipidemia. J Cardiovasc Nurs 1988;5:55–57.
115. Bruce SL, Grove SK. The effect of a coronary artery risk evaluation program on serum lipid values and cardiovascular risk levels. Appl Nurs Res 1994;7:67–74.
116. Cofer LA. Aggressive cholesterol management: role of the lipid nurse specialist. Heart Lung 1997;26: 337–344.
117. DeBusk RF, Miller NH, Superko HR, et al. A case-management system for coronary risk factor modification after acute myocardial infarction. Ann Intern Med 1994;120:721–729.
118. Gerber J. Implementing quality assurance programs in multigroup practices for treating hypercholesterolemia in patients with coronary artery disease. Am J Cardiol 1997;80(8B):57H–61H.
119. Dunn PJ, Ryan MJ Jr, Hiebert M. Strategic and cost effective role for preventive cardiology. J Cardiovasc Manag 1998;9:13–20.
120. Dunn PJ, Superko HR, Halbrook M, et al. Setting up a preventive cardiology program in the real world. J Cardiovasc Manag 1998;9:16–21.

18 Pharmacoeconomics of Cardiovascular Medicine

Melanie Oates, PHD, MBA, RN, William F. McGhan, PHARMD, PHD, and Ron Corey, PHD, MBA, RPH

INTRODUCTION

The growth of managed care in the 1980s and 1990s and the resulting emphasis on cost containment have impacted the practice of cardiovascular medicine as we enter the twenty-first century. In this age of limited economic resources, it is no longer appropriate to embrace all advancements, however minor, in health care technology. Instead, today's physician often must choose treatments with a careful consideration of the expected improvement in patient outcomes compared to the added costs to both patients and third-party payers. This frame of reference does not imply a reduction in quality of care. Instead, it implies an awareness of the quality of health care offered per dollar spent.

From: *Contemporary Cardiology: Preventive Cardiology:*
Strategies for the Prevention and Treatment of Coronary Artery Disease
Edited by: J. Foody © Humana Press Inc., Totowa, NJ

CARDIOVASCULAR DISEASE

Cardiovascular disease (CVD) resulted in over 959,000 deaths in the United States in 1996, and is the leading cause of death in this country. Coronary heart disease (CHD) was responsible for 476,124 of those deaths *(1)*. The American Heart Association estimated that in 1996, 58.8 million Americans suffered from some form of CVD. According to the National Center for Health Statistics, in 1993 nearly 633 yr of potential life were lost to heart disease for every 100,000 persons under 65 yr of age *(2)*. The economic burden of heart disease is also high, with 1999 direct costs plus indirect costs for CVD plus stroke in the United States estimated to exceed $286 billion *(3–5)*.

HEALTH ECONOMIC ANALYSIS

Health economic analysis employs tools for comprehensively examining the economic impact of alternative drug therapies and other medical interventions. Health economics identifies, measures, and compares the costs and consequences of medical products and services. The health care system is facing a multitude of economic challenges. The realizations of limited resources and the impact of cost containment is causing administrators and policy makers in the managed care field, and throughout the health system, to vigilantly apply health economic principles in examining the costs and benefits of both proposed and existing drugs and services. With health care reform, all health service sectors will experience increasing pressure and demands that all patient care interventions be evaluated in terms of clinical and social outcomes related to costs incurred.

All of the following groups may have differing agendas and it is important in health economic evaluations to consider these various perspectives. It must be kept in mind, in considering all these perspectives, that the most important perspective to include in all health economic evaluations is that of society as a whole. Some of the various health economic perspectives include (1) Individual patients, (2) Employers, (3) HMOs, (4) Hospitals, (5) Insurance companies, and (6) Medicaid and Medicare (Government).

In considering the foregoing points of view, it is of course important to consider who pays the cost of the intervention and who gets the benefits. For example, an employer may be very interested in a new therapy (e.g., for treating migraine or asthma) that decreases the loss of work days, but the HMO may be concerned about an increase in the pharmacy drug budget. Because Medicare's diagnosis-related groups (DRGs) do not include quality-of-life or outcome adjustments, some people have expressed concern that the federal government is allowing budgetary considerations to override the individual patient's desire for improved quality of life and long-term health outcomes.

QUANTITATIVE TOOLS

Health economics brings to the health arena sophistication in the types of quantitative tools that are available to assist health care managers and providers in making decisions for their patients, including (1) Cost of illness, (2) Cost minimization, (3) Cost benefit, (4) Cost effectiveness, and (5) Cost utility *(6)*.

All health economic principles can be framed in the traditional paradigm of comparing inputs versus outputs. The inputs are the resources consumed (i.e., the cost of therapy, health care program, etc.) and the health improvements. The outputs are often effectiveness measures, such as changes in blood pressure (BP) or cholesterol, and utility scales,

Table 1
Comparison of Evaluation Techniques Regarding Inputs and Outputs

Technique	Inputs	Outputs
Cost of illness	Dollars	N/A
Cost-effectiveness analysis	Dollars	Natural Units
Cost-benefit analysis	Dollars	Dollars
Cost-utility analysis	Dollars	Utilities/Preferences
Cost-minimization analysis	Dollars	Assumed Equal

N/A = not applicable.

Table 2
Cost-Minimization Analysis: Example Applied to Drug Therapy

		Cost of therapies ($)	
		Drug A	Drug B
Costs			
Acquisition cost		250	350
Administration		75	0
Monitoring		75	25
Adverse effects		100	25
	Subtotal	500	400
Outcomes			
Drug effectiveness		90%	90%
	Result = cost of drug A > cost of drug B		

In cost minimization, both interventions (drugs) are considered to be equally effective; and in this example, the cost minimization question is answered by stating that drug B is $100 less than drug A.

which are comparisons between healthy states and patient assessments of care. The most difficult step is translating all this activity in dollars, as is required in cost benefit analysis. Table 1 compares the evaluation techniques and the different sets of inputs and outputs.

Assigning a dollar value to each step in care of a patient can be complicated. There are obvious costs such as the drug costs, hospital costs, and clinic costs. But what about the costs of patient's waiting time travel time, or even cholesterol changes? The answer to these questions depends on the health economic methodology chosen.

1. *Cost-of-illness studies* are important because they help policy makers and planners to identify what diseases and health problems should be targeted. These studies are basically cost identification studies that can take place at national or local levels. Cost studies have been done on most diseases including asthma, arthritis, depression, CVD, and migraine.
2. *Cost-minimization analysis* compares costs for comparable treatments with the same clinical effectiveness, such as me-too situations. When competing choices have equal effectiveness, the cost-minimization objective is finding the least expensive way to reach an identical endpoint in therapy. Table 2 describes a "me-too" ACE analysis where effectiveness is presumed equal.
3. *Cost-benefit analysis* measures costs and consequences only in dollars. This can be a complex analysis because all outcomes, such as BP changes, must be assigned a dollar value. Table 3 compares different formulas for cost-benefit calculations, and Table 4 provides an example of a cost-benefit analysis.

Table 3
Sample Comparison Using Three Different Cost-Benefit Equations

	Costs (t1)	Benefits (t1)	1 Cost benefit ratio (B/C)	2 Net present value (B − C)	3 Internal rate of return $\frac{(B − C)}{C}$
A	$10,000	$15,000	1.5:1	$5,000	50%
B	$100,000	$180,000	1.8:1	$80,000	80%

Table 4
Cost-Benefit Analysis: Example Applied to Drug Therapy

		Cost of therapies ($)	
		Drug A	Drug B
Costs			
Acquisition cost		300	400
Administration		50	0
Monitoring		50	0
Adverse effects		100	0
	Subtotal	500	400
Benefits			
Days at work ($)		1000	1000
Extra months of life ($)		2000	3000
	Subtotal ($)	3000	4000
Benefit–cost ratio:		3000/500 = 6:1	4000/400 = 10:1

4. *Cost-effectiveness analysis* measures costs in relation to therapeutic objectives. For example, the benefits of a hypertension medication may be the percentage reduction in diastolic blood pressure. Table 5 illustrates how cost-effectiveness ratios can be used to rank therapies.

5. *Cost-utility analysis* measures costs and therapeutic objects against intervention preferences by the patient. Thus, the total costs of cancer chemotherapeutic agents would be adjusted by the number of years of life gained and the patient's preference for various health states. Table 6 provides an example of a cost-utility analysis.

Another limitation is the economic confusion that can surround the terms "direct costs" and "indirect costs." Direct costs are the ones that can usually be related to writing a check or monitored by standard health care billing procedures. Direct costs can include hospital or clinic expenses, health professional fees, product costs, and administration overhead. These costs are usually the ones targeted for reductions in health care costs.

Indirect costs are the more intangible factors such as the days that the patient is too sick to work, an early death that reduces lifelong wage earnings, or even time spent waiting for the doctor. These expenses are usually not measured from hospital bills, yet they can account for as much as 60% of the total costs of an illness. Morbidity, the days lost from work, generally accounts for about 22%. Premature mortality, which is permanent loss from the work force, is about 38% *(7)*. These numbers significantly affect total health

Table 5
Cost-Effectiveness Analysis: Example Applied to Drug Therapy

		Cost of therapies ($)	
		Drug A	Drug B
Costs			
Acquisition cost		300	400
Administration		50	0
Monitoring		50	0
Adverse effects		100	0
	Subtotal	500	400
Outputs			
Extra years of life		1.5	1.6
Cost-effectiveness ratio:		500/1.5	400/1.6
		= $333	= $250
		per extra year of life	

Table 6
Cost-Utility Analysis: Example Applied to Drug Therapy

		Cost of therapies ($)	
		Drug A	Drug B
Costs			
Acquisition cost		300	400
Administration		50	0
Monitoring		50	0
Adverse effects		100	0
	Subtotal	500	400
Utilities			
Extra years of life		1.5	1.6
Quality of life		.33	.25
QALYs[a]		0.50	0.40
Cost-utility ratio:		500/0.5	400/0.4
		= $1000	= $1000
		per extra quality of life year	

[a]QALYs = Quality-adjusted life years.

care costs yet are not often considered fully in health care debates. In the context of total health expenditures in the US, we are already spending more than $1 trillion for health care. This nationally reported statistic only represents direct costs. So if we estimate that this is half of the total cost of illness in the US, illness in this country would include another $1 trillion in indirect costs from lost productivity and early death for a total cost of illness of $2 trillion. Health economic analysis allows us to evaluate the impact of new health interventions as illustrated in Fig. 1. The point illustrated in this circle is that we want to develop health interventions that decrease the total costs of illness, even though the direct expenditures may have to increase. For example, we could certainly reduce the direct costs of care if we denied paying for polio vaccine, but we certainly would risk dramatic increases in indirect and thus total costs of illness.

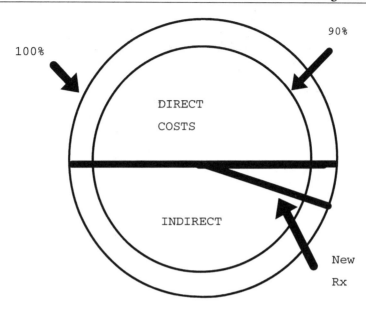

Fig. 1. An increase in direct costs with new therapy may decrease indirect costs and total costs.

HEALTH ECONOMICS
AND OUTCOMES MANAGEMENT

Health economics is a central component of the outcomes model. As in continuous quality improvement, the health economic outcomes model is a continuous process with six recursive steps: (1) setting outcome goals, with treatment protocols and standards; (2) designing clinical and economics evaluations that are implemented through randomized control trials, postmarketing epidemiology, or individual patient monitoring; (3) implementing the interventions; (4) measuring (collecting data on) the patients' clinical and economic outcomes; (5) analyzing the outcomes data; and (6) the final continuous, recursive step is translating these analyses and feedback into improved procedures, protocols, and guidelines.

In a health economic outcomes program the inputs and outcomes are illustrated as follows:

1. Specific input parameters
   a. Acquisition costs
   b. Efficacy
   c. Side effects
   d. Compliance
   e. Administration costs
   f. Acquisition costs
   g. Monitoring costs
2. Outcome parameters: impact on total system
   a. Changes in cost of illness
   b. Potential increases in productivity
   c. Improved quality of life
   d. Other outcomes

GENERAL STEPS IN A HEALTH ECONOMIC STUDY

When evaluating or planning a health economic study, there are several steps that should have to be addressed in the specific health economic methodology (e.g., cost effectiveness versus cost benefit).

To illustrate this, the steps associated with cost effectiveness analysis are listed as follows.

Step 1: Prior to incorporating health economic evaluations into any research project, the investigator must first establish the *perspective* from which to evaluate the various costs, benefits, and outcomes. That is, will the costs and consequences be those of society, specific patients, a third-party payer, HMO, or hospital? Depending on whose perspective is taken, the results may vary greatly.

Step 2: Describe/specify the *treatment alternatives*. The alternatives included in a health economic evaluation should be those acceptable to the patient and practitioners. The competing alternatives should be dosed at comparable levels.

Step 3: For each treatment alternative, specify the *possible outcomes* (i.e., patient pathways) and their probabilities. This can be retrospective, using information from clinical studies, medical literature, and/or expert panels. It can also be a product of a current clinical trial. The pathways can often be clearly presented in the form of decision trees or similar diagrams.

Step 4: Specify and monitor the *health care resources* that are consumed in each pathway. Resources include: drugs, physician services, hospital "hotel," and ancillary services, lab tests, and the like. This can be done retrospectively or concurrently with a clinical trial. If this is done retrospectively, each patient pathway is described in terms of the health care resources that are likely to be consumed. If concurrent with a clinical trial, the "artificial" use of services—required by the trial's protocol—must be considered.

The perspective of the study (e.g., insurer, hospital, society) affects the resources that are included in a study. For instance, a DRG-paid hospital is not concerned with the increased intensity of nursing home care that may be associated with shorter hospital stays.

Step 5: Assign *dollar values* to the resources consumed. Dollar values are assigned to each resource. In drug studies, hospital services require special attention because of their relative magnitude. Also, drug prices need to be selected carefully because of their availability.

Step 6: Specify and monitor *non-health-care resources* consumed in each pathway. Generally, this is not a concern in drug studies. Often these resources, such as the economic impact a patient's treatment has on the family, are difficult to measure. The resources should be estimated or at least noted and brought into discussion as a caveat when reporting the results of the study. The qualitative endpoints can support the quantitative analysis.

Step 7: Specify the unit of *effectiveness*. The appropriate unit depends on the disease/condition and the results of treatment. Some possibilities are patient lives saved, year of life added, or reduction in morbidity attributed to the disease. (These data are derived from the clinical portion of the trial.)

Step 8: Specify other *noneconomic attributes* of the alternatives (e.g., pain, side effects). These may be difficult to quantify and may lead to employing quality-of-life determination and cost-utility analysis.

Step 9:   Analyze the data employing the appropriate health economic *methodology* (e.g., cost-effectiveness analysis, cost-minimization analysis). The appropriate analysis will be determined by how the study was set up, the perspective, and the type and quality of the data gathered.

Step 10: Conduct a *sensitivity analysis*. Ratios are recalculated, using different values for those items not known with certainty. Sensitivity analysis essentially defines a range of confidence for the results of the study.

CHALLENGES AND OPPORTUNITIES

There are many challenges that we must face in the future, including (1) dealing with health care reform, (2) supporting research on new drugs and paying for appropriate use of new or unapproved uses of current drugs, and (3) including individual patient variation and patient preferences into drug protocols.

The standard tools for health economic analyses make it possible to ask basic questions like "how much does illness cost in my organization" and "what is the most cost-beneficial way to treat the illness?" Final, conclusive answers, however, can be difficult to find because there is a need for continuing data collection on the cost of treating many illnesses, especially when new drugs or procedures affect older therapies. We need further economic research on how to account for factors such as stress on the family, home health care intervention, life extension based on quality of life years, and so on.

This section of the chapter has provided a general overview of health economic analyses in health care. In the following sections we review the economic factors in the treatment or prevention of selected cardiovascular conditions.

ECONOMIC CONSIDERATIONS
IN COMMON CARDIOVASCULAR CONDITIONS

Economic evaluations of cardiovascular treatment programs have employed the variety of analytic methods discussed above. Comparison of the costs and effectiveness of one treatment relative to another can help decision makers determine the appropriate allocation of scarce resources. Numerous pharmacoeconomic evaluations of cardiovascular treatments have been conducted during the past 20 yr. Summarized as follows are some of the more recent and relevant examples. Although this is not an exhaustive review, it provides the reader with insight into the previous research conducted.

MYOCARDIAL INFARCTION:
THROMBOLYTIC THERAPY

Myocardial infarction (MI) occurs in over 1 million persons per year in the US, with about one-third of the victims dying. More than 250,000 of these deaths occur before the patient reaches the hospital, within one hour of the onset of symptoms *(4,5)*. An estimated 4 million people across the globe die each year from MI *(8)*.

MI imposes a substantial economic burden on the US health care system. The costs (1993 dollars) of treating an acute MI range from $14,470 to $31,397 for a patient who dies soon after the event, according to a 1995 report issued by the Office of Technology Assessment. The figure escalates to $74,217 (at a 5% discount rate) for a patient who survives for 5 yr *(9,10)*.

The high death rate from acute MI plus the substantial treatment costs incurred even among patients who expire leads to consideration of the acceptable costs to prevent death in some of these patients. In theory, no cost is too great to save a life, but in practice, finite resources dictate that limits must be set. The decision to employ or to not employ a new or expensive treatment regimen is often made by comparing the costs per year of life gained (YLG) or the costs per quality-adjusted life year gained (QALY) for the new treatment to that of currently accepted standards of treatment. An arbitrary upper limit of acceptable expenditure may be set based on community standards. There is no absolute standard for acceptable treatment costs, as ability and willingness to pay will vary depending on wealth as well as cultural factors. Expert opinion is that health care interventions that cost less than $20,000/QALY are acceptable, whereas interventions with costs that exceed $100,000/QALY are inappropriate (8). It is in this context of acceptable costs per life year gained that economic analyses of treatments for acute MI must be viewed.

Treatment of acute MI includes reperfusion techniques such as percutaneous transluminal coronary angioplasty (PTCA), CABG, and intravenous thrombolytic therapy with agents such as streptokinase, alteplase (recombinant tissue plasminogen activator, rt-PA), anistrepase, reteplase, and saruplase. Thrombolysis has become the treatment of choice for eligible patients (8). Clinical trials have demonstrated the survival benefit of thrombolysis, which has been shown to result in an 18% proportional reduction in mortality when the thrombolytic agent is administered within 24 h of the infarct (11). The least expensive of the thrombolytic drugs is streptokinase, which was the first thrombolytic agent to be widely used in MI.

Pharmacoeconomic studies have shown thrombolytic therapy with streptokinase to be cost effective for the treatment of acute MI in a number of circumstances. Early computer models of thrombolytic cost effectiveness suggested that the routine administration of either streptokinase or rt-PA was likely to increase the volume of coronary angioplasty and coronary artery bypass surgery performed in the US (12).

However, subsequent studies did not find this to be an economic disincentive to thrombolysis. Simoons et al. (13) studied 533 patients from the Netherlands Interuniversity Trial of Streptokinase and concluded that thrombolysis improved survival after MI without substantially increasing the need for other costly revascularization procedures such as CABG or PTCA. A lack of consensus among cardiologists about the benefits of streptokinase for older patients prompted a 1992 investigation by Krumholz et. al. (14). Pooled clinical data from trials in elderly patients indicated that administration of streptokinase within 6 h of symptom onset would reduce mortality by 13%. Using a decision analytic model, the authors estimated that the cost of streptokinase treatment for an 80-yr-old patient would be $21,200 per year of life saved, whereas the cost of treating a 70-yr-old would be $21,600 per year of life saved. Both figures are less than an arbitrary cost-effectiveness cutoff point of $55,000 per life year saved (14).

The value of streptokinase therapy may depend on the site of the infarct. Midgette et al. (15) investigated the effects of infarct location on the cost effectiveness of streptokinase for acute MI. The authors combined a meta-analysis of short-term survival data from clinical trials of streptokinase with a simple decision tree model. They determined that the marginal cost effectiveness (dollars per life saved) of thrombolytic therapy varies depending on infarct site. For definitively diagnosed acute MI, the cost per life saved was calculated to be $9900, $56,600, and $28,400, respectively, for anterior, inferior, and other infarcts. The marginal costs increased as the diagnosis of acute MI became less certain, approaching $132,000 per life saved when the probability of an inferior infarct was 50%. Nevertheless, the authors concluded that given a societal willingness to pay of $250,000 per life saved, streptokinase therapy should be administered in most cases of suspected acute MI *(15)*.

The cost effectiveness of thrombolysis with rt-PA was evaluated by Levin and Jonsson *(16)*, who analyzed data from 314 patients in the Anglo-Scandanavian Study of Early Thrombolysis (ASSET) trial. Although the direct plus indirect costs for the rt-PA patient group was 8% higher (5700 Swedish kroner [SEK]) than that of the placebo group, the 12-mo survival rate for the rt-PA patients was 7.1% higher. The authors concluded that the cost effectiveness of thrombolysis treatment is high compared with other treatments for CHD, due to the benefit of increased survival *(16)*.

The use of rt-PA rather than streptokinase increases the cost of thrombolytic therapy, as the acquisition cost of rt-PA may be 5–15 times greater than that of streptokinase *(8)*. An important recent evaluation of the comparative cost effectiveness of streptokinase and rt-PA was conducted by Mark et al. *(17)* using data from the Global Utilization of Streptokinase and Tissue Plasminogen Activator for Occluded Coronary Arteries (GUSTO) study. The 41,021-patient GUSTO study found a statistically significant relative decrease of 15% and absolute decrease of 1% in 30-d mortality among patients treated with an accelerated rt-PA regimen (administration of the drug over a period of 1½ h rather than the conventional 3-h administration) compared with patients treated with streptokinase. The investigators concluded that the $32,678 extra cost per year of life saved by the use of rt-PA was in line with the costs of other routine therapies, including coronary bypass surgery. The use of rt-PA rather than streptokinase was shown to produce one extra disabling stroke per 1000 patients treated. When the increased risk of stroke was considered, the cost per year of life saved increased to $32,538–$42,400, depending on assumptions for the level of poststroke care. These figures were still below the investigators' $50,000 per year-of-life saved (YLS) benchmark for cost effectiveness. Although the routine substitution of rt-PA for streptokinase would cost the US health care system almost $500 million per year, the authors calculated that this substitution would also offer an additional 3.5 million years of life for MI patients *(17)*.

In reviewing the GUSTO cost-effectiveness study, Gillis and Goa *(8)* noted that the added costs of rt-PA may be a decision factor for some hospital formularies. Furthermore, Stanek et al. *(18)* determined that rt-PA was preferred by potential patients when there was a zero-cost assumption, but that potential patients' preference shifted toward streptokinase when they were asked to pay for the drug themselves *(18)*.

PRIMARY PREVENTION: HORMONE REPLACEMENT THERAPY IN POSTMENOPAUSAL WOMEN

The direct plus indirect costs of CHD in the US are estimated to approach $100 billion per year, according to the American Heart Association *(1–5)*. As discussed previously, the estimated costs of treatment for MI, a life-threatening consequence of CHD, are as high as $74,217 per patient *(9,10)*. Prevention of the development of CHD, therefore, makes economic, as well as medical, sense.

The most common cause of death among women as well as men in the United States is CHD *(9,10)*. However, the risk profile for women differs from that of men. Premenopausal women face a lower risk of CHD than do men of the same age. This is believed to be due to the cardioprotective effects of endogenous estrogen, which offers a number of benefits including a positive impact on plasma lipid levels *(19)*. At menopause the advantage for women begins to disappear, and by 70 yr of age, women are as likely to die of CHD as men *(20)*.

Numerous observational studies since 1970 have indicated that estrogen replacement therapy (ERT) reduces the risk of CHD among postmenopausal women. Pooled data indicate this reduction in risk to be about 35% among women who have never had CHD. In one meta-analysis, the pooled risk of death from CHD was estimated at 0.63 among women who had ever used estrogen compared to women who had never used estrogen *(21)*.

Nabulsi et al. *(22)* analyzed retrospective data from the Atherosclerosis Risk in Communities study. Their investigation of 4958 postmenopausal women from a community-based cohort showed that current users of hormone replacement therapy had higher mean levels of HDL-C and lower mean levels of LDL-C. The authors estimated that their findings would translate into a reduction of 42% in the risk of CHD. Their findings also indicated that users of estrogen with a progestin (PERT) had a favorable TG profile compared to users of estrogen alone (ERT), suggesting that PERT users would derive even greater benefit than ERT users *(22)*.

The conclusions of Nabulsi et al. *(23)* regarding a greater cardioprotective benefit of PERT compared to ERT were called into question by the results of the Postmenopausal Estrogen/Progestin Interventions (PEPI) trial. This three-year, randomized, double-blind, placebo-controlled trial evaluated 875 healthy postmenopausal women. The PEPI investigators concluded that estrogen alone or in combination with a progestin improves lipid profiles. However, the PEPI results provided unequivocal evidence that ERT has a more favorable effect on HDL levels than PERT. The authors noted that the increased risk of endometrial cancer in women on ERT makes the addition of a progestin prudent unless a woman has had a hysterectomy, and that the addition of a progestin still preserves the bulk of the benefit of estrogen on HDL. Unlike the Nabulsi study, all hormone-treated women in the PEPI trial showed increased levels of TGs that did not differ between the ERT and PERT groups *(23)*.

Prior to the release of the PEPI report, several authors concluded that the cost effectiveness of hormone replacement therapy (HRT) was most sensitive to the regimen's impact on cardiovascular disease. Cheung and Wren *(24)* showed that short-term use of HRT was economically inefficient, and that cost effectiveness depended upon the magnitude of cardiovascular effect. Similarly, a comprehensive model developed by Daly et al. *(25)* demonstrated that the effects of HRT on cardiovascular disease would have the greatest impact on the health benefits of the regimen. They concluded that HRT compared favorably to other accepted health care interventions in terms of cost per quality-adjusted life years (QALY) *(25)*.

The United States Office of Technology Assessment (OTA) in August 1995 released the most thorough evaluation of the economics of HRT. The Monte Carlo model used by OTA included the risks and costs of breast cancer, endometrial cancer, and other potential adverse effects of HRT, as well as the impact of therapy on the incidence of hip fracture and heart disease. As in earlier evaluations, OTA determined that the cost effectiveness of HRT is most sensitive to the treatment effect upon the risk of heart disease. The OTA recommended lifelong postmenopausal administration of HRT as cost-effective preventive medicine *(9,10)*.

PRIMARY AND SECONDARY PREVENTION:
CHOLESTEROL AND LIPID REDUCTION

Pooled data from studies of secondary prevention of ischemic heart disease and CHD suggest that each 1% reduction in serum cholesterol levels results in a 1.9% reduction in recurrent CHD events *(26)*. Early studies of the cost effectiveness of cholesterol-lowering agents focused on the drugs cholestyramine and colestipol. In general, the studies reported that these cholesterol-lowering drugs were less cost effective than other common treatment regimens *(26)*. For example, a 1988 study by Kinosian and Eisenberg reported that cholestyramine and colestipol cost over $60,000 per life year saved except when used by smokers, for whom costs were only $51,500 per life year saved *(27)*. However, the newer "statin" drugs (HMG-CoA reductase inhibitors) have been shown to be much more cost effective. A review of treatment costs in the British National Health Service demonstrated that annual costs per 10% drop in cholesterol levels were more than three times lower for simvastatin or pravastatin compared to cholestyramine *(28)*.

Several large-scale, placebo-controlled trials have demonstrated the survival benefit of the statins. These studies demonstrated the need for further research on morbidity and mortality outcomes, not just clinical endpoints like % LDL reduction.

The Scandinavian Simvastatin Survival Study, or 4S Study, conducted in 1987, was designed to test whether lipid-lowering therapy could decrease mortality in CAD. This landmark study demonstrated the true outcome associated with this therapy was not just lowering the amount of cholesterol in the blood but impacting mortality and morbidity *(29)*.

The West of Scotland Coronary Prevention Study, or WOSCOPS, was conducted using pravastatin to investigate the effectiveness of the drug in preventing coronary events in men with moderate hypercholesterolemia and no history of MI. Results of this trial among 6595 subjects showed that pravastatin reduced the risk of fatal and nonfatal coronary events by approximately 30% compared with placebo. In addition, the need for coronary angiography and revascularization procedures was significantly lower among men who received pravastatin. There were no excess deaths from noncardiovascular causes among the pravastatin patients *(30)*.

Goldman et al. *(26)* evaluated the cost effectiveness of HMG-CoA reductase inhibitors in the primary and secondary prevention of CHD. Using a computer simulation called The Coronary Heart Disease Policy Model, the authors estimated the risk-specific incidence of heart disease and the risk of recurrent coronary events in persons with pre-existing coronary disease. The Coronary Heart Disease Policy Model takes the perspective of society as a whole, rather than that of the individual patient. The model was used to estimate the costs and effectiveness of the HMG-CoA reductase inhibitor lovastatin among specific subsets of the population. Lovastatin 20 mg/d was demonstrated to be cost effective for secondary prevention of CHD among patients with moderate or severe hypercholesterolemia, with costs (1989 dollars) below $20,000 per life year saved for men and women of all ages. Increasing the dosage to 40 mg/d added costs ranging from $8600–$38,000 for men, and $29,000–$49,000 for women. Increasing the dosage to 80 mg/d added incremental costs of over $70,000 per year of life saved. For men with cholesterol levels below 250 mg/dL, the costs for lovastatin 20 mg were calculated to range from $16,000–$38,000 per year of life saved. The secondary prevention costs for women with the same pretreatment cholesterol levels ranged from $23,000 per year of life saved for women 75–84 yr of age, to $210,000 per year of life saved for women 35–44 yr of age.

The use of lovastatin for primary prevention was cost effective only for selected groups such as men aged 35–44 who also had hypertension, smoked, and were more than 13% above ideal weight. In general, the lovastatin study indicated that cost effectiveness of drug therapy was higher for men, older patients, and patients with higher risk of CHD (26).

Additional morbidity/mortality studies have been conducted or are in progress with other statins (fluvastatin, atorvastatin, cerivastatin). All economic analyses of the statins have shown that appropriate use translates to economic savings (31).

HYPERTENSION

Hypertension is the most common cardiovascular condition in the United States, afflicting an estimated 50 million persons (1–5). The American Heart Association estimates that the total direct costs plus indirect costs for the treatment of hypertension in the United States exceeds $33 billion per year (1–5). Hypertension medication accounts for up to 81% of direct costs by the third year of treatment (32).

Hypertension is a notable risk factor for the development of a number of diseases. A 15-yr follow-up of the nearly 350,000 men in the Multiple Risk Factor Intervention Trial (MRFIT) demonstrated that the relative risk of stroke mortality among men with stage 4 hypertension is more than 18 times the risk of men with optimal blood pressure (33). Hypertension also contributes to the development of CHD, with relative risks of CHD mortality 6.9 times higher for men with stage 4 hypertension than for men with optimal BP. The major cause of the development of congestive heart failure (CHF) is hypertension, according to the Framingham Heart Study (34).

Meta-analysis of hypertension treatment trials demonstrated that treatment of hypertension reduces the incidence of CHF by 52% (35). Meta-analysis also demonstrated a positive impact on stroke mortality, with the risk of fatal stroke reduced by 45% with the treatment of hypertension (36). Epidemiological studies show that a 35–40% decline in stroke risk was associated with lowering diastolic BP by 5–6 mmHg. The risk of CHD fell by 20-25% for the same decrease in BP (37).

Modern economic analysis of hypertension treatment began with Weinstein and Stason's 1976 study (38), which evaluated the costs of treatment per quality adjusted life year (QALY). The model developed by Weinstein and Stason indicated that hypertension treatment is more cost effective with increasing age and with higher pretreatment BP levels. Although some of the assumptions used by Weinstein and Stason have been shown to be in error, the analysis is still considered to be among the best in the field (39).

Edelson and colleagues (40) estimated that one-third of the US population has hypertension. The authors evaluated the cost effectiveness of hypertension treatment using the Coronary Heart Disease Policy Model, which is a computer simulation of overall mortality, morbidity, and cost of CHD in the US population. Estimated antihypertensive and anticholesterol effects of various antihypertensive regimens were derived from a meta-analysis of 153 reports in a literature search for studies that met prospectively determined criteria. Cost of medication was estimated from average wholesale price (AWP) (plus 10% markup and $2 pharmacy fee/100 units) in the 1987 Redbook (40a). A 5% yearly discount rate was used. For 20 yr of simulated therapy from 1990 through 2010, the cost per year of life saved was projected to be $10,900 for propranolol HCL, $16,400 for hydrochlorothiazide, $31,600 for nifedipine, $61,900 for prazocin HCL, and $72,100 for captopril. Propranolol was the preferred initial option under most assumptions in this study (40).

Several recent studies have investigated the cost effectiveness of drug treatment for hypertension. The cost effectiveness of hypertension treatment appears to be highly sensitive to the price of the medications *(41)*. In general, the older, less expensive drugs such as diuretics and beta blockers were found to be more cost effective. As in the study by Edelson *(40)*, ACE inhibitors and other newer drug products are more costly and therefore were usually found to be less cost effective. For example, Pearce and associates *(42)* calculated the cost effectiveness of antihypertensives in the prevention of MI, stroke, or death. Drug acquisition costs to prevent one major adverse event in middle-aged patients ranged from $4730 for the diuretic hydrochlorothiazide to $346,236 for nifedipine gastrointestinal therapeutic system (GITS), a calcium channel blocker. Enalapril, an ACE inhibitor, cost $156,520 for prevention of one major adverse event *(42)*. Hoerger et al. *(41)* found that a combination of hydrochlorothiazide and bisoprolol, a beta blocker, was more cost effective than amlodipine, a calcium channel blocker, or enalapril. It was estimated that the acquisition cost *(40a)* of enalapril would have to decrease by 57.9% and that of amlodipine by 50.9% to equal the cost effectiveness of the hydrocholorothiazide/bisoprolol combination. Similarly, Griebenow et al. *(43)* found a 50% difference in cost per mmHg blood pressure reduction for a combination of reserpine and clopamide vs. enalapril.

Cost effectiveness of antihypertensive medication is also influenced by patient age. For example, in the Pearce *(42)* study, the cost of preventing one adverse event in the elderly was only $1595 with hydrochlorothiazide and $52,780 with enalapril. Johannesson *(44)*, in a review of 19 hypertension cost-effectiveness trials, demonstrated by regression analysis that the average cost per life year gained for men with a diastolic blood pressure of 95 decreased from $83,333 at age 40 to $5000 at 70 yr of age. Costs for women were slightly higher, declining from $85,000 at age 40 to $8333 at 70 yr of age. Schueler *(45)* reviewed the cost-effectiveness literature for hypertension and concluded that a treatment approach characterized by therapeutic restraint is warranted. Therapeutic restraint implies the use of less expensive medications, initiated at older ages and only after high diastolic BPs are measured. Under the assumptions of therapeutic restraint, the use of diuretics alone or with beta blockers is recommended as initial therapy for hypertension.

It must be noted, however, that the conditions of daily practice may not match the ideal conditions of a clinical trial. A medication that the patient does not take will not be cost effective, no matter how inexpensive the drug. Compliance with therapeutic recommendations is an issue in the treatment of hypertension, which is usually an asymptomatic disorder. A medication or treatment regimen that is not tolerable to the patient, perhaps due to side effects or inconvenience, may be discontinued or used suboptimally, leading to reduced effectiveness. Rizzo and colleagues performed multivariate analysis of compliance with ACE inhibitors, calcium antagonists, beta blockers, and diuretics. They found that higher rates of compliance were associated with ACE inhibitors and calcium antagonists. Poor compliance was associated with higher health care costs *(46)*. Clinicians' choice of antihypertensive therapy must be guided, therefore, not only by drug acquisition cost but also by patient preferences and individual needs.

CONGESTIVE HEART FAILURE

Congestive heart failure (CHF) is the leading diagnosis among older adults who are hospitalized in the United States, afflicting almost 5 million Americans *(47)*. Approximately 400,000 patients are diagnosed with CHF each year *(48)*, and more than 46,000 annual deaths may be attributed to the disorder *(47)*. Annual costs for the treatment of CHF in the United States exceed $10 billion *(49)*.

Mortality from congestive heart failure averages 50% over 5 yr, with an annual death rate of 10% *(49)*. Despite progress in treatment, the mortality of CHF remains high, although recent analyses suggest that the yearly age-adjusted death rates are dropping among patients ≥65 yr of age. Although the age-adjusted death rates for CHF increased throughout most of the 1980s, the period from 1988–1995 showed a 1.1% average annual decline in deaths due to CHF among Americans over 65 yr of age *(47)*.

Experts at the Centers for Disease Control and Prevention suggest that this improvement may be due to new treatment strategies and earlier detection of heart disease or its precursors, such as hypertension. However, the incidence and prevalence of heart failure is likely to grow as the population ages. Aging of the cardiovascular system, hypertension, CAD, and valvular heart disease are more prevalent among adults over 65 yr of age, leading to an increased incidence of heart failure in this age group *(50)*. Moreover, a 1982 follow-up of the Framingham Study showed that the incidence of heart failure more than doubled every 10 yr for persons between the ages of 45 and 75 yr *(51)*. As a result of growth in the population of older Americans, the total death toll from CHF is expected to continue to increase *(47)*.

CHF is most often a consequence of the conditions discussed in the previous sections of this chapter. Hypertension is the leading cause of CHF in the United States *(34)*. Treatment of hypertension reduces the incidence of heart failure by 52% *(35)*. Myocardial infarction is the second major cause of CHF *(52)*. The economics of therapies for the prevention of CHF are, therefore, identical to the economics of therapies for the prevention and control of the major risk factors for CHF, hypertension, and MI.

Although drug therapy is the mainstay of CHF treatment, nondrug interventions including surgical options, nursing interventions, and implantable cardiac devices are also employed. Heart transplantation is indicated for adults with life threatening CHF that has not responded adequately to more conservative treatment. The American Heart Association reported that about 40,000 Americans age 65 or below could benefit from a heart transplant in a given year, but that only 2290 of these procedures were actually performed in 1997 (the most recent year of AHA statistics). Aravot and associates *(53)* investigated the impact of heart transplantation on patients 60 yr of age or older. Quality of life was evaluated using the Nottingham Health Profile, a validated, generic quality of life instrument. At 1 yr after transplantation, 84% of the patients (21/25) were still alive, and quality of life among the survivors was improved compared with pretransplant levels *(53)*. A 1986 study by Evans calculated the cost effectiveness for heart transplantation as $23,500 per life year saved, a figure that compares favorably to other major medical-surgical interventions *(54)*.

CONCLUSION

The impact of cardiovascular disease can be measured in economic and noneconomic terms. The direct and indirect costs associated with cardiovascular disease are very high. Physicians need to balance these costs when making treatment decisions. The efficacy of these treatment alternatives may need to be balanced by the economic outcomes.

This chapter discussed the various economic approaches used to measure the health economic impact of treatment choices. Cost effectiveness is the most widely used method to balance the inputs (costs) and outputs (outcomes) of these choices. Applying these techniques can assist the clinician in making more efficient use of the limited health care resources.

The second part of this chapter presented a review of the economic analyses of several cardiovascular diseases. The objective is to introduce the previous research as the beginning of the quest for more efficient clinical decisions.

As the population ages and the cost of health care increases, the clinician in all practice settings needs to understand the balance between effectiveness and cost effectiveness in order to make the difficult treatment decisions required in this environment.

REFERENCES

1. American Heart Association. Cardiovascular Disease Statistics. In: Science and Professional Statistics. http:\\www.americanheart.org., 1999.
2. National Center for Health Statistics. Highlights of a new report from the National Center for Health Statistics (NCHS). Monitoring Health Care in America. Quarterly Report, March 1996.
3. American Heart Association. Cardiovascular Diseases. http:\\www.americanheart.org., 1999.
4. American Heart Association. Economic Cost of Cardiovascular Diseases. http:\\www.americanheart.org., 1999.
5. American Heart Association. Heart Transplants and Statistics. http:\\www.americanheart.org., 1999.
6. Bootman JL, Townsend RJ, McGhan WF. Principles of Pharmacoeconomics, 2nd ed. Harvey Whitney Books, Cincinnati, OH, 1996.
7. Rice DP, Cost of illness studies: fact or fiction. Lancet 1994;344;1519–1520.
8. Gillis JC, Goa KL. Streptokinase: a pharmacoeconomic appraisal of its use in the management of acute myocardial infarction. Pharmacoeconomics 1996;10(3):281–310.
9. US Congress, Office of Technology Assessment, Effectiveness and Costs of Osteoporosis Screening and Hormone Replacement Therapy, Volume I: Cost Effectiveness Analysis, OTA-BP-H-160, US Government Printing Office, Washington, DC, August 1995.
10. US Congress, Office of Technology Assessment, Effectiveness and Costs of Osteoporosis Screening and Hormone Replacement Therapy, Volume II: Evidence on Benefits, Risks, and Costs, OTA-BP-H-144, US Government Printing Office, Washington, DC, August 1995.
11. Fibrinolytic Therapy Trialists (FTT) Collaborative Group. Indications for fibrinolytic therapy in suspected acute myocardial infarction: collaborative review of early mortality and major morbidity from all randomized trials of more than 1000 patients. Lancet 1994;343:311–322.
12. Steinberg EP, Topol EJ, Sakin JW, et. al. Cost and procedure implications for thrombolytic therapy for acute myocardial infarction. J Am Coll Cardiol 1988;12(6):58A–68A.
13. Simoons ML, Vos J, Martens LL. Cost-utility analysis of thrombolytic therapy. Eur Heart J 1991;12: 694–699.
14. Krumholz HM, Pasternak RC, Weinstein MC, et. al. Cost effectiveness of thrombolytic therapy with streptokinase in elderly patients with suspected acute myocardial infarction. N Engl J Med 1992;327(1): 7–13.
15. Midgette AS, Wong JB, Beshansky JR, et. al. Cost-effectiveness of streptokinase for acute myocardial infarction: a combined meta-analysis and decision analysis of the effects of infarct location and of likelihood of infarction. Medical Decision Making 1994;14(2):108–117.
16. Levin LA, Jonsson B. Cost-effectiveness of thrombolysis—a randomized study of intravenous rt-PA in suspected myocardial infarction. Eur Heart J 1992;13:2–8.
17. Mark DB, Hlatky MA, Califf RM, et. al. Cost effectiveness of thrombolytic therapy with tissue plasminogen activator as compared with streptokinase for acute myocardial infarction. N Engl J Med 1995; 332(21):1418–1424.
18. Stanek EJ, Cheng JW, Peeples PJ, et. al. Patient preferences for thrombolytic therapy in acute myocardial infarction. Medical Decision Making 1997;17(4):464–471.
19. Thorneycroft IH. HRT and cardiovascular protection. Menopausal Management 1992;Sept/Oct:10–16.
20. Whittington R, Faulds D. Hormone replacement therapy II: a pharmacoeconomic appraisal of its role in the prevention of postmenopausal osteoporosis and ischemic heart disease. Pharmacoeconomics 1994;5(6): 513–554.

21. Grady D, Rubin SM, Petitti DB, et al. Hormone therapy to prevent disease and prolong life in postmenopausal women. Ann Intern Med 1992;117:1016–1037.
22. Nabulsi AA, Folsom AR, White A, et. al. Association of hormone-replacement therapy with various cardiovascular risk factors in postmenopausal women. N Engl J Med 1993;328(15):1069–1075.
23. Writing Group for the PEPI Trial. Effects of estrogen or estrogen/progestin regimens on heart disease risk factors in postmenopausal women. JAMA 1995;273(3):199-208.
24. Cheung AP, Wren BG. A cost-effectiveness analysis of hormone replacement therapy in menopause. Med J Aust 1992;156:312–316.
25. Daly E, Roche M, Barlow D, et al. HRT: an analysis of benefits, risks and costs. Br Med Bull 1992;48: 368–400.
26. Goldman L, Weinstein MC, Goldman PA, Williams LW. Cost-effectiveness of HMG-CoA reductase inhibition for primary and secondary prevention of coronary heart disease. JAMA 1991;265(9):1145–1151.
27. Kinosian BP, Eisenberg JM. Cutting into cholesterol: cost-effective alternatives for treating hypercholesterolemia. JAMA 1988;259:2249–2254.
28. Reckless JPD. Cost-effectiveness of hypolidaemic drugs. Postgrad Med J 1993;69(Suppl 1):S30–S33.
29. Pederson TR. Coronary artery disease: The Scandinavian Simvastatin Survival Study experience. Am J Cardiol 1998;82(10B):55T–56T.
30. Shepherd J, Cobbe SM, Ford I, et. al. Prevention of coronary heart disease with pravastatin in men with hypercholesterolemia. N Engl J Med 1995;333:1301–1307.
31. Hay JW, Yu WM, Ashraf T. Pharmacoeconomics of lipid-lowering agents for primary and secondary prevention of coronary artery disease. Pharmacoeconomics 1999;15(1):47–74.
32. Odell TW, Gregory MC. Cost of hypertension treatment. J Gen Intern Med 1995;10(12):686–688.
33. Stamler J. The INTERSALT study: background, methods, findings and implications. Am J Clin Nutr 1997;65(2 Suppl):626S–642S.
34. Kannel WB, Castelli WP, McNamara PM, et. al. Role of blood pressure in the development of congestive heart failure: the Framingham Study. N Engl J Med 1972;287(16):781–787.
35. Moser M, Herbert PR. Prevention of disease progression, left ventricular hypertrophy and congestive heart failure in hypertension treatment trials. J Am Coll Cardiol 1996;27(5):1214–1218.
36. Collins R, Peto R, MacMahon S, et. al. Blood pressure, stroke, and coronary heart disease. Part 2. Short term reductions in blood pressure: overview of randomised drug trials in their epidemiological context. Lancet 1990;335(8693):827–838.
37. MacMahon S, Peto R, Cutler J, et. al. Blood pressure, stroke, and coronary heart disease. Part 1. Prolonged differences in blood pressure: prospective observational studies corrected for the regression dilution bias. Lancet 1990;335(8692):765–774.
38. Weinstein MC, Stason WB. Hypertension: A Policy Perspective. Harvard University Press, Cambridge, MA, 1976.
39. Johannesson M, Jonsson B. A review of cost-effectiveness analyses of hypertension treatment. Pharmacoeconomics 1992;1(4):250–264.
40. Edelson JT, Weinstein MC, Tosteson ANA, et. al. Long-term cost-effectiveness of various initial monotherapies for mild to moderate hypertension. JAMA 1990;263(3):407–413.
40a. Redbook, vol. 6. Montvale, NJ, Medical Economics Company, 1987.
41. Hoerger TJ, Bala MV, Eggleston JL, et. al. A comparative cost-effectiveness study of three drugs for the treatment of mild-to-moderate hypertension. P&T 1998;23(5):245–267.
42. Pearce KA, Furberg CD, Psaty BM, Kirk J. Cost-minimization and the number needed to treat in uncomplicated hypertension. Am J Hypertens 1998;11(5):618–629.
43. Griebenow R, Pittrow DB, Weidinger G, et. al. Low-dose reserpine/thiazide combination in first-line treatment of hypertension: efficacy and safety compared to an ACE inhibitor. Blood Pressure 1997;6(5): 299–306.
44. Johannesson M. The impact of age on the cost-effectiveness of hypertension treatment: an analysis of randomized drug trials. Medical Decision Making 1994;14(3):236–244.
45. Schueler K. Cost-effectiveness issues in hypertension control. Can J Public Health 1994;85(Suppl 2): S54–S56.
46. Rizzo JA, Simons WR. Variations in compliance among hypertensive patients by drug class: implications for health care costs. Clin Ther 1997;19(6):1446–1457.
47. Centers for Disease Control and Prevention. Changes in mortality from heart failure—United States, 1980–1995. MMWR 1998;47:633–637.
48. Patterson JH, Adams KF. Pathophysiology of heart failure. Pharmacotherapy 1993;13:73S–81S.

49. Konstam MA, Dracup K, Baker DW, et al. Heart failure: evaluation and care of patients with left-ventricular systolic dysfunction. Clinical Practice Guideline No. 11. AHCPR Publication No. 94-0612. Rockville, MD: Agency for Health Care Policy and Research, Public Health Service, U.S. Department of Health and Human Services, June 1994.
50. Rich MW. Epidemiology, pathophysiology, and etiology of congestive heart failure in older adults. J Am Geriatr Soc 1997;45(8):968–974.
51. Kannel WB, Savage D, Castelli WP. Cardiac failure in the Framingham Study: twenty-year follow up. In: Braunwald E, Mock MB, Watson JT, eds. Congestive Heart Failure: Current Research and Clinical Applications. Grune & Stratton, New York, 1982, pp. 15–30.
52. Vasan RS, Levy D. The role of hypertension in the pathogenesis of heart failure. A clinical mechanistic overview. Arch Intern Med 1996;156(16):1789–1796.
53. Aravot DJ, Banner NR, Khaghani A, et al. Cardiac transplantation in the seventh decade of life. Am J Cardiol 1989;63(1):90–93.
54. Evans RW. Cost-effectiveness analysis of transplantation. Surg Clin North Am 1986;66:503–517.

INDEX

A

ABCD, *see* Appropriate Blood Pressure in Diabetes
ACADEMIC trial, 57, 58
ACE inhibitors, *see* Angiotensin-converting enzyme inhibitors
ACES, *see* Azothromycin Coronary Events Study
AFCAPS/TEXCAPS, *see* Air Force/Texas Coronary Atherosclerosis Prevention Study
Air Force/Texas Coronary Atherosclerosis Prevention Study (AFCAPS/TEXCAPS), 70–72, 126, 207
ALLHAT, *see* Antihypertensive and Lipid Lowering Treatment to Prevent Heart Attack Trial,
Amlodipine,
    antioxidant activity, 32–34
    indications, 34, 36
Angina, aspirin trials, 262
Angiography, efficacy in atherosclerosis quantification, 7, 8
Angiotensin-converting enzyme (ACE) inhibitors,
    angiotensin-converting enzyme, endothelial production and dysfunction, 21
    heart failure studies, 247, 248
    hypertension management,
        agent selection factors,
            congestive heart failure, 106, 107
            costs, 112, 352
            demographics, 110
            isolated systolic hypertension, 109, 110
            postmyocardial infarction, 108
            quality of life, 111
            renal parenchymal disease, 107, 108
        algorithm, 104
        combination therapy, 105, 106
        initial therapy, 103, 105, 106
    post-myocardial infarction benefits, 245, 246
Anticoagulation therapy,
    combination with antiplatelet agents, 273, 274
    post-myocardial infarction, 247
Antihypertensive and Lipid Lowering Treatment to Prevent Heart Attack Trial (ALLHAT), 129
Antioxidants, *see also specific vitamins,*
    amlodipine activity, 32–34

Antioxidants (*cont.*),
    atherosclerosis treatment,
        epidemiological studies, 40–42
        preclinical studies, 39, 40
    carvedilol activity, 36
    endothelial dysfunction protection, 25, 40
    enzymes and free radical protection, 32
    women and therapy, 210
Appropriate Blood Pressure in Diabetes (ABCD), 129
ARIC, *see* Atherosclerosis Risk in Communities
Aspirin,
    adverse effects, 263
    benefit overview, 275
    combination therapy with thienopyridines, 266, 267
    historical perspective, 258, 259
    mechanisms of action, 259, 260
    prevention of myocardial infarction,
        evolving infarction benefits, 262, 263
        primary prevention, 244, 260, 261
        secondary prevention, 244, 245, 261, 262
    resistance,
        clinical consequences, 272, 273
        dosing, 272
        etiology, 271
        gender differences, 272
        prevalence, 271
    stable angina trials, 262
    unstable angina trials, 262
    warfarin combination therapy, 273, 274
Atherosclerosis, *see also* Plaque,
    antioxidants in treatment,
        epidemiological studies, 40–42
        preclinical studies, 39, 40
    coronary artery remodeling, 6, 304
    ideal screening test, 304, 305
    imaging, *see* Electron beam tomography
    infection role,
        chicken virus models, 54
        Chlamydia pneumoniae, 55–58
        cytomegalovirus, 54
        Helicobacter pylori, 54
    inflammatory response,
        complex lesions, 49
        C-reactive protein as marker, 49–53
        early lesions, 48, 49
        intermediate lesions, 49
        overview, 47, 48